The world needs this book—today more than ever. By reframing the discussion of mental health to brain health, Dr. Daniel Amen obliterates the concept that mental health issues are someone's fault, or that people should just deal with them any differently than they would the flu or a broken arm. Most important, Dr. Amen gives everyone not just the permission but the validation and hope to seek help for a better tomorrow.

> **DARRIA LONG GILLESPIE, MD,** emergency physician; national TV expert and host; author of bestselling book *Mom Hacks*

The End of Mental Illness is a radical new way to overhaul psychiatry, using the lessons from neuroimaging in the context of a whole-person functional medicine approach. My family has benefited from Dr. Amen's work, and I hope you will too.

> **MARK HYMAN, MD,** Pritzker Foundation Chair in Functional Medicine, Cleveland Clinic Lerner College of Medicine; director of the Cleveland Clinic Center for Functional Medicine

Dr. Amen's approach has revolutionized our understanding of the causes and therefore the treatment of mental illness.

> **DAVID PERLMUTTER, MD,** author of the #1 *New York Times* bestseller *Grain Brain* and *Brain Wash*

This is a great book. It presents a radical challenge to the psychiatric status quo and represents the best of the clinical transformative traditions. Dr. Amen makes disciplined observations and pursues them to the end for the sake of his patients without regard to the dense (and increasingly toxic) academic politics that make psychiatry impotent to accomplish much.

> **MANUEL TRUJILLO, MD,** clinical professor in the department of psychiatry; director of the Public Psychiatry Fellowship program at New York University School of Medicine

Through his vast experience with neuroimaging, Dr. Amen has learned that the "wiring diagram" of our brain is not fixed but constantly changes depending on our choices, environmental factors, and experiences. By recommending that we balance our choices in the biological (diet and exercise), psychological (stress control), social (relationships), and spiritual components of our lives, he provides a desperately needed road map to maximize brain health and prevent or reverse many of the epidemic mental afflictions that are often poorly treated in our medical system.

> **JOSEPH C. MAROON, MD,** vice chairman of neurosurgery, University of Pittsburgh Medical Center; team neurosurgeon, the Pittsburgh Steelers; author of *Square One: A Simple Guide to a Balanced Life*

A truly revolutionary work, at least I certainly hope it will be! Books like this challenge and change the existing paradigm of mental health and brain health. A fantastic and comprehensive approach for patients and healthcare providers alike.

ANDREW NEWBERG, MD, bestselling author of *How God Changes Your Brain*; director of research at the Marcus Institute of Integrative Health at Thomas Jefferson University Hospital; adjunct professor of psychology at the University of Pennsylvania School of Medicine

A timely must-read that will change the way we think about brain health.

DR. MIKE DOW, *New York Times* bestselling author of *The Sugar Brain Fix*

Mental illness is a complex and often confusing world. There is a lack of certainty on what is going wrong and what to do about it. Dr. Amen's new contribution is a thoughtful and well-planned approach to looking at the actual brain's health as a fundamental aspect of maintaining a vibrant life in emotions, relationships, and career.

JOHN TOWNSEND, PhD, *New York Times* bestselling author of Boundaries series, *Leading from Your Gut*, and *People Fuel*; psychologist and leadership consultant; founder of The Townsend Institute for Leadership and Counseling

Daniel Amen, a staunch advocate for mental health and one of today's most important neuropsychiatrists, provides an insightful challenge to the mental illness industry: Focus on brain health rather than deficits! Read this book carefully. Reclaim your brain; reclaim your life.

JEFFREY K. ZEIG, PhD, The Milton H. Erickson Foundation

The End of Mental Illness is a powerful new book that directly attacks the outdated mental health paradigm of making diagnoses based on symptom clusters without any biological data. In simple, straightforward language, Dr. Amen shows readers how to optimize the physical functioning of their brains to improve their minds. It is brilliant, and I highly recommend it!

STEVEN MASLEY, MD, FAHA, FACN, FAAFP, CNS, author of *The Mediterranean Method*

Daniel Amen has been one of the real pioneers in using imaging technology to correlate brain blood flow and activity patterns with various types of mental health issues. More important, he has developed innovative dietary and lifestyle techniques that can improve these patterns with significant improvement for his patients. *The End of Mental Illness* extends his leadership. If you want to keep the most complex organ in the body in top condition, this book provides the technical information to do so. I recommend it highly.

BARRY SEARS, PhD, author of *The Zone* and *The Resolution Zone*

Dr. Amen's book *The End of Mental Illness* is a defining mark in the history of psychiatry. Scientific research has completely eliminated the notion that nutritional deficiencies and nutritional supplements are a form of alternative medicine. Those of us who have practiced integrative medicine for many years understand that objective, biological testing is simply good medicine. Our current symptomatic treatment model in the field of psychiatry has been inadequate for those struggling with mental illness. Dr. Amen captures the essence of hope and healing by transforming a model of mental illness into a model of brain health. Please read *The End of Mental Illness* and make sure your doctors understand how neuroscience can redefine our current models of treatment.

JAMES GREENBLATT, MD, founder of Psychiatry Redefined; chief medical officer of Walden Behavioral Care

The End of Mental Illness offers a wealth of vital information, including fascinating SPECT imaging results, about how to create optimal mind-body-spirit health and overcome the stigma of "mental illness." Dr. Amen offers a multitude of options to create a healthy brain and a healthy, happy life.

JUDITH ORLOFF, MD, psychiatrist; author of *Emotional Freedom*

By outlining the compelling research he and his colleagues have published in peer-reviewed journals, and by including a myriad of elucidating case studies, Dr. Amen provides an optimistic yet realistic approach to life that demonstrably improves brain health. Given his prescience in collecting what is now surely one of the largest databases of brain scans and behavioral, cognitive, and emotional data, we can expect to see even clearer science and more comprehensive lifestyle and medical suggestions in the near future.

J. GALEN BUCKWALTER, PHD, research psychologist and CEO of psyML

As Dr. Amen helps us reframe the discussion from mental health to brain health, people will see their problems as medical, not moral. This new perspective decreases shame and guilt for those who suffer and increases forgiveness, patience, and compassion from their families. *The End of Mental Illness* will give you a totally new way of thinking about and getting help for anxiety, depression, bipolar disorders, ADHD, addictions, OCD, PTSD, schizophrenia, and even personality disorders. Thank you, Dr. Amen.

DR. DERWIN GRAY, former NFL player; lead pastor at Transformation Church

When someone has a broken ankle, they don't call it "motion sickness," but sadly, when the brain malfunctions, we have used the stigma-filled and shaming term *mental illness*. Dr. Daniel Amen takes the focus off outdated labels and places it properly on the injured and damaged organ by looking at the way it functions, rather than just the symptoms it produces. The path set by Dr. Amen really could be the end of focusing on mental illness and the beginning of creating brain health, which is exactly what Dr. Amen has done for me.

STEPHEN ARTERBURN, MEd, *New York Times* bestselling author of *Take Your Life Back*; host of *New Life Live!*

Dr. Daniel Amen has made the natural progression from psychiatrist to brain imaging researcher to neuroendocrinologist in his quest for a greater understanding of the relationship between one's emotional constitution and the traumas encountered during life. Addressing the underlying inflammation precipitated by these traumas can lead to a normalization of the brain's function and a return to a life without mental illness. Dr. Amen has unraveled the code that decrypts the means by which illness can become wellness.

MARK L. GORDON, MD, neuroendocrinology, Millennium-TBI Centers, Encino, California

I have conducted research with and known Daniel Amen for many years. With *The End of Mental Illness*, he delivers an inspiring tour de force on brain health. This book will educate people, make them question the status quo as they seek to know their brains better, and inspire them to change their lives so that they might change their brains . . . for the better.

THEODORE A. HENDERSON, MD, PhD, child, adolescent, and adult psychiatrist; cofounder of Neuro-Luminance Inc. Brain Health Centers; president of the International Society of Applied Neuroimaging

The End of Mental Illness blends cutting-edge brain science with progressive regenerative medicine to deliver revolutionary treatment for anyone suffering from a brain illness. The therapies work—I have witnessed firsthand the tremendous improvements in both my family and clients. Thank you, Dr. Amen, for showing how we can better care for our precious brains.

DR. MARK CALARCO, national medical director for clinical diagnostics, Addiction Labs of America

My dream is that, in future years, after seeing more mental health tragedies, we don't find ourselves saying, "We should have listened closer to Dr. Daniel Amen's call for a paradigm shift in the treatment of mental illness. His scientific leadership could have prevented so many of our personal and national disasters." Dr. Amen lays out proven science-based solutions to this in his book *The End of Mental Illness*.

JIM FAY, coauthor of *Parenting with Love and Logic*

Audacious claims and revolutionary ideas come from "out of the box" thinkers like Dr. Daniel Amen. He is leading the way in the fight to end mental illness, and he's doing it based on solid science and extensive clinical expertise.

WILLIAM S. HARRIS, PhD, president of OmegaQuant Analytics, LLC; professor of medicine, University of South Dakota

As usual, Dr. Amen is on point about mental illness and the use of advanced technologies to help diagnose and treat them. I applaud Dr. Amen's attention to SPECT scans, genetics, QEEG, and other modern technologies as tools to aid the prescriber. The day is coming soon when not using these techniques will be considered out of the norm, if not malpractice.

DANIEL A. HOFFMAN, MD, FAPA, retired neuropsychiatrist

The End of Mental Illness is a courageous, science-based approach to tackling our society's most pressing problems. Every day we read about suicide, drug addiction, and abnormal behavior ending in horrific crime. This book helps us understand these difficult behaviors and, most important, gives clear solutions. The book is very aptly titled and is a superb read.

ANDREW W. CAMPBELL, MD, editor-in-chief of *Alternative Therapies in Health and Medicine*; editor-in-chief of *Advances in Mind-Body Medicine*; editor of *Integrative Medicine: A Clinician's Journal*

Dr. Amen brings a functional medicine approach to mental health so you can learn how to support your brain health, reclaim your mood, and take care of yourself naturally. By sharing how the brain works and what we need to do to care for it, Dr. Amen hopes to end the stigma of mental health issues and replace it with compassion and understanding.

ALISA VITTI, HHC, author of *In the FLO*; founder of FLOliving.com

Having lost a brother to suicide and dealing with the life struggles of more than 14,000 students who attend my schools each year, I found in *The End of Mental Illness* the empowerment I need to bravely move forward without the shame and stigma associated with mental health issues. Dr. Amen delivers this valuable information with his neuroscience knowledge, but he is also a brilliant storyteller, which makes his message both relevant and relatable. In addition to a solid plan, *The End of Mental Illness* provides hope—a commodity rarely offered in the world of psychiatry today.

WINN CLAYBAUGH, dean and cofounder, Paul Mitchell Schools; author of *Be Nice (Or Else!)*

Dr. Amen is again well ahead of his time with this comprehensive, insightful, and compelling book. This book is a must-read for any individual or mental health professional who desires to obtain a more clear understanding of how to heal our brains for a happier and healthier life. Dr. Amen's refreshing biological and brain-based approach to understanding and resolving brain-related issues has the power to revolutionize the mental health industry.

DR. KRISTY HODSON, EdD in organizational change and leadership from the University of Southern California

A SAMPLE OF OTHER BOOKS BY DANIEL AMEN

Feel Better Fast and Make It Last, Tyndale, 2018

Memory Rescue, Tyndale, 2017

Stones of Remembrance, Tyndale, 2017

Captain Snout and the Super Power Questions, Zonderkidz, 2017

The Brain Warrior's Way, with Tana Amen, New American Library, 2016

The Brain Warrior's Way Cookbook, with Tana Amen, New American Library, 2016

Time for Bed, Sleepyhead, Zonderkidz, 2016

Change Your Brain, Change Your Life (revised), Harmony Books, 2015, *New York Times* Bestseller

Healing ADD (revised), Berkley, 2013, *New York Times* Bestseller

The Daniel Plan, with Rick Warren, DMin, and Mark Hyman, MD, Zondervan, 2013, #1 *New York Times* Bestseller

Unleash the Power of the Female Brain, Harmony Books, 2013

Use Your Brain to Change Your Age, Crown Archetype, 2012, *New York Times* Bestseller

The Amen Solution, Crown Archetype, 2011, *New York Times* Bestseller

Unchain Your Brain, with David E. Smith, MD, MindWorks, 2010

Change Your Brain, Change Your Body, Harmony Books, 2010, *New York Times* Bestseller

Magnificent Mind at Any Age, Harmony Books, 2008, *New York Times* Bestseller

The Brain in Love, Three Rivers Press, 2007

Making a Good Brain Great, Harmony Books, 2005, Amazon Book of the Year

ADD in Intimate Relationships, MindWorks, 2005

Preventing Alzheimer's, with William R. Shankle, MS, MD, Penguin, 2004

Healing Anxiety and Depression, with Lisa Routh, MD, Putnam, 2003

New Skills for Frazzled Parents, MindWorks, 2000

The Most Important Thing in Life I Learned from a Penguin!?, MindWorks, 1995

DANIEL G. AMEN, MD

THE **END** OF **MENTAL ILLNESS**

HOW NEUROSCIENCE IS TRANSFORMING PSYCHIATRY AND HELPING PREVENT OR REVERSE

MOOD AND ANXIETY DISORDERS, ADHD, ADDICTIONS, PTSD, PSYCHOSIS, PERSONALITY DISORDERS, AND MORE

TYNDALE
MOMENTUM®

The Tyndale nonfiction imprint

Visit Tyndale online at www.tyndale.com.

Visit Tyndale Momentum online at www.tyndalemomentum.com.

Visit Daniel G. Amen, MD, at http://www.amenclinics.com.

TYNDALE, *Tyndale Momentum,* and Tyndale's quill logo are registered trademarks of Tyndale House Publishers. The Tyndale Momentum logo is a trademark of Tyndale House Publishers. Tyndale Momentum is the nonfiction imprint of Tyndale House Publishers, Carol Stream, Illinois.

The End of Mental Illness: How Neuroscience Is Transforming Psychiatry and Helping Prevent or Reverse Mood and Anxiety Disorders, ADHD, Addictions, PTSD, Psychosis, Personality Disorders, and More

Designed by Libby Dykstra

Published in association with the literary agency of WordServe Literary Group, www.wordserveliterary.com.

Scripture quotations are taken from the *Holy Bible,* New Living Translation, copyright © 1996, 2004, 2015 by Tyndale House Foundation. Used by permission of Tyndale House Publishers, Carol Stream, Illinois 60188. All rights reserved.

For information about special discounts for bulk purchases, please contact Tyndale House Publishers at csresponse@tyndale.com, or call 1-800-323-9400.

Library of Congress Cataloging-in-Publication Data
Names: Amen, Daniel G., author.
Title: The end of mental illness : how neuroscience is transforming
   psychiatry and helping prevent or reverse mood and anxiety disorders,
   ADHD, addictions, PTSD, psychosis, personality disorders, and more /
   Daniel G. Amen, MD.
Description: Carol Stream, Illinois : Tyndale Momentum, the nonfiction
   imprint of Tyndale House Publishers, [2020] | Includes bibliographical
   references and index.
Identifiers: LCCN 2019042700 (print) | LCCN 2019042701 (ebook) |
   ISBN 9781496438157 (hardcover) | ISBN 9781496438171 (kindle edition) |
   ISBN 9781496438188 (epub) | ISBN 9781496438195 (epub)
Subjects: LCSH: Mental health–Popular works. | Mental
   illness–Treatment–Popular works. | Mental illness–Popular works.
Classification: LCC RA790 .A52 2020 (print) | LCC RA790 (ebook) | DDC
   616.89–dc23
LC record available at https://lccn.loc.gov/2019042700
LC ebook record available at https://lccn.loc.gov/2019042701

Printed in the United States of America

26   25   24   23   22   21   20
7   6   5   4   3   2   1

To Alizé and Amelie.

Your history is not your destiny.

Let's end mental illness with your generation.

Contents

Before You Begin

Daniel Amen, MD, believes that brain health is central to all health and success. When your brain works right, he says, you work right, and when your brain is troubled, you are much more likely to have trouble in your life. His work is dedicated to helping people have better brains and better lives.

Sharecare.com named him the web's #1 most influential expert and advocate on mental health, and the *Washington Post* called him the most popular psychiatrist in America.

A military-trained psychiatrist, he spent 10 years on active duty in the US Army—first as an infantry medic and X-ray technician and later as an officer in the Medical Corps. He is board-certified in child and adolescent psychiatry and general psychiatry. He holds active medical licenses in nine states.

He was given the Marie H. Eldridge Award for research by the American Psychiatric Association for his work on suicide, and he received the Distinguished Fellow Award from his peers at the American Psychiatric Association (the highest award given to members). He has presented his research and clinical work at scientific meetings around the world, including Harvard's Learning & the Brain conference and the National Science Foundation.

Discover magazine listed his research using brain SPECT imaging to accurately distinguish post-traumatic stress disorder from traumatic brain injury as one of the top 100 stories in science for 2015.

He is the principal investigator on the first and largest brain imaging and rehabilitation study on active and retired NFL players, showing high levels of damage but also the possibility of recovery for many, using the principles in this book. He was a consultant on the 2015 movie *Concussion* starring Will Smith.

Amen Clinics, which he founded in 1989, has the world's largest database of functional brain scans (SPECT and QEEG) related to behavior, totaling more than 170,000 scans on patients from 121 countries. Amen Clinics has some of the best published outcomes on complex psychiatric patients. On average, their patients have 4.2 diagnoses and have failed 3.3 providers and

5 medications. At the end of 6 months, 75 percent report being better; 84 percent if they maintained treatment at Amen Clinics.

Dr. Amen has hosted 14 public television specials about the brain, which have aired more than 110,000 times across North America during the past 12 years. He is passionate about brain health education.

Together with Pastor Rick Warren and Dr. Mark Hyman, Dr. Amen is also one of the chief architects of The Daniel Plan, a program designed to help people all around the world get healthy through religious organizations. This program has already been put in place in thousands of churches, mosques, and synagogues.

Dr. Amen and Professor Jesse Payne created the high school and college course Brain Thrive by 25, which has students from 7 countries and all 50 states. Independent research has found the program decreases drug, alcohol, and tobacco use; decreases depression; and improves self-esteem in teens.

In November 2017, a video of Dr. Amen's passion story (six minutes) was anonymously posted and now has more than 40 million views.[1]

No doubt Dr. Amen and his colleagues at Amen Clinics are disrupting psychiatry, the only medical specialty that virtually never looks at the organ it treats.

Dr. Amen has published more than 70 peer-reviewed scientific articles, including some of the largest brain imaging studies ever done on 21,000, 46,000, and 62,000 SPECT scans. If you type in "brain SPECT" in the search tool at the National Library of Medicine's website, www.pubmed.gov, it will return more than 14,000 scientific abstracts.

More than 10,000 mental health and medical professionals have referred patients to Amen Clinics, and more than 3,000 have been trained in his brain health coaching certification course.

Scientists in Canada have replicated his brain imaging work, publishing studies showing it improved diagnoses and outcomes.[2]

Dr. Amen does not work for or hold stock in any pharmaceutical companies, yet he believes in using psychiatric medications when necessary. However, they are usually not his first choice because, once started, they are often very hard to stop.

Dr. Amen owns BrainMD, a nutraceutical company he founded after seeing on brain imaging studies the negative effects of some medications he had prescribed. He believes in the principle taught to all first-year medical students: "First, do no harm."

LOOK FOR THESE ICONS

As you read *The End of Mental Illness*, keep an eye out for the three icons below.

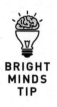

BRIGHT MINDS TIP

BRIGHT MINDS TIPS: Tips will highlight essential information.

BRAIN LOVE STORIES: When one person falls in love with their brain and optimizes how it functions, it tends to lead to many other people falling in love with their brains and a cascade of healing. When "brain love" goes viral, whole family, work, and community systems improve. We call these "brain love stories."

TINY HABITS: Helping people change has been Dr. Amen's passion for more than 40 years, so he partnered with BJ Fogg, director of the Persuasive Tech Lab at Stanford University, and his sister Linda Fogg-Phillips to learn the latest change technology. They believe creating "tiny habits" is the most effective way to facilitate big change: making small, incremental changes over time that evolve into big ones.

Introduction

WHY I HATE THE TERM *MENTAL ILLNESS* AND YOU SHOULD TOO

In times of profound change, the learners inherit the earth, while the learned find themselves beautifully equipped to deal with a world that no longer exists.
ERIC HOFFER

Stuck at a traffic light midday at the corner of Hollywood and Vine in Hollywood, California, on my way to record a podcast with storyteller and social media phenom Jay Shetty, I saw a thirtysomething man, about 5′10″, with dirty blond hair, ripped clothes, and blood on his face, talking to himself while gesturing wildly in the air. He seemed oblivious to everyone around him, and those walking on the street paid him no mind. After all, this was Hollywood and Vine. Most of my colleagues would have diagnosed him with schizophrenia or unstable bipolar disorder and wondered why he wasn't taking his medication to help the voices and visions stay away. When I saw him, I wondered when he'd had his last brain injury, if he had been exposed to mold or environmental toxins, if he suffered with severe gut-health issues, or whether he had an infectious disease like Lyme or toxoplasmosis ravaging his brain.

We are on the cusp of a new revolution that will change mental health care forever. *The End of Mental Illness* discards an outdated, stigmatizing paradigm that taints people with disparaging labels, preventing them from getting the help they need, and replaces it with a modern brain-based, whole-person program rooted in neuroscience and hope. No one is shamed for cancer, diabetes, or heart disease, even though they have significant lifestyle contributions. Likewise, no one should be shamed for depression, panic disorders, bipolar disorder, addictions, schizophrenia, and other brain health issues.

Over the last 30 years, my colleagues and I have built the world's largest database of brain scans related to behavior. We have performed more than 160,000 brain SPECT (single photon emission computed tomography) scans, which measure blood flow and activity patterns, and over 10,000

QEEGs (quantitative electroencephalograms), which measure electrical activity, on patients from 9 months old to 105 years from 121 countries. Our brain imaging work has completely disrupted how we help our patients get well, and this information can help you, even if no one ever looks at your brain. The human brain is an organ just like your heart and all your other organs, and you can only be as mentally healthy as your brain is functionally healthy.

It has become crystal clear to us that, as psychiatrists, we are not dealing with *mental health* issues, but we are dealing with *brain health* issues; and this one idea has changed everything we do to help our patients.

> **We are not dealing with mental health *issues, but we are dealing with* brain health *issues; and this one idea has changed everything.***

I have come to hate the terms *mental illness* and *psychiatric disorders*, and you should too. They place emphasis in the wrong domain (the mind or the psyche), when our imaging work teaches us that we must *first* focus on the brain. "Mental illness" and "psychiatric disorders" conjure up stigmatizing images of lunacy in people who are mad, disturbed, unbalanced, or unstable, even though these adjectives apply to an extremely small percentage of people who struggle with brain health/mental health issues.

Being diagnosed with a mental illness or a psychiatric disorder insidiously taints or stains everyone who struggles with perceived issues of the mind, making them less likely to ever want to seek help for fear they'll be diminished in the eyes of others. Just look at what happened to 1972 vice-presidential nominee Thomas Eagleton. The up-and-coming senator from Missouri, who had been the Show-Me State's youngest-ever attorney general, a devout Catholic, and a fiery opponent to the Vietnam War, was tapped to be presidential candidate George McGovern's running mate and was considered a perfect choice.[1] But when it was discovered that he had been treated for depression, he was asked to step down from McGovern's political ticket only 18 days after his nomination. Ever since this dark national memory, mental health issues have been considered lethal in political circles.

Yet, according to biographer Joshua Wolf Shenk, Abraham Lincoln "fought clinical depression all his life, and if he were alive today, his condition would be treated as a 'character issue'—that is, as a political liability. His condition was indeed a character issue: It gave him the tools to save the nation."[2] Shenk argues that because of depression, Lincoln knew how to suffer and how to rise above his bad feelings in difficult times. Of note, Lincoln had a serious head injury at age ten, when he was kicked in the head by a horse and left unconscious.[3] You will see that head injuries are a common and often overlooked cause of emotional and behavioral problems.

[Lincoln's depression] was indeed a character issue:
It gave him the tools to save the nation.

By labeling these issues as mental health or psychiatric instead of brain health, people suffer in silence because of the shame they feel. Consider the rash of celebrity suicides and deaths by overdose of people who were too embarrassed or ashamed to ask for help (from Ernest Hemingway, Judy Garland, and Junior Seau to Robin Williams, Mindy McCready, Philip Seymour Hoffman, Anthony Bourdain, and Kate Spade). On the outside, they seemed as if they had everything; on the inside, they were suffering.

If we do not erase—or at least lower—the stigma for these brain health issues, many more people will unnecessarily suffer and die without getting the help they need. We must do better because:

- About every 14 minutes, someone dies by suicide in the United States. Suicide is the 10th leading cause of death overall and the second leading cause of death for those 10 to 34 years of age.[4] Since 1999, suicide has increased 33 percent, decreasing overall life expectancy, while during the same period of time cancer has decreased 27 percent.[5] The last time America experienced a decrease in life expectancy was in the early 20th century, when the Spanish influenza and World War I killed nearly one million people. I've been surrounded by suicide, with an aunt who killed herself, as did my adopted son's biological father, and my son-in-law's father. The pain of suicide is unlike any other loss because people see it as a choice, rather than as a consequence of an illness.

- Every eight minutes, someone dies of a drug overdose,[6] and the recent opiate crisis in America is only getting worse year after year. In 2017, there were more than 70,000 drug overdoses, with 67 percent of them from opiates (an increase of 45 percent from 2016).[7]

- In 2017, teens and young adults in the United States were more prone to depression, distress, and suicide compared with millennials when they were the same age.[8]

- Thirty-six percent of girls will experience clinical depression during their teenage years, compared to 13 percent of teenage boys.[9] Both numbers are unacceptable.

- Twenty-three percent of women between the ages of 40 and 59 are taking antidepressant medication.[10]

- According to a large epidemiological study, 50 percent of the US population will struggle with a mental health issue at some point in their lives.[11] Anxiety disorders (28 percent), depression (21 percent), impulse control disorders (25 percent), and substance use disorders (15 percent) are the most common. Half of all cases start by age 14, and 75 percent start by age 24.

- According to the World Health Organization, 25 percent of all health-related disability is due to mental health and substance use conditions—eight times more than disability caused by heart disease and 40 times more than cancer.[12]

Shame holds people back from getting the help they need. No one is shamed for cancer, diabetes, or heart disease; likewise, no one should be shamed for depression, panic disorders, bipolar disorder, and other brain health issues.

Even though I have loved being a psychiatrist for the past 40 years, I am not a fan of my professional label because psychiatrists are often dismissed as unscientific and scorned by other medical professionals and the general public. In 1980, when I told my father, a highly intelligent and successful entrepreneur, that I wanted to be a psychiatrist, he asked me, "Why don't you want to be a 'real' doctor? Why do you want to be a nut doctor and hang out with nuts all day long?" At the time, his words upset me, but 40 years later, I have a deeper understanding of why he was concerned. In a similar vein, I've heard countless patients say, "I'm not going to see a psychiatrist because I'm not crazy." Stigma reigns. I prefer the term *clinical neuroscientist* to psychiatrist.

REIMAGINING *MENTAL* HEALTH AS *BRAIN* HEALTH CHANGES EVERYTHING

Early in my career, I learned that very few people *want* to see a psychiatrist. No one wants to be labeled as defective or abnormal, but once people learn about the importance of their brain, everyone wants a better one. What if *mental health* was *brain health*? That is what the brain imaging work we are doing at Amen Clinics teaches us daily. Think of it this way. Your brain can have problems just as your heart can have problems. Most people who see cardiologists, however, have never had a heart attack. They are there because they have risk factors—a family history of heart disease, high blood pressure, or too much abdominal fat—and they want to *prevent* a heart attack. To end mental illness, we must develop a similar way of thinking.

Reframing the discussion from mental health to brain health changes everything. People begin to see their problems as *medical*, not *moral*. It decreases shame and guilt and increases forgiveness and compassion from their families. Reframing the discussion to brain health is also more accurate and elevates hope, increases the desire to get help, and increases compliance to make the necessary lifestyle changes. Once people understand that the brain controls everything they do and everything they are, they want a better brain so they can have a better life.

Reframing the Discussion from Mental Health to Brain Health Changes Everything

- People see their problems as medical, not moral.
- It decreases stigma, shame, and guilt.
- It increases compassion and forgiveness from families.
- It is a more accurate description of the biology involved.
- It elevates hope.
- It increases compliance with treatment plans.

The End of Mental Illness will give you a completely new way to think about and treat brain health/mental health issues, such as anxiety, depression, bipolar disorders, attention deficit disorder/attention deficit hyperactivity disorder (ADD/ADHD), addictions, obsessive-compulsive disorder (OCD), post-traumatic stress disorder (PTSD), schizophrenia, and even personality disorders. It is based on a very simple premise: *Get your brain right, and your mind will follow.* In study after study, improving the physical functioning of the brain improves the mind.[13]

YOUR BRAIN'S HISTORY IS NOT YOUR DESTINY

The reason I dedicated this book to my two nieces, Alizé (15) and Amelie (10), is that they were born into a family plagued by mental illness—multiple suicides, major depression, schizophrenia, drug abuse, manic depressive behavior, OCD, anxiety and panic disorders, ADD/ADHD, body dysmorphia, and criminal behavior. Their genetic vulnerability for mental illness was incredibly high from before birth. In addition, they were born into chaos, with parents who struggled with addictions, depression, and behavioral issues. In 2016, Child Protective Services, who deemed they were living in a dangerous situation, took them from their parents. The two girls still vividly remember the panic and horror of police taking them from their mother.

At the time, my wife, Tana, was estranged from her half-sister, Tamara, the girls' mother, but when we found out that the children were taken into foster care, we knew we must act. We wrapped brain health/mental health services around Tamara (at the time, the father refused to get help), and she was able to gain control over her addiction, depression, ADHD, and past head trauma (19 car accidents). Thanks to this progress, she was reunited with her children on Mother's Day 2017. Since that time, using the principles in this book, Tamara, Alizé, and Amelie have thrived. Like all people who experience this type of chaos, they have had ups and downs, but Tamara is gainfully employed at a job she loves, and the girls are both A students, happy, social, and purposeful. At the time of this writing, Alizé is an honor society student and participates in cross country and track and field. In the last year, she has been awarded Language Arts, Life Science, and Automation and Robotics Student of the Year.

Tana, Tamara, and I are committed to ending the cycle of mental illness in the girls as well as in their future children and grandchildren. This book is our blueprint. It is your blueprint too. The end of mental illness starts with you and the people close to you.

ALIZÉ (RIGHT) AND AMELIE

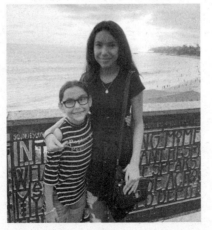

THIS BOOK IS YOUR BLUEPRINT

Part 1 will briefly introduce you to the history of psychiatry and mental health treatment. To illustrate this, I will reveal some of the surprising and downright shocking ways one of my patients, Jarrett, would have been treated throughout the ages. I'll help you reframe mental illness. We'll discard an outdated diagnostic paradigm based solely on symptom clusters and replace it with a brain-centered paradigm based on symptoms *plus* neuroimaging, genetics, and a personalized medicine approach to brain/body health. Then I'll share the 12 major lessons we've learned from our brain imaging work that completely changed the way we think about and help our patients. You will be introduced to the Amen Clinics Four Circles BRIGHT MINDS Program to end mental illness, which reveals the simple yet very powerful concept that, in order to have a healthy mind, you must first have a healthy brain. To do that, you must optimize the four circles of a whole life (biological, psychological, social, and spiritual), as well as prevent or treat the 11 major risk factors that damage the brain and steal your mind.

In part 2, you will learn how to create or eliminate mental illnesses. If you know how they're created, you will have the prescriptions to avoid and treat them. Here you'll discover the enormous impact that modern society has had on the exploding brain health/mental health crisis in America. This section will also explore the 11 BRIGHT MINDS risk factors that steal your mind and show you how to avoid them. I wrote about these risk factors extensively in my book *Memory Rescue* but only as they relate to memory; these same factors greatly influence other brain health/mental health problems. BRIGHT MINDS stands for:

Blood Flow

Retirement/Aging

Inflammation

Genetics

Head Trauma

Toxins

Mind Storms (abnormal brain electrical activity)

Immunity/Infections

Neurohormone Issues

Diabesity

Sleep

As you will see, once you reduce your risk factors, your brain—and mind—will be healthier.

In part 3, I'll share many practical strategies on how to boost your brain and optimize your mind, including how to think about psychiatric medicines versus nutritional supplements (nutraceuticals), the important health numbers to check every year, and the critical importance of your food. In addition, the final chapter summarizes the strategies on how to create and end mental illness.

BRIGHT MINDS TIP

Get your brain right, and your mind will follow. It's time to get the help you need by discarding an outdated, stigmatizing, unscientific paradigm.

Here's an example of why we need to discard the current outdated paradigm in favor of our new model.

 ## HOW CHASE ELIMINATED HIS "MENTAL ILLNESS" BY HEALING HIS BRAIN

Chase was a smart, successful young man fresh out of college with a great job. But inside, he was suffering. Chase struggled with severe anxiety, uncontrollable mood swings, negative thought patterns, crippling panic attacks, a bad temper, and disrupted sleep. He had difficulty with work relationships and making friends. He couldn't talk to people and always seemed to be in a bad mood. He also lacked a clear sense of any purpose.

As a teenager, he saw a psychiatrist, who after asking him to fill out a questionnaire, diagnosed Chase with bipolar disorder (a severe mood disorder in which people cycle between depression and mania) as well as ADHD and intermittent explosive disorder (IED). Chase also had a family history of depression and addictions.

Over the years, he jumped from one medication to the next, trying to find something that worked. The side effects only made things worse, and he gained more than 80 pounds. This young man, who already had social anxiety, now had even more reasons to isolate himself. Chase's brain and body finally gave up; he had a nervous breakdown and was unable to work.

Chase's stepmother, Terry, suggested he come to our clinic in New York

City for an evaluation. Terry's daughter had struggled with learning and anxiety attacks but had a dramatic turnaround after coming to our clinic. That inspired Terry to visit one of our clinics, which helped her improve her own troubled brain to become a better businesswoman. Subsequently, Terry sent many other members of her family to our clinics for help.

As we do with all our patients, we did a comprehensive evaluation of Chase. As part of our diagnostic process, we took a detailed history, performed neuropsychological tests, ran a lab workup (Chase had low levels of vitamin D and testosterone), and scanned his brain to assess blood flow and activity patterns in the brain. SPECT looks at how the brain works. It is different than CAT scans and MRIs, which are anatomy studies that look at the structure of the brain. SPECT looks at brain function and, in my opinion, is much more helpful for people with complex brain health/mental health problems, like ADD/ADHD and bipolar disorder. You will learn much more about our work with SPECT in chapters 2 and 3.

Chase's SPECT scan (see images on the following pages comparing his scan to a healthy scan) showed significantly low overall blood flow to his brain, especially to his prefrontal cortex (a brain region associated with focus, forethought, judgment, planning, empathy, and impulse control) and his temporal lobes (a brain region associated with mood stability, learning, memory, and temper control). His scan was consistent with past head trauma and toxicity, which caused us to ask Chase more pointed questions to try to understand why his brain looked so troubled.

It turned out that his family owned a NASCAR speedway, and Chase had been racing cars since he was a child, spending a lot of time around and breathing in toxic gasoline fumes. He'd had a number of significant concussions, including one from racing. Many people are misdiagnosed with bipolar disorder (mental illness) after they have had a significant concussion (brain illness) that affects their prefrontal cortex and temporal lobes.

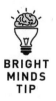

BRIGHT MINDS TIP

Many people are misdiagnosed with bipolar disorder after they have had a significant concussion. The right diagnosis is critical to effective treatment.

HEALTHY SPECT

CHASE'S SPECT

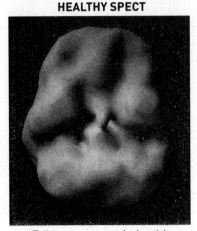

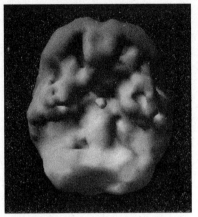

Full, even, symmetrical activity

Low activity (areas that look like indentations), especially in prefrontal cortex and temporal lobes

CHASE PLOWS INTO A WALL

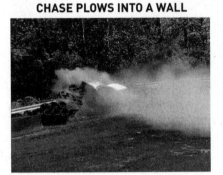

After seeing his scans and understanding the story of Chase's life, it was clear he did not have bipolar disorder, ADHD, and IED but, rather, the long-term effects of concussions and toxic exposure to the gasoline fumes, giving him these symptom clusters. We stopped his medications, gave him brain supportive supplements, and went to work rehabilitating his brain using the Amen Clinics Four Circles BRIGHT MINDS Program, which will be laid out in detail in upcoming chapters. As part of the program, we completely changed Chase's diet, encouraging him to only eat foods that served his brain health rather than ones that hurt it. Plus, he started exercising daily. Chase did everything we asked him.

CHASE'S BEFORE SPECT

AFTER SPECT

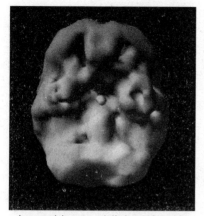

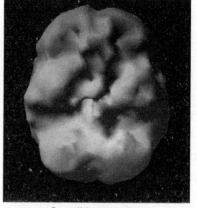

Low activity, especially in prefrontal cortex and temporal lobes

Overall improvement

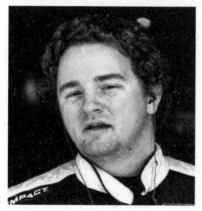

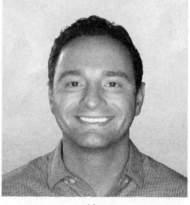

Before

After

In just a few months, his confidence soared. Several months later, his brain showed significant improvement. (His skin also cleared up, and he had lost 80 pounds—other signs that his brain was healthier.) Now he has an even better job where he says he has great working relationships, lots of friends outside the office, loves trying new things, and is in a committed relationship.

After learning about his brain, Chase still loves watching car racing but says he'll personally never race again. And not just because of the concussions but also because of the toxins he was inhaling: gas, oil, burned rubber, and all the other chemicals he does not want inside his body.

Chase desperately needed a radical new approach; both his physical and mental health were going the wrong way.

Chase had been given three major psychiatric diagnoses—bipolar disorder, ADHD, and IED—from his psychiatrist, who used checklists and groups of related symptoms, known as symptom clusters, from the American Psychiatric Association's Diagnostic and Statistical Manual of Mental Disorders (DSM), and his treatment was doing him more harm than good. Yes, on the surface, it is much easier to try different medications, hoping for a quick fix, and not have to bother with changing your life. But the medications we use in psychiatry are often insidious, meaning once you start them, they are very hard to stop. They change your brain to need them in order for you to feel normal. In the long run, it is generally easier to do a bit of work to change your habits, so you need fewer medications or, in some cases, none at all.

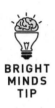

BRIGHT MINDS TIP

On the surface, it's easier to try different medications, hoping for a quick fix, and not have to bother with lifestyle changes. But psychiatric medications are often insidious, meaning once you start them they are very hard to stop. They change your brain to need them in order for you to feel normal.

The way we evaluated and helped Chase is very different from the typical way most people are diagnosed and treated for "mental illnesses." In 2020, if you suspect you have a mental health issue, you are likely to visit a psychiatrist or primary care physician (who prescribe 85 percent of psychiatric medications), who will ask you to describe your symptoms. In most cases, your doctor will listen, do an examination, then look for symptom clusters. Based on this, they will give you a diagnosis and treatment plan, usually involving one or more psychiatric medications.

For example, if you are anxious, you usually get an "anxiety disorder" diagnosis and end up with a prescription for an anti-anxiety medication, which has been found in some studies to be associated with an increased incidence of dementia.[14] If you have attention problems, you may end up with a diagnosis of ADHD and a prescription for stimulant medication, such as Ritalin or Adderall. These medications can help many people, but it's important to be aware that they can also make some people worse.

Or you may say, "I'm depressed." Your doctor will then label you with a diagnosis that has the same name as your symptoms—depression, in this example—without taking any biological information into consideration. Treatment is typically an antidepressant medication.

According to psychiatrist Thomas Insel, the former director of the National Institutes of Mental Health (NIMH), "For the antidepressants . . . the rate of response continues to be slow and low. In the largest effectiveness study to date, with more than 4,000 patients with major depressive disorder in primary care and community settings, only 31 percent were in remission after 14 weeks of optimal treatment. . . . In most double-blind trials of antidepressants, the placebo response rate hovers around 30 percent . . . The unfortunate reality is that current medications help too few people to get better and very few people to get well."[15] This is consistent with what Insel's predecessor, Steve Hyman, former director of the NIMH, wrote in 2018, that in the last half century we have failed to progress significantly in medications to treat psychiatric illnesses.[16]

A typical example of this outdated diagnostic method is for people who have temper problems, like Chase, and who explode intermittently. They often get diagnosed with IED, which is an ironic acronym. These people are often prescribed anger management classes or any number of medications.

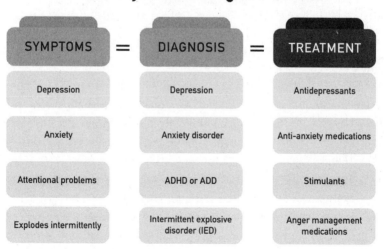

Current Psychiatric Diagnostic Model

SYMPTOMS	=	DIAGNOSIS	=	TREATMENT
Depression		Depression		Antidepressants
Anxiety		Anxiety disorder		Anti-anxiety medications
Attentional problems		ADHD or ADD		Stimulants
Explodes intermittently		Intermittent explosive disorder (IED)		Anger management medications

From our experience with tens of thousands of patients at Amen Clinics and after 40 years in the field, I'm convinced that making diagnoses solely based on DSM symptom clusters, such as anxiety, depression, temper outbursts, or a short attention span, is inadequate and disrespectful to patients.

Symptoms don't tell us anything about the underlying biology of the problems our patients have. All other medical professionals look directly at the organs they treat, but psychiatrists are taught to *assume* what the underlying biological mechanisms are for illnesses—such as depression, ADD/ADHD, bipolar disorder, and addiction—without ever looking at the brain, even though our patients are every bit as sick as those with heart disease, diabetes, or cancer.

> *Making diagnoses solely based on DSM symptom clusters, such as anxiety, depression, temper outbursts, or a short attention span, is inadequate.*

An explosive 2019 study in *Psychiatry Research* confirms what I've been saying for decades: Making psychiatric diagnoses based solely on symptom clusters is scientifically meaningless and disingenuous. The study, led by University of Liverpool researchers, focused on a meticulous analysis of five chapters in DSM-5: anxiety disorders, depressive disorders, trauma-related disorders, bipolar disorder, and schizophrenia. Their main findings highlight many of the shortcomings of the current diagnostic paradigm:[17]

- There is a major overlap of symptoms among diagnoses.
- Many diagnoses overlook the role of psychological trauma and head trauma.
- The current approach rarely takes the individual into account.

This study's deep dive into the numbers shows just how murky and inconsistent the diagnostic model is. For example, "there are almost 24,000 possible symptom combinations for panic disorder in DSM-5, compared with just one possible combination for social phobia." Equally concerning is their finding that "two people could receive the same diagnosis without sharing any common symptoms." And the sheer number of combinations of symptoms makes the ability to arrive at an accurate diagnosis nearly impossible. Take this stunning fact, for instance: "In the DSM-5 there are 270 million combinations of symptoms that would meet the criteria for both PTSD and major depressive disorder, and when five other commonly made diagnoses are seen alongside these two, this figure rises to one quintillion symptom combinations—more than the number of stars in the Milky Way." The researchers conclude that following a different approach may be more effective than remaining committed to what they called a "disingenuous categorical system."[18]

Rest assured, it doesn't have to be this way. Reframing the way we think about "mental illnesses" by looking at them as brain health issues is more accurate. It is this discovery that completely changed the way we approach diagnosing and treating our patients at Amen Clinics. It is also the underlying reason why Amen Clinics has one of the highest published success rates for complex patients, who have failed an average of 3.3 providers and five medications.[19] In fact, 84 percent of the complex, treatment-resistant patients we treat at Amen Clinics report feeling better after six months.

This book will share some of those stories and provide the steps to end mental illness now, not just in the lives of Alizé and Amelie, but also in your own life and in the lives of your children and grandchildren.

1. Eliminate the term *mental illness* and replace it with the term *brain health/mental health issues.*

2. Discard an outdated diagnostic paradigm based solely on symptom clusters and replace it with a brain-centered paradigm based on symptoms *plus* neuroimaging, genetics, and a personalized medicine approach to brain/body health (chapters 1–3).

3. Assess and treat whole people in four circles—biological, psychological, social, and spiritual (chapter 4).

4. Prevent or treat the 11 major BRIGHT MINDS risk factors that damage the brain and steal the mind (chapters 5–15).

5. First, do no harm. Know the science comparing "mind meds" versus nutraceuticals. Nutraceuticals have more scientific support than most people know and are often an evidence-based option (chapter 16).

6. Know your important health numbers and re-check them on a yearly basis to help prevent brain health/mental health issues before they start (chapter 17).

7. Eat foods that enhance brain health rather than those that accelerate brain/mind illnesses (chapter 18).

8. Provide brain health/mental health education in schools, businesses, churches, and anywhere people congregate (chapter 19).

PART 1

REFRAMING MENTAL HEALTH AS BRAIN HEALTH CHANGES EVERYTHING

CHAPTER 1

FROM DEMON POSSESSION TO THE 15-MINUTE MED CHECK

A BRIEF HISTORY OF MENTAL ILLNESS DIAGNOSES AND TREATMENTS

The first known use of "headshrinker" as a slang term for a psychotherapist appeared in the Nov. 27, 1950 issue of Time *magazine, which asserted that anyone who had predicted the phenomenal success of the television Western* Hopalong Cassidy *would have been sent to a "headshrinker." The article explained in a footnote that headshrinker is Hollywood slang for a psychiatrist. . . . The headshrinker metaphor arguably reflects the feelings of fear, mystery, and hostility traditionally associated with the profession. Another theory holds that it implicitly refers to shrinking a patient's narcissistic, inflated sense of self. Although many mental-health professionals have come to accept the term with self-deprecating humor, it has also been criticized as a relic of an outmoded therapeutic approach that reduces people to mere causes and symptoms rather than regarding them as complex individuals.*[1]

When one person gets better, it can cause a cascade of help across generations of people. When I first met my wife, Tana, in 2006, I really, really liked her. Having been divorced for six years, I had told myself that before I ever married again, I would need to see the woman's brain scan before going to the next level. About three weeks after we met, I invited Tana to the clinic. She was a neurosurgical intensive care nurse, and we bonded over our love of the brain, so it wasn't that weird. Her brain was beautiful, and two-and-a-half years later we were married. Over the years, that one scan changed many other brains.

A few months after Tana was scanned, a neurologist diagnosed Tana's estranged father with Alzheimer's disease, but when I scanned her dad, his

SPECT scan showed he did not have Alzheimer's disease but, rather, depression masquerading as it. We prescribed natural dietary supplements for him, and several months later, he was able to teach a six-hour seminar at a local church. Then Tana's mother and uncle were fighting at work, so I evaluated and scanned them. It turned out they both had terrible attention deficit hyperactivity disorder (ADHD). On medication they got along much better, and their business improved. Then, a friend of Tana's from her early 20s saw us on a public television show together and reached out to Tana because her son, Jarrett, was really struggling.

 ## JARRETT

Jarrett was diagnosed with ADHD in preschool. His mother said he was driven by a motor that was revved way too high. He was hyperactive, hyperverbal, restless, and impulsive, and he couldn't focus. He also didn't sleep well and interrupted everyone all the time. He had no friends—his classmates avoided him, and their parents kept their children away from him. His third-grade teacher said he would never do well in school and cautioned his parents to lower their expectations. He had seen five doctors and was prescribed five stimulant medications for ADHD. All of them made Jarrett worse, triggering mood swings and terrible rages. He put holes in the walls of their home and scared his siblings. His behavior had gotten so bad that his last doctor wanted to put him on an antipsychotic medication. This is when his mother brought him to see us. Jarrett's brain SPECT scan clearly showed dramatic overactivity in a pattern we call "the ring of fire." No wonder stimulants didn't work; it was like pouring gasoline on a fire. Our published research shows that stimulants make this pattern worse 80 percent of the time.[2]

On a group of natural supplements to calm his brain—together with parent training and structured, brain-healthy habits—Jarrett's behavior dramatically improved. His grades went up, the rages stopped, and he was able to make friends. He has now been on the honor roll for eight straight years. After searching for so long, his parents are grateful to have found the correct treatment plan for him, which has completely altered the course of his life. There is no telling what the future would have held for Jarrett if he had stayed on his previous path.

JARRETT AND DR. AMEN

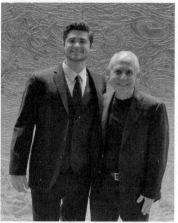

HOW WOULD JARRETT HAVE BEEN TREATED THROUGHOUT HISTORY?

The word *psychiatry* originates from the Medieval Latin *psychiatria*, meaning "healing of the soul."[3] Many societies have viewed mental illness as a form of divine punishment or demon possession. This chapter will walk you through history to show you some of the strange and unsettling things that would have been prescribed in an attempt to heal Jarrett.

Ancient civilization

In ancient Indian, Egyptian, Greek, and Roman writings, mental illness was often seen as a religious or personal failure. As early as 6,500 BC, prehistoric skulls and cave art showed evidence of trepanation, a surgical procedure that involved drilling or scraping a hole in the skull to release evil spirits thought to be trapped inside.[4]

Treatment: Religious leaders may have attempted an exorcism for Jarrett or drilled a hole in his skull to release the evil spirits.

TREPANATION TO ALLOW TRAPPED EVIL SPIRITS TO ESCAPE

HIPPOCRATES

The Greek physician Hippocrates (460–370 BC) believed all mental illnesses came from the brain.[5] He wrote, "Men ought to know that from the brain, and from the brain only, arise our pleasures, joy, laughter, and jests, as well as our sorrows, pains, despondency, and tears. . . . And by the same organ we become mad and delirious, where fears and terrors assail us. . . . All these things we endure from the brain, when it is not healthy."[6]

Recognized as the "father of medicine," Hippocrates proposed one of the first classifications of mental disorders, including mania, melancholy, phrenitis (brain inflammation, fever, delirium), insanity, disobedience, paranoia, panic, epilepsy, and hysteria. Some of those terms are still used today. The renowned physician did not view mental illness as shameful; he believed that mentally ill people were not responsible for their behavior and advocated that their family care for them at home. He was a pioneer in treating mentally ill people with more rational techniques, focusing on changing a person's diet, environment, or occupation and adding medications, exercise, music, art therapy, and even divine solicitation.

It's incredible to consider that nearly 2,500 years ago, Hippocrates was already suggesting that mental illnesses should be treated as physical medical illnesses and treated with lifestyle changes (the main point of this book).[7] However, he also theorized that physical and medical illnesses were caused by an imbalance of four essential bodily fluids or humors (blood, yellow bile, black bile, and phlegm), which is partly to blame for the practices of bloodletting and purging (similar to taking laxatives to empty the bowels).

Treatment: Likely, Hippocrates would have had Jarrett exercise, listen to music, create art, and focus on an occupation that fit his restless nature. He may have also bled him to release excess blood and had him take some natural supplements.

GALEN

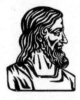

Galen (AD 130–201), another Greek physician during the Roman Empire and ultimately one of the most influential physicians in history, agreed with Hippocrates' four-humor theory of illness and associated them to four temperaments:

- Sanguine (blood: extroverted, social, risk-taking)
- Phlegmatic (phlegm: relaxed, peaceful, easy-going)
- Choleric (yellow bile: take-charge, decisive, goal-oriented)
- Melancholic (black bile: creative, kind, and introverted)

Like Hippocrates, Galen believed no difference existed between mental and physical illness[8] and noted that psychological stress could cause mental health issues. He is credited with the development of a tripartite theory of the soul, attempting to localize where the three parts were housed in the body: rational (brain), spiritual (heart), and appetitive (liver). In his book, *On the Diagnosis and Cure of the Soul's Passion*, Galen discussed how to treat psychological problems, which some have called an early attempt at psychotherapy.[9] He directed people with psychological issues to share their deepest passions and secrets, which can help them feel better.

Treatment: Galen would have prescribed Jarrett a treatment plan similar to Hippocrates, with the addition of talk therapy.

Middle Ages

By the Middle Ages, supernatural explanations of mental illnesses resurfaced in Europe in an attempt to explain natural disasters, such as plagues and famines. In the 13th century, mentally ill people, especially females, were treated as demon-possessed witches. In the 16th century, Dutch physician Johann Weyer and Englishman Reginald Scot tried to persuade their populations that those accused of witchcraft were actually people with mental illnesses in need of help, but the Catholic Church's Inquisition banned their writings. This practice did not decline until the 17th and 18th centuries. In the largest set of witch trials in America, between February 1692 to May 1693, more than 200 people were accused of being witches in Salem, Massachusetts; 20 were executed (14 females and 6 males), and others died in prison.

In the 16th and 17th centuries, asylums were created to house the mentally ill against their will. Inmates, many of whom were chained and beaten, often lived in squalor. Sometimes they were even exhibited to those willing to pay a fee. They were also subjected to a host of arcane medical practices, such as purging, blistering, or bloodletting.[10]

Treatment: Religious leaders may have attempted an exorcism on Jarrett, or physicians may have placed him in an asylum, where he would have been blistered, bled, or given laxatives.

18th and 19th centuries

In 1789, King George III of England descended into madness. His doctors were unable to say if he would recover or if someone else should replace him.[11] This crisis triggered physicians at England's insane asylums to begin looking into the inheritance patterns of mental illness. Long before the discovery of DNA, doctors started collecting family histories of the insane, criminals, and those with intellectual disabilities among those in the asylums, prisons, and schools for "feebleminded" children. At the time, physicians who specialized in mental illness were called alienists because they treated people who were alienated from society. Some alienists thought stress caused mental illness, but most ascribed to the belief that it was transmitted through families by heredity.

Asylum directors started using family trees and surveys to study and track down affected relatives of their patients and institutionalized them as well, believing these people should be discouraged from reproducing. Asylum superintendents, legislators, and social reformers embarked on a deeply mis-guided eugenics movement to improve society by passing sterilization laws that were eventually supported by the US Supreme Court (1927 Buck vs. Bell case). They passed in 32 states and formed part of the rationale for Nazi Germany's atrocities. This movement continued into the 1960s, with more than 60,000 Americans undergoing sterilization.[12]

In 18th-century Europe, protests broke out over the conditions in the asylums, and reformers aimed to end the abusive practices. They took the patients out of chains and encouraged good hygiene, recreation, and occupa-tional training.[13] In the United States, one of the signers of the Declaration of Independence, physician Benjamin Rush, who is considered the father of American psychiatry, established a more benevolent approach, unshackling patients, forbidding beatings, and lobbying for improved living conditions in Pennsylvania.

This doesn't mean that all of Rush's therapies were helpful. In his book, *Medical Inquiries and Observations upon the Diseases of the Mind*, he wrote that hypochondriasis, a form of melancholia or modern-day depression, needed to be treated by "direct and drastic interferences" that involved "assaulting the patient's mind and body" in an attempt to reset their constitution.[14] He recommended that doctors "plumb" patients' systems by bleeding (leeches), blistering, and cupping (similar to the current cupping trend that reached national attention when swimmer Michael Phelps was spotted at the 2016 Olympics with the telltale purple blotches on his back that arise from the treatment[15]). Rush also prescribed drugs, like mercury, arsenic, and strychnine—now known to be poisonous—to induce vomiting and diarrhea and suggested fasting for two or three days.[16] Once the body was cleaned out, he recommended stimulants, such as tea and coffee, ginger, and black pepper in large doses; magnesia, mustard rubs; hot baths to induce sweating followed by cold baths; and exercise.

When Abraham Lincoln was severely depressed in January 1841, his physician Dr. Anson Henry subscribed to Rush's aggressive theories and likely subjected the future president to these punishing treatments. After Lincoln spent a week alone with Dr. Henry, he described himself "as the most miserable man living."[17]

Rush also believed many psychiatric illnesses were the result of blocked circulation. To improve brain blood flow in schizophrenic patients, Rush would strap them into the "gyrating chair," a device that spun them around until they became dizzy. It didn't work.

In the 1770s, Europe was influenced by German physician Franz Anton Mesmer, who attempted to treat the "energy blockages" he believed were at the root of mental illness. He thought all illnesses could be attributed to an insufficient flow of what he called "animal magnetism." By putting patients into a trance-like state and then probing certain body parts to restore energy flow, Mesmer drove his patients to states of crisis (delirium or seizures). In some patients, symptoms miraculously vanished after the treatment, rocketing Mesmer to celebrity status. In 1843, Scottish physician James Braid coined the term *hypnosis* for a technique originally derived from animal magnetism to induce hypnotic trances.

Treatment: Jarrett may have been institutionalized and sterilized, if not euthanized, and his family placed under suspicion. American physician Rush might have prescribed blistering and poisonous drugs like arsenic, followed by hot and cold baths. Germany's Mesmer might have hypnotized Jarrett to relieve the blockage of energy.

FREUD AND PSYCHOANALYSIS

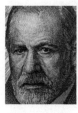

In the late 19th century, Viennese physician Sigmund Freud voyaged to Salpêtriere Hospital in Paris, where he studied with the founder of modern neurology Jean-Martin Charcot, who was best known for his work with hysteria and hypnosis. Charcot used hypnosis as a cathartic energy release to enable healing. Freud later abandoned hypnosis in favor of psychoanalysis, the talking cure, which dominated psychiatry for the first half of the 20th century.

Freud, a neurologist, was determined to understand the human mind. He tried to understand it from a neuroscience or brain perspective, but gave up in 1895, when he concluded that the science of his time was not up to the task of explaining patients' symptoms. Eventually, he came to believe in the power of the subconscious, which could not be accessed during wakefulness but could be accessed in hypnotic trances and later through psychoanalysis. For Freud, the mind was like an iceberg—the largest part was unconscious and hidden from sight. He argued that the mind had three parts: (1) the id (child self, selfish desires, and instincts), (2) ego (adult self that helps control the id to make more rational decisions), and (3) superego (moral self that is the voice in your head judging your actions).

He developed the "talking cure" of psychoanalysis to help rid mentally ill patients of the internal conflicts between their id, ego, and superego, which he viewed as the cause of many mental illnesses. For example, if a man wants to steal from his employer (id), he may sublimate the desire by writing crime stories or deny the desire altogether. But what if these defense mechanisms (sublimation and denial) are not strong enough? Freud hypothesized the person may develop a psychiatric disorder. By encouraging people to talk about their hidden fears and desires, Freud believed he could lead them to a cure. He encouraged his patients to talk about everything that came to mind, including their dreams, then he would psychoanalyze them. He believed many conflicts typically started in childhood. Psychoanalysis provided the launching pad for hundreds of schools of psychotherapy and "talking cures" still in existence today, including behavior therapy; cognitive behavioral therapy; psychodynamic therapy; and marital, family, and group therapy.

Treatment: Freud may have had Jarrett lying on the psychiatrist's couch four or five times a week, attempting to work out his internal conflicts.

KRAEPELIN AND THE BIOLOGICAL CAUSES OF MENTAL ILLNESS
A contemporary of Freud's, German psychiatrist Emil Kraepelin believed the primary cause of mental illness was biological with a strong genetic component. His theories were influential during the early 20th century and reemerged at the end of the 20th century when psychoanalysis fell out of favor. Viewing psychiatry as a branch of medicine, he began developing the modern classification system for mental disorders. He also protested against the inhumane treatments in psychiatric asylums and argued against alcoholism and capital punishment. He emerged as an advocate for the treatment, rather than the imprisonment, of the insane and rejected Freud's psychoanalytical theories as unscientific, especially those suggesting that early sexual urges were the cause of mental illness.

Treatment: Kraepelin would have diagnosed Jarrett with a brain that was misfiring and attempted to find a biological cure.

Early 20th century

FEVER, INSULIN SHOCK, ECT, AND LOBOTOMY CURES

Austrian physician Julius Wagner-Jauregg experimented with curing psychosis by inducing fevers. Misguided, he infected his patients with a by-product of the bacteria that causes tuberculosis. It was not successful. Undeterred, he began to use malaria parasites in 1917 to treat psychotic patients suffering from syphilis. Fifteen percent of them died, and the rest contracted malaria, but the fevers did temporarily decrease their symptoms. Wagner-Jauregg was awarded the Nobel Prize for his research in 1927.

In 1927, another Austrian psychiatrist, Manfred Sakel, administered large doses of insulin to purposely cause seizures in psychotic patients. Researchers discovered that if blood glucose levels went too low, people fell into a coma or experienced seizures, and this could temporarily alleviate symptoms. Unfortunately, the treatment was associated with negative side effects, such as obesity, and more severe consequences, including brain damage and even death.

In 1938, Italian neurologists Ugo Cerletti and Lucino Bini were the first to deliver electric shocks to patients to induce seizures. They found that electroconvulsive therapy (ECT) had more lasting benefits than insulin-shock therapy with fewer side effects. ECT is still used today to treat severe cases of schizophrenia, depression, mania, and serious suicidal thoughts.[18] With anesthesia, muscle relaxants, and more targeted dosing, it can be an effective technique, but it can also cause memory problems, confusion, headaches, and muscle aches.

In 1935, Portuguese neurologist António Egas Moniz drilled holes into the skulls of 20 mentally disturbed patients and used a wire in 13 of them to sever the connections in the brain's frontal lobes. Moniz was hoping the procedure, called a lobotomy, would calm his patients, who suffered from anxiety, depression, and schizophrenia. It worked! Patients became more compliant, spurring wide adoption of the procedure, which was subsequently used on thousands of patients. Over time, however, it became apparent that it destroyed personalities and turned people into zombie-like beings. Despite these alarming side effects, Moniz also received a Nobel Prize for his work.

Treatment: Wagner-Jauregg would have given Jarrett malaria in an attempt to heal him. Sakel would have tried insulin-shock therapy on Jarrett. Cerletti and Bini would have subjected Jarrett to electric shock therapy to reset his brain. Moniz would have performed a frontal lobotomy on Jarrett, calming his aggression but permanently damaging his personality.

Today, there is a renaissance of surgical techniques for psychiatric illnesses, but they are very different from the frontal lobotomy of old. Very precise, nondamaging surgical interventions can be used to turn off or on certain circuits in the brain. This approach has been effective in Parkinson's disease and has shown some efficacy for obsessive-compulsive disorder (OCD) and some patients with refractory depression.

LOBOTOMY: SURGICALLY DAMAGING FRONTAL LOBES

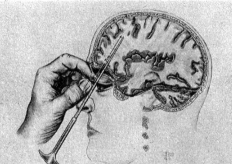

The late 20th century
THE MIND MEDICATION REVOLUTION

Despite psychoanalysis and the other techniques listed above, there was little hope for a cure for serious mental illnesses until the 1950s, when a host of psychiatric medications became available to practitioners and patients. The first effective medication for schizophrenia (chlorpromazine, brand name Thorazine) was developed in 1951 to treat nausea and allergies and to calm patients before surgery. When it was administered to a hospitalized violent young man, it immediately calmed him and caused such an improvement in his behavior, he was discharged a few weeks later. Chlorpromazine and subsequently other antipsychotic medications, which reportedly block excessive dopamine in the brain, led to dramatic improvements for many psychotic patients and ultimately to a significant reduction in state hospital populations.

The 1950s also saw the release of methylphenidate (Ritalin), which soon was prescribed to help hyperactive children; chlordiazepoxide (Librium), the first benzodiazepine, for anxiety disorders; and imipramine (Tofranil) for severe depression. The age of psychopharmacology had begun in earnest, with medications for bipolar disorder, OCD, and other disorders flooding the market in the decades that followed.

While I was in medical school, Xanax was released for panic disorders with the erroneous notion that it was less addictive than Librium and the other benzodiazepines. Since it was new, psychiatric residents prescribed it a lot, which is something I later regretted when I saw what it did to SPECT scans. Plus, whenever I prescribed it to patients, I found it was incredibly hard for them to get off it.

In 1987, with the FDA approval of the blockbuster antidepressant Prozac (fluoxetine), the mind drug revolution began to dominate psychiatry. Reportedly, Prozac had fewer side effects than imipramine and medications like it, leading to other selective serotonin reuptake inhibitor (SSRIs) antidepressant medications being approved for depression. Since Prozac was introduced, antidepressant use in the United States has increased 400 percent, and more than one in 10 Americans now takes one. Only medications to lower cholesterol are prescribed more often than antidepressants in the United States.[19]

After the global success of Prozac, the "chemical imbalance" theory of mental illness burst into the public consciousness, and many people began proactively asking their doctors to fix their down moods. Famously, after actress Carrie Fisher was cremated, her ashes were placed in a green and white Prozac-pill shaped urn.

Since Prozac was introduced, antidepressant use in the United States has increased 400 percent, and more than one in 10 Americans now takes one.

Taking pills may seem like an easier and quicker solution to bad moods than taking the time and effort to develop brain-healthy habits, build skills, or change troublesome behavior. Yet there is a dark side to the mind-meds that is often overlooked. Thousands of lawsuits claim that Prozac and other psychiatric medications increase violent or suicidal behavior. Virtually all antidepressants and antipsychotic medications have black box warnings, which, in simple terms means the FDA cautions patients in the strongest terms to pay close attention to potentially extremely harmful or dangerous threats to their health.

In 1991, just when I was beginning to use brain SPECT imaging, reports surfaced suggesting Prozac increased violent behavior. When it happened to one of my patients, it horrified me. It caused us to start reviewing scans to see if we could predict which scan patterns were associated with medications making patients worse, such as the negative reaction Jarrett had on multiple stimulants. We have published papers on ADD/ADHD[20] and depression,[21] revealing the SPECT patterns that are associated with both positive and negative responses to medications.

Despite the problems, the pharmaceutical industry is incredibly successful at marketing psychiatric medications to doctors and the general public.

From 1997 to 2016, the industry increased direct-to-consumer prescription drug advertising from $1.3 billion to $6 billion.[22] Prescription drug ads often do not adequately explain side effects, and because of repeated exposure, many people tune out those statements at the end of TV commercials, often delivered in a rapid-fire manner, such as, "This drug may cause permanent liver damage, seizures, an allergic reaction that leads to fatal throat swelling and suicidal tendencies." Patients in the United States are more than twice as likely to ask for drugs seen in ads compared with those in Canada, where most direct-to-consumer advertising is prohibited.[23]

There is no doubt in my mind that psychiatric medication saves lives, especially for people who have the more serious brain-health/mental-health disorders, such as bipolar disorder and schizophrenia. Yet we should all be cautious with meds because, once they are started, they are hard to stop,[24] and they do not just reset your brain; they change it. An Oxford University study found most SSRIs—such as Prozac, Paxil, Zoloft, and Lexapro—do not just decrease negative emotions; they reduce all emotions, including love, happiness, and joy. Participants felt separated from their surroundings and cared less about important things in their daily lives. They felt like their personalities had changed.[25]

Treatment: Even though Jarrett had failed five prescription medications before seeing us, other doctors would continue the trial and error method of trying to get his symptoms under control.

THE DSM: A MORE SCIENTIFIC APPROACH?

In an effort to adopt a more objective and scientific approach and to increase standardization in a field that struggled with credibility, in 1952, the American Psychiatric Association (APA) released the first version of the Diagnostic and Statistical Manual of Mental Disorders (DSM-I), which categorized all mental disorders. Initially modeled after diagnostic tools used by the military and Veterans Administration, the DSM has since undergone revisions resulting in five subsequent editions (DSM-II 1968, DSM-III 1980, DSM-IIIR 1987, DSM-IV 1994, and DSM-V 2013). The DSM has had great success and nearly all mental health professionals in the United States and many around the world use it. Yet it is not without controversy.

In a 2005 lecture at the annual meeting of the APA, Thomas Insel, one of the most powerful psychiatrists in the world at the time as director of the National Institutes of Mental Health, caused an uproar when he announced the DSM was 100 percent reliable . . . but zero percent valid, meaning if you make a diagnosis with the criteria today for a certain disorder, like depression, you will make it again tomorrow, but zero percent valid because it is not based on any underlying neuroscience.

After the DSM-V was released in 2013, Insel posted a blog:

> The goal of this new manual, as with all previous editions, is to provide a common language for describing psychopathology. While DSM has been described as a "Bible" for the field, it is, at best, a dictionary, creating a set of labels and defining each. The strength of each of the editions of DSM has been "reliability"—each edition has ensured that clinicians use the same terms in the same ways. The weakness is its lack of validity. Unlike our definitions of ischemic heart disease, lymphoma, or AIDS, the DSM diagnoses are [not] based on . . . any objective laboratory measure. . . . Patients with mental disorders deserve better.[26]

After using a number of the DSM versions on thousands of patients over the past 40 years, it is clear to me that it can help us categorize illnesses such as depression, bipolar disorder, schizophrenia, panic disorder, or borderline personality disorder, but it doesn't tell us anything about what causes them or how to predict which treatments will work because, as Insel suggested, it is not based on any underlying neuroscience.

What's more, each new version of the DSM adds additional mental disorders, which leads to an increase in the number of people diagnosed with problems—a concept called medicalization, where, in a given year, about one in five Americans will suffer from at least one DSM disorder.[27] Contrast that with rates from the 1950s when far fewer people were being diagnosed each year. The more disorders that are included in the DSM, and the more lenient their definitions, the easier it is to diagnose healthy people as having a problem. Predictably, the increase in "sick" people correlates with an increase in treatment, especially medications.

Treatment: Jarrett had been diagnosed with DSM-IV ADHD since the age of three, but none of the standard medications recommended had worked. In fact, they all made him worse.

THE 15-MINUTE MED CHECK

When I was in training in the late 1970s to mid-1980s, psychiatrists were able to spend time with patients. If patients needed to be hospitalized, psychiatrists could treat and stabilize them over weeks or months. In outpatient settings, psychiatrists performed both psychotherapy and medication management, often seeing patients one to two times a week. In the early 1990s, when managed health care became more popular, insurance companies began to dictate how long patients could stay in the hospital and how many sessions they could have with therapists. Having been in the trenches at the time, it seemed to me that many of their decisions were based not on patient need but on attempts to optimize company profits.

Over the years, professionals have been squeezed to see more patients in less time in order to make enough money to pay back their student loans and support their families. Less trained and less expensive professionals were doing more therapy and psychiatrists were relegated to 15-minute monthly med checks. As med checks increased, so did the use of psychiatric medication, in part because it was the unique tool psychiatrists had in their toolboxes. As a side effect of the 15-minute med check, psychiatrists became more disconnected from the intimate details of patients' lives.

Treatment: Jarrett and his parents had seen 5 different doctors who all practiced with the 15-minute med check model. It was not helpful.

The 21st century
NONPSYCHIATRIC PHYSICIANS, NURSE PRACTITIONERS, AND PHYSICIAN ASSISTANTS ARE NOW WRITING MOST OF THE PRESCRIPTIONS TO MANAGE YOUR MIND

One of the most disturbing trends is that nearly 85 percent of psychiatric medications are prescribed by primary care physicians, nurse practitioners, and physician assistants in short office visits, and 72 percent of these prescriptions are accompanied by no diagnosis in the charts.[28] These medical professionals often do not have the time or the specialized training to develop comprehensive treatment plans or to tell you about safer and more natural solutions. Some primary care physicians do a wonderful job handling mental health issues, while others cause more harm than good.

Treatment: Many patients like Jarrett start by getting prescriptions from their family physicians or pediatricians. Sometimes this is helpful, sometimes not.

TRANSCRANIAL MAGNETIC STIMULATION (TMS)

TMS is a newer treatment to change the brain for the better. It uses brief magnetic pulses to stimulate activity in the areas of the brain known to affect mood, anxiety, and pain. This is *not* the same as ECT from the 1930s. TMS does not require anesthesia, plus it's less expensive and has fewer side effects than ECT. An Israeli study showed that TMS and ECT have similar efficacy.[29] The FDA has approved TMS for the treatment of resistant depression, but new evidence shows it can enhance memory and potentially help improve a wide range of other brain-related issues, including depression;[30] anxiety;[31] addiction;[32] smoking cessation;[33] post-traumatic stress disorder (PTSD);[34] OCD;[35] cognitive problems, memory, and dementia;[36] and tinnitus (ringing in the ears).[37] At Amen Clinics, we use TMS differently than most of our colleagues. We change the settings based on what we see from our brain imaging work. Doing the same treatment settings for everyone is like giving every depressed patient the same medication, which seems to work about as well as giving a placebo.

Treatment: Jarrett may have tried a course of TMS.

MARIJUANA AND PSYCHEDELICS

The current trend, besides pharmaceutical medication, is using marijuana and psychedelic drugs—such as LSD, ketamine, psilocybin mushrooms, ecstasy, ayahuasca, and ibogaine—to treat psychiatric illnesses. At the time of this writing, using marijuana for at least medical purposes is legal in 30 states, with more on the way. As the perception of the danger of a drug goes down, its use goes up. Many clinicians are now prescribing marijuana and CBD (cannabidiol, one of the ingredients of the marijuana and hemp plants) oil to help patients with anxiety, depression, irritability, and aggression despite limited research. This new market has made many marijuana millionaires with an exuberance rarely seen. The FDA recently approved a cannabidiol solution, Epidiolex, for two seizure disorders.

Our brain imaging work over the last 30 years has given me pause in regard to marijuana, and at the time of this writing, the jury is still out for me on CBD. Over the last 30 years, I've seen thousands of SPECT scans of patients who were regular marijuana users. In 2016, my colleagues and I published a study on more than 1,000 marijuana users and showed that virtually every area of the brain was lower in blood flow compared to healthy scans, especially in the hippocampus, one of the brain's major memory centers.[38] In 2018, we published the world's largest brain imaging study on 62,454 SPECT scans on how the brain ages. Marijuana was associated with accelerated aging in the brain.[39] So caution is needed.

Other professionals are also studying and using psychedelics for addictions and depression, especially ketamine. Due to its hallucinogenic effects, ketamine has a reputation as a popular and illicit party drug, going by the nickname "Special K." It dulls pain and users often feel detached or dissociated from their own body. First developed in the 1960s, ketamine was administered as an anesthetic and given to soldiers during the Vietnam War. In 2000, researchers started studying ketamine as a treatment for depression and discovered that it improves mood much faster than traditional antidepressant medications, and sometimes works when other drugs have failed. More than a hundred studies have shown that ketamine has antidepressant effects.[40] Unlike antidepressants, which work by enhancing neurotransmitters like serotonin and dopamine, ketamine is thought to change the way brain cells talk to each other—similar to a computer reboot or hardware fix. Ketamine is showing potential, but a new study argues for caution. It showed that the antidepressant effects of ketamine were eliminated with the opiate blocker naltrexone, meaning it worked by activating the opiate centers of the brain.[41] In the long run, could it have similar damaging effects as other opioids and be causing more harm than good?

Treatment: As Jarrett became an adult, his doctor may have treated him with marijuana or ketamine.

INSANITY IS OFTEN DESCRIBED AS DOING THE SAME THING AND EXPECTING A DIFFERENT RESULT:
The Psychiatric Diagnostic and Treatment System Needs a New Paradigm

When President Barack Obama called for more mental health services[42] after 20-year-old Adam Lanza murdered his mother and went to the Sandy Hook Elementary School in Newtown, Connecticut, where he fatally shot 20 six- and seven-year-old children and six adults, I knew that if we spent more money using the same symptom-based diagnostic and treatment model, we would still get the same disturbing results. Like Lanza, a number of our nation's most notorious mass shooters had seen psychiatrists or mental health professionals and had received "standard of care" treatment before their crimes, including Kip Kinkel (Springfield, OR, 1998), Eric Harris (Columbine, CO, 1999), Seung-Hui Cho (Virginia Tech, 2007), James Holmes (Aurora, CO, 2012), and Nikolas Cruz (Parkland, FL, 2018).

We do not need more of the same. We need a completely different paradigm rooted in neuroscience and hope. A new way forward in psychiatry will require ending the paradigm of mental illness, because psychiatric issues really are so much more. Your brain creates your mind. The issues that affect our minds stem from our brains, our bodies, our thoughts, our social and work interactions with others, and our deepest sense of meaning and purpose. We were able to help Jarrett change the trajectory of his life by addressing all of these factors in an integrative way. It started by looking at his brain, because if you never look, you never really know.

CHAPTER 2

MAKING INVISIBLE ILLNESSES VISIBLE

HOW LOOKING AT THE BRAIN DISRUPTS AN OUTDATED PARADIGM AND CHARTS A NEW PATH FORWARD

The significant problems we face cannot be solved at the same level of thinking we were at when we created them.

ALBERT EINSTEIN

If you have crushing chest pain, your doctor will scan your heart; but if you have crushing depression, no one will ever look at your brain.

If you are sick to your stomach, your doctor will image your abdomen; but if you are sick with anxiety, no one will ever look at your brain.

If you have stabbing back pain, your doctor will order an MRI; but if you have urges to stab others, no one will ever look at your brain.

If you have persistent knee pain, your doctor will image your knees; but if you have persistent heartache, no one will ever look at your brain.

If you have a chronic cough, your doctor will x-ray your chest; but if alcoholic behavior is ruining your life, no one will ever look at your brain.

If you have tormenting hip pain, your doctor will scan your hip; but if you torment your spouse so much that he or she leaves you, no one will ever look at your brain.

If you are paralyzed from an accident, your doctor will scan your spine; but if you are paralyzed with obsessive thoughts, no one will ever look at your brain.

If you develop a runaway tachycardia, your doctor will scan your heart; but if your teenager runs away and lives on the street, no one will ever look at his or her brain.

You have heard it said that a picture is worth 1,000 words, but a map is worth 1,000 images. Without a map, you are lost. If you are lost in the wilderness without a map, you unnecessarily suffer and are at risk of dying. Likewise, many people are lost in the morass of psychiatric care, and lack of proper diagnosis and treatment costs many people their lives. In 2020 this is simply unacceptable. Here is an example.

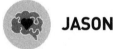 ## JASON

Jason was 18 and in his first year of college at the University of Rhode Island when he first started hearing voices and having visual hallucinations. Based on his symptoms, the university psychiatrist diagnosed him with schizophrenia and told his parents he would need to be on antipsychotic medication for the rest of his life, but the medication triggered suicidal thoughts. Horrified, his mother called me. She and I had worked together at a large public television station. I told her I wanted to see Jason immediately.

Jason's brain SPECT scan showed evidence of a past brain injury affecting his left temporal lobe, which when damaged is often involved in mood instability, dark thoughts, and hallucinations, and it also revealed low activity in his frontal lobes (where focus, forethought, and planning occur). When he was five years old, Jason had jumped headfirst into an empty bathtub and was unconscious for a brief period. He had also sustained several concussions while wrestling and playing soccer. Since the age of five, Jason had struggled with low-grade depression. His symptoms worsened when he was 12 years old and experienced bullying at school. While at college, Jason started hearing voices. They constantly made mean comments about him and others. Often, the voices would speak at the same time. In addition, he began seeing gory visions of his own death, including being strangled by a snake.

HEALTHY SPECT

JASON'S SPECT

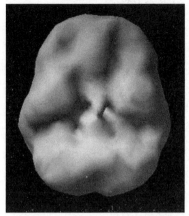 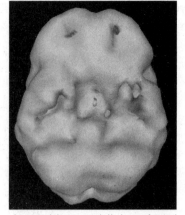

Full, even, symmetrical activity

Low activity, especially in prefrontal cortex and temporal lobes

After meeting with Jason and reviewing his SPECT brain scans, my conclusion was that he did not have schizophrenia; rather, he had a psychotic depression, which had been made worse by the prior brain injury, undisciplined thought patterns, and chronic stress. I took him off his antipsychotic medication, supported his brain recovery with healing nutrients, and had him do cognitive-behavioral therapy (you'll find out more about this simple method to eliminate ANTs—automatic negative thoughts—in an upcoming chapter) and hyperbaric oxygen therapy (HBOT) to help heal his prior brain injury. Within four months, he was remarkably improved. The following year, he was back at school. Subsequently, we have also helped many people in Jason's family, including his mother, father, nephew, and cousin.

HOOKED ON BRAIN IMAGING

When we first started our brain imaging work, we were so excited because it added incredibly useful information to help our patients, as in Chase's case in the introduction and Jarrett's case in chapter 1. Once I knew people were getting better faster because of what we learned about them through our brain imaging work, I was hooked on SPECT, despite the fierce criticism that would eventually come my way. When I started to talk about our work at national psychiatric meetings, academic psychiatrists chastised me and my colleagues for using these tools in our clinics, saying they were only for research—not immediate application to people's lives. But, for me, once my patients got better faster, there was no going back.

After giving all-day courses on SPECT for several years in the early 1990s, the APA dismissed the use of SPECT and related neuroimaging because it did not match their diagnostic bible (the DSM, which it owns and profits from).[1] Unfortunately, the APA's position completely missed the point on how doctors and patients benefit from brain imaging tools, leaving psychiatrists as the only medical specialists who virtually never look at the organ they treat, condemning them to make diagnoses of complex cases based only on talking to the patients, looking at them, and looking for symptom clusters, similar to how Dr. Anson Henry diagnosed Lincoln with melancholia back in 1841.

Without imaging, psychiatrists still make symptom-cluster diagnoses, similar to how Dr. Anson Henry diagnosed Lincoln with melancholia in 1841.

Those of us who use functional brain imaging know that scans will never match the DSM because the DSM was not based on any underlying neuroscience and was developed before there was access to functional assessment tools, such as SPECT and QEEG. Experienced clinicians can tell if someone is *likely* to have attention deficit disorder/attention deficit hyperactivity disorder (ADD/ADHD), obsessive compulsive disorder (OCD), or bipolar disorder without the benefit of these tools. But *what clinicians cannot do, and will never be able to do, without functional brain imaging is to know the underlying brain biology of the patients they treat.* Without imaging your brain, your doctor cannot tell if your inattention, depression, or aggression is from:

- Low blood flow from vascular disease
- A premature aging process
- An inflammatory process, related to low omega-3 fatty acids or gut problems
- A genetic abnormality
- Lasting physical trauma from playing football in high school
- Toxic exposure to carbon monoxide or mold, which needs to be treated
- Seizure activity
- A brain infection
- Nutrient or neurohormone abnormalities
- Blood sugar abnormalities
- Undiagnosed sleep apnea
- A brain that is working too hard and needs to be calmed down
- A brain that is not working hard enough and needs to be stimulated

If we don't look at the brain, we are unnecessarily flying blind. That can lead us to miss important diagnoses, give the wrong treatment plan, and hurt the people entrusted to us to help.

If we don't look at the brain, we are unnecessarily flying blind,
which can hurt the people entrusted to us to help.

WHY DON'T ALL PSYCHIATRISTS USE BRAIN IMAGING?

If I'm right, then why isn't the whole of psychiatry on board? Because this new way of thinking completely changes the diagnostic and treatment paradigm that has been taught in medical schools and psychiatric residency training programs for more than 50 years. Functional brain imaging takes psychiatry from a generalized symptom-cluster diagnostic and treatment specialty without any biological evidence to a more objective specialty, one that is solidly based on using state-of-the-art brain mapping tools to help optimize the patient's brain function.

Besides completely changing the way we diagnose brain health/mental health, functional imaging leads to entirely different treatment protocols to improve brain function. These include strategies that are often more natural and lifestyle-based and more directly accessible to patients. These types of protocols are not taught in medical schools and are not underwritten by the pharmaceutical industry that has dominated the financial support of the psychiatric establishment. (One only has to attend psychiatric meetings or read most psychiatric journals to see the massive advertising funded by the pharmaceutical industry.)

When my colleagues began attacking me for our brain imaging work, it initially made me anxious and upset. Then I realized anyone who tries to change a paradigm invites vitriol. In the 16th century, the Italian politician Niccolò Machiavelli explained, "There is nothing more difficult to plan, more doubtful of success, nor more dangerous to manage than a new system. For the initiator has the enmity of all who would profit by the preservation of the old institution." Yet, by functionally imaging Chase's, Jarrett's, and Jason's brains and then developing treatments personalized for them, we were able to positively change the trajectory of their lives.

Thomas Kuhn: The Structure of Scientific Revolution

In 1962, scientific historian and philosopher Thomas Kuhn wrote that scientific revolutions typically occur in five stages.

STAGE I: THE DISCREPANCIES SHOW

In the first stage, the revolution is started when the standard paradigm begins to fail. For example, I would diagnose patients with major depression or ADD/ADHD based on DSM criteria, put them on standard treatments—such as Prozac or Ritalin—and then see them become suicidal or aggressive. This was a paradigm-based failure that occurred far too often and was emotionally traumatic for my patients, as well as for me.

STAGE II: THE DISAGREEMENTS START

Once the paradigm begins to fail, experts begin to look for ways to fix their theories, but they resist discarding their old models entirely and instead look for small fixes. Over time, the failing model splinters into many competing schools of thought. More than 250 types of psychotherapies and myriad medications exist to treat mental illnesses. Kuhn wrote that no matter how wrong their models have become, the leaders maintain their beliefs and continue trying to tweak their ideas to preserve their power and influence. This makes me think of the six versions of the DSM, which has been tweaked but not substantially overhauled since 1980.

STAGE III: THE REVOLUTION

Over time, a new paradigm emerges that resolves many of the problems in the field. A new paradigm—such as "Get your brain right, and your mind will follow"—reinterprets existing knowledge, retaining the best of the old thinking and integrating the latest knowledge into a fresh model, a paradigm shift.

STAGE IV: THE REJECTION

The new paradigm is then rejected and ridiculed by the leaders in the field. This is one of the most reliable stages of a scientific revolution. The old guard becomes frustrated that the new idea did not come from them and because they hold tightly to their own theories, this period may last for decades until they retire or die. Nobel Prize–winning physicist Max Planck wrote, "A new scientific truth does not triumph by convincing its opponents and making them see the light, but rather because its opponents eventually die, and a new generation grows up that is familiar with it."[2] Science advances through funerals.

STAGE V: THE ACCEPTANCE

The new theory is adopted gradually as younger, more open-minded scientists accept it early in their careers and later become the leaders of the field. Kuhn also noted that professionals who are outsiders and not wed to the status quo are often the ones who champion new paradigms. It takes courage to be on the outside, but in the long run it pays off because everyone gets better care. Currently, thousands of young psychiatrists and brain health practitioners have been trained in our work, and we're training more of them all the time. We and others are also publishing landmark research articles with the new paradigm in respected scientific journals.

BRAIN SPECT IMAGING MADE RIDICULOUSLY SIMPLE

The brain SPECT imaging work we do at Amen Clinics has revolutionized my life and is an important part of the foundation for *The End of Mental Illness*. Throughout this book you'll see many more SPECT scans, so it is important to know a bit about the science and how to look at the images.

First, let me give you the brief backstory on how I fell in love with brain imaging, which I've written about in *Change Your Brain, Change Your Life*. In 1972, I joined the US Army and became an infantry medic, which is when my love of medicine was born. After about 18 months, I was retrained as an X-ray technician and developed a passion for medical imaging. As our professors used to say, "How do you know unless you look?" In 1979, when I was a second-year medical student, someone I loved tried to kill herself, and I took her to see a wonderful psychiatrist. Over time, I realized that if he helped her, which he did, it would not just help her; it would eventually help her children and even her future grandchildren as they would be shaped by someone who was happier and more stable. I fell in love with psychiatry because I realized it had the potential to help generations of people. I have loved it every day for the past 40 years.

Yet I fell in love with the only medical profession that almost never looks at the organ it treats. As you saw in the opening to this chapter, cardiologists image the heart; gastroenterologists image the stomach and intestines; and orthopedic doctors image bones. Virtually every other medical specialty images the organs it treats, but psychiatrists don't look at the brain. Rather, they are trained to make diagnoses based on symptom clusters and to make educated guesses about treatment needs. Early in my career, I knew there had to be a better way and began searching for it.

In 1991, I went to a lecture on brain SPECT imaging by Jack Paldi, MD, who was the chief of medicine at the hospital where I worked. Dr. Paldi told us that SPECT was a tool to give psychiatrists more information to help their patients. SPECT looks at blood flow and activity. It looks at how the brain works. It is different from MRI and CT studies that look at *brain structure*. SPECT looks at *brain function*. He said SPECT basically tells us three things about the activity in each area of the brain: *if it is healthy, underactive, or overactive.*

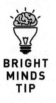

BRIGHT MINDS TIP

SPECT basically shows three important things about each area of the brain: if it is healthy, underactive, or overactive.

To help you understand our brain imaging work, look at the following examples of common brain SPECT patterns. A surface SPECT scan helps us see areas that have healthy activity and those with low activity on the outside surface of the brain. The surface scans show the top 45 percent of activity in the brain. Any areas that fall below that percentage look like a hole or indentation on the scan. These "holes" are not actually missing brain structures but, rather, a sign of too little activity. An active SPECT scan reveals inner areas of the brain where there is too much activity. Following are examples of common brain SPECT patterns, looking down from the top of the head.

Surface SPECT Scans

The first scan is a healthy one, showing the outside surface of the brain. It shows full, even, symmetrical activity and blood flow.

HEALTHY SURFACE SCAN
(looking from the top down)

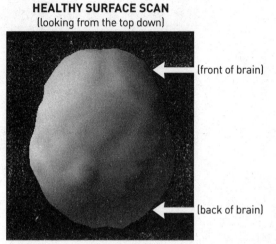

(front of brain)

(back of brain)

Full, even, symmetrical activity

Now compare the healthy brain to that of a woman who had two strokes.

TWO STROKES

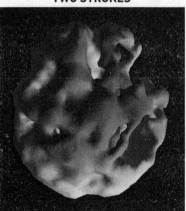

Holes indicate low or missing activity

Based on the level of activity, SPECT can see how much tissue can be improved or rehabilitated.

ALZHEIMER'S DISEASE

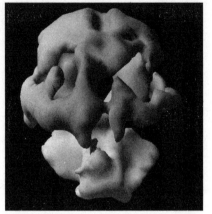

Back half of brain is dying

Alzheimer's disease starts years, even decades, before people develop any symptoms. This 59-year-old woman likely had negative changes in her brain in her 20s.

BRAIN TRAUMA

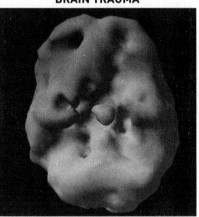

Soccer head trauma

Brain trauma is a major cause of mental health issues, but few psychiatrists know it because they rarely image the brain.

TOXICITY FROM DRUG AND ALCOHOL ABUSE

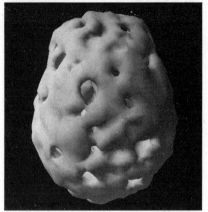

Scalloping or overall low activity

The real reason not to use drugs or much alcohol is because they damage the brain.

Active SPECT scans

In an active SPECT scan, the gray background represents average activity; white represents the top 15 percent. In a healthy scan, the most activity typically appears in the back, bottom part of the brain, in an area called the cerebellum (Latin for "little brain"), because this area contains 50 percent of the brain's neurons.

HEALTHY ACTIVE SCAN
(looking from the top down)

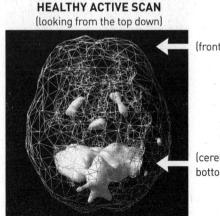

(front of brain)

(cerebellum, back, bottom of brain)

Gray is average activity; white is top 15 percent showing most active areas of the brain

OBSESSIVE COMPULSIVE TRAITS

Marked increased activity in frontal lobes

POST-TRAUMATIC STRESS DISORDER

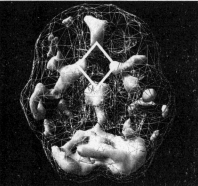

Diamond pattern of increased activity in deep emotional part of brain (diamond)

SEIZURE ACTIVITY

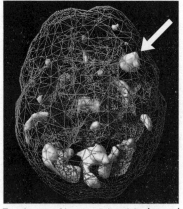

Focal area of increased activity (arrow)

THE RESEARCH ON SPECT

SPECT was originally developed more than 50 years ago to evaluate living tissue. SPECT is a nuclear medicine study that uses very small pieces of light called photons to look at living tissue. Because SPECT is a nuclear medicine procedure, there is some radiation exposure with it. It is about the same as a head CT, which was ordered 19 million times in the US in 2006.[3] Michael Devous, PhD, the past president of the Society of Nuclear Medicine, wrote, "SPECT . . . procedures have no more risk than MRI-based procedures. . . . Indeed, there are no data demonstrating harm to humans by radiation exposure at diagnostic imaging levels."[4]

Since the 1970s, brain SPECT has been used to evaluate strokes, seizures, and brain tumors.[5] In the 1980s, scientists were also using it to study Alzheimer's disease, head trauma, schizophrenia, depression, ADD/ADHD, and substance abuse. Today, physicians around the world typically order brain SPECT scans to look at the following conditions:[6]

- Alzheimer's disease and other types of dementia
- Seizures
- Strokes
- Head trauma
- Chemical exposure
- Lyme disease
- Brain inflammation
- Drug toxicity

The research on brain SPECT is vast, with more than 14,000 scientific research articles on it listed on www.pubmed.com. Below is a listing of the number of scientific articles for some common neurological and psychiatric conditions.

CONDITION	SCIENTIFIC ARTICLES	CONDITION	SCIENTIFIC ARTICLES[7]
Strokes	> 1,300	Infections	> 270
Dementia	> 2,200	Anxiety disorders	> 250
Alzheimer's disease	> 1,500	OCD	> 150
Seizures and epilepsy	> 1,600	ADD/ADHD	> 120
Depression	> 850	Bipolar disorder	> 120
Schizophrenia	> 570	Autism	> 75
Head trauma	> 350	Eating disorders	> 70
Drug abuse	> 310	PTSD	> 50
Alcohol abuse	> 280		

The first 10 cases where I ordered SPECT scans completely changed the way I help my patients and created a revolution in how I practice psychiatry and even how I live my life. I care about my brain as never before. Since 1991, Amen Clinics has built the world's largest database of SPECT scans for psychiatric issues, totaling nearly 160,000 scans on patients from 121 countries. We have studied and used SPECT to help us with complex psychiatric patients and have published 70 peer-reviewed scientific studies on SPECT, including those on:

- ADD/ADHD[8] and predicting treatment response to stimulants in ADD/ADHD[9]
- Aging[10]
- Aggression[11] and murder[12]
- Alzheimer's disease[13]
- Anxiety[14]
- Autism[15]
- Depression, predicting treatment response in depression[16] and mania[17]
- Distinguishing depression from dementia[18]
- Gender differences[19]
- Distinguishing PTSD from a traumatic brain injury (TBI) in veteran and general populations[20] (*Discover* magazine listed this research as one of the top 100 stories in science [#19] for 2015)
- Marijuana[21]
- Meditation[22]
- Omega-3 fatty acids[23]
- Obesity[24]
- Suicide[25]
- TBI[26]
- Impact of playing football in the NFL[27]
- Rehabilitating brain trauma in NFL players[28]
- HBOT in TBI[29]

Based on our experience, a number of common SPECT patterns guide diagnosis and treatment decisions. Here are several of the common patterns.

COMMON SPECT PATTERNS THAT GUIDE DIAGNOSIS AND TREATMENT

1. Scalloping/overall decreased perfusion on surface SPECT

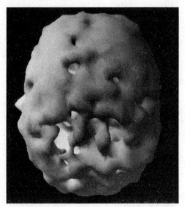

This pattern shows overall low activity and blood flow,
which look like waves or scallops on a surface SPECT scan

This pattern is most commonly seen with:

- Drug or alcohol abuse
- Chemotherapy or radiation exposure
- Environmental toxins, such as mold
- Heavy metal exposure
- Carbon monoxide poisoning
- Anoxia (lack of oxygen for several minutes, e.g., from a heart attack or near drowning)
- Infections, such as Lyme disease or herpes
- Hypothyroidism
- Severe anemia (SPECT looks at blood flow)

When this pattern is seen, we consider the following treatments:

- Finding and stopping the toxin or infection if present
- Treating any medical causes
- Brain rehabilitation program is essential. Components include:
  - Avoiding anything that hurts the brain
  - Engaging in regular brain healthy habits
  - Neurofeedback
  - HBOT
  - Targeted nutraceuticals and medications

SCALLOPING EXAMPLES

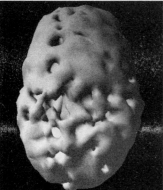

Moderate to severe scalloping
from inhalant abuse

Moderate to severe scalloping from
chemotherapy and radiation

SCALLOPING: BEFORE AND AFTER TREATMENT

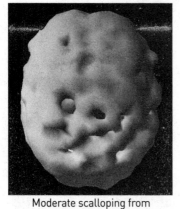
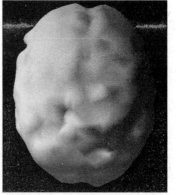

Moderate scalloping from
arsenic poisoning

Marked improvement 11 months
after treatment

2. Overall increased activity on active SPECT

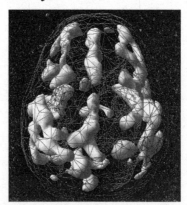

This pattern shows overall increased activity on scans

This pattern is most commonly seen with:

- Bipolar disorder/mania
- Autoimmune or inflammatory processes, such as acute allergies, infections, or lupus
- ADD/ADHD—when we see this in people with ADD/ADHD, we call it the "ring of fire." Stimulants make this pattern worse in 80 percent of cases.[30]

When this pattern is seen, we consider the following treatments:

- Investigating and treating potential causes of inflammation, such as lupus or food allergies
- Eliminating allergens
- Treating any underlying conditions
- Calming interventions, such as magnesium, gamma-aminobutyric acid (GABA), or antiseizure medication

OVERALL INCREASED ACTIVITY EXAMPLES

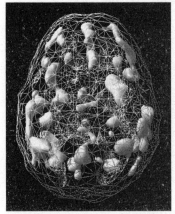

Overall increased activity: bipolar disorder, manic

Overall increased activity: lupus flare

OVERALL INCREASED ACTIVITY EXAMPLES (continued)

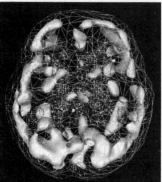

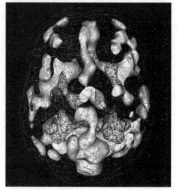

Overall increased activity:
ring of fire ADD/ADHD

Overall increased activity:
obsessional psychotic state

3. Traumatic brain injury (TBI) patterns on surface SPECT

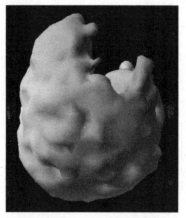

There are many TBI patterns

We suspect a TBI if the following patterns are present:

- Low activity in one or more areas of the brain
- One side looks worse than the other
- Flattening of the frontal lobes
- Decreased activity in the poles (front portion) of the temporal lobes
- Damage seen in both the front and back of the brain (coup contrecoup injury)

When this pattern is seen, we consider the following treatments:

- Brain rehabilitation program—components include:
  - Avoiding anything that hurts the brain
  - Engaging in regular brain-healthy habits
  - Neurofeedback
  - HBOT
  - Targeted nutraceuticals and medications

TBI EXAMPLES

Underside View

Underside View

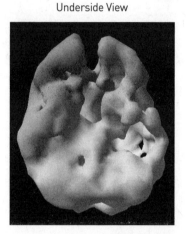 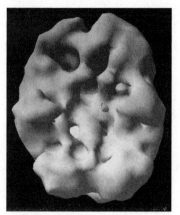

Frontal and left temporal lobe damage: fall from roof

Damage to whole right side of brain: motorcycle accident

Top-Down View

Top-Down View

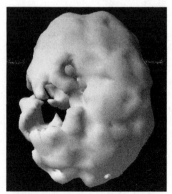 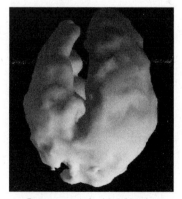

Damage to left parietal lobe: blunt force trauma from assault

Damage to left side of brain: fall down stairs

**TBI: BEFORE AND AFTER TREATMENT
(NFL PLAYER ANTHONY DAVIS, USC AND LA RAMS)**

Underside View   Underside View

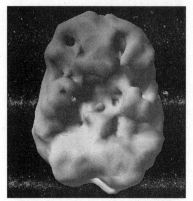 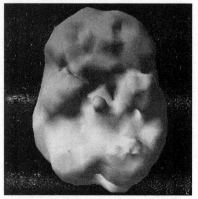

Damage to left frontal/temporal lobe: Marked improvement:
multiple concussions   10 years later, after treatment

4. Hyperfrontality on active SPECT

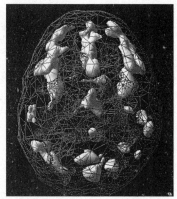

This pattern shows increased activity in the front part of the brain.

This pattern is most commonly seen with:

- OCD
- Obsessive compulsive personality disorder
- Oppositional defiant disorder[31]
- Autistic spectrum disorders
- People who are worried, rigid, and inflexible and get stuck on negative thoughts
- Types of anxiety, depression, ADD/ADHD, and addictions where people get stuck on negative thoughts or negative behaviors

When this pattern is seen, we consider the following treatments:

- Increasing serotonin to calm the front part of the brain
  - Exercise
  - Supplements such as 5-hydroxytryptophan (5-HTP), saffron, or St. John's wort for anxiety or depression
  - Selective serotonin reuptake inhibitors (SSRIs), such as Lexapro, Zoloft, or Prozac for anxiety or depression
  - Antipsychotics, such as Risperdal, for psychosis

HYPERFRONTALITY EXAMPLES

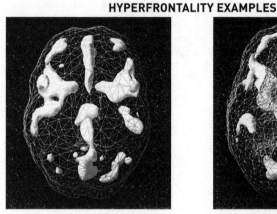

Hyperfrontal pattern: OCD

Hyperfrontal pattern: anxiety with obsessive thoughts

HYPERFRONTALITY: BEFORE AND AFTER TREATMENT (BUSINESS OWNER WITH OCD PERSONALITY)

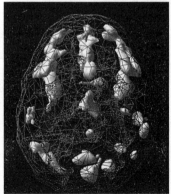
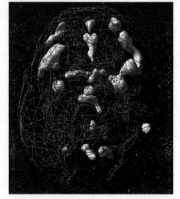

Hyperfrontal pattern: OCD personality traits

Calming of hyperfrontal pattern: improved personality, work relationships, and marriage

5. *Hypofrontality on surface SPECT*

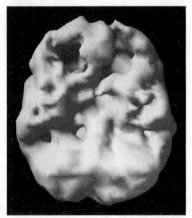

This pattern shows decreased activity in the front part of the brain

This pattern is most commonly seen with:

- ADD/ADHD
- Schizophrenia
- TBI
- Alcoholics at risk of relapse
- Lack of conscientiousness
- Forms of depression
- Types of anxiety, ADD/ADHD, and addictions where people struggle with short attention spans, distractibility, disorganization, and impulse control issues

When this pattern is seen, we consider the following treatments:

- Increasing dopamine to increase frontal lobe activity
    - Exercise
    - Stimulating supplements, such as green tea, L-tyrosine, or rhodiola
    - Stimulants for ADD/ADHD
    - Stimulating antipsychotics if needed, such as Abilify
    - Stimulating antidepressants, such as Wellbutrin, or s-adenosyl methionine (SAMe) if depressed
    - Brain rehab if needed

HYPOFRONTALITY EXAMPLES

Underside View   Underside View

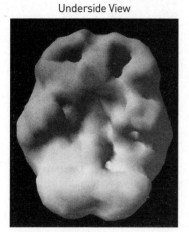 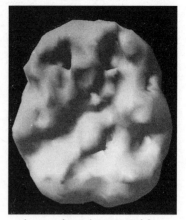

Low prefrontal cortex activity: Low prefrontal cortex activity:
sex addiction   classic ADD/ADHD

HYPOFRONTALITY: BEFORE AND AFTER TREATMENT (SCHOOL FAILURE)

Underside View   Underside View

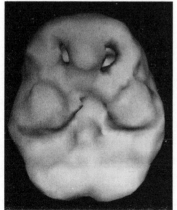 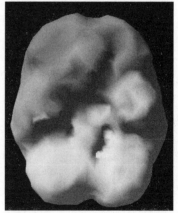

Low prefrontal cortex activity: Marked improvement: after six
college failure   months of treatment

6. Diamond pattern on active SPECT

Underside View

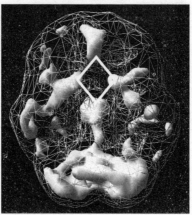

This pattern shows increased activity in anterior cingulate (top of diamond), basal ganglia (sides of diamond), and deep thalamus (bottom of diamond)

This pattern is most commonly seen with:

- PTSD
- Past unresolved trauma
- Types of anxiety, depression, and addictions where people get stuck on negative thoughts or negative behaviors, which make them anxious and sad

When this pattern is seen, we consider the following treatments:

- EMDR for PTSD to calm unresolved past trauma
- Increasing serotonin and GABA to calm the front part of the brain
  - Exercise
  - Supplements such as 5HTP, saffron, GABA, and magnesium
  - SSRIs, such as Lexapro, Zoloft, or Prozac
  - Anticonvulsants, such as Neurontin, Trileptal, or Lamictal

DIAMOND PATTERN EXAMPLES

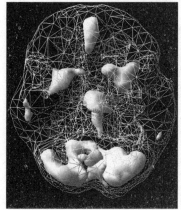

Diamond pattern: PTSD

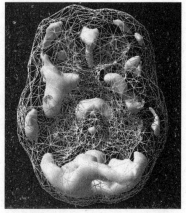

Diamond pattern: does not meet criteria for PTSD, but patient grew up in abusive alcoholic home and struggles with anxiety and worry

DIAMOND PATTERN (PTSD):
BEFORE AND AFTER TREATMENT (EMDR THERAPY)

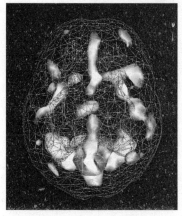

Diamond pattern: PTSD

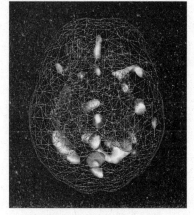

Calming of diamond pattern, improved sleep and anxiety

7. Temporal lobe hypoperfusion on surface SPECT

TEMPORAL LOBE HYPOPERFUSION

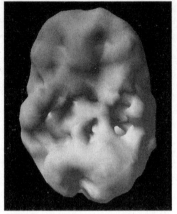

This pattern shows decreased activity in one or both of the temporal lobes.

The temporal lobes are involved with memory, learning, mood stability, and emotional reactions.

This pattern is most commonly seen with:

- Memory problems
- Forms of dementia
- Temporal lobe epilepsy
- Dyslexia and other learning disabilities
- Mood instability
- Intermittent explosive disorder (IED)
- Types of anxiety, depression, ADD/ADHD, and addictions where people struggle with mood instability, irritability, dark thoughts, and memory and learning

When this pattern is seen, we consider the following treatments:

- Ketogenic diet
- Neurofeedback
- GABA-enhancing nutraceuticals or medications, such as antiseizure medications, for mood instability or irritability
- Memory-enhancing nutraceuticals, such as gingko, vinpocetine, or huperzine A, or memory-enhancing medications, such as Namenda or Aricept, for memory of learning issues

TEMPORAL LOBE EXAMPLES

Underside View | Underside View

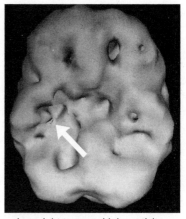

Low prefrontal cortex and left and right temporal lobe activity (arrows): intermittent explosive disorder

Low right temporal lobe activity: social skills issues; trouble reading social cues

INTERMITTENT EXPLOSIVE DISORDER
Underside View

SOCIAL SKILLS ISSUES (TROUBLE READING SOCIAL CLUES)
Underside View

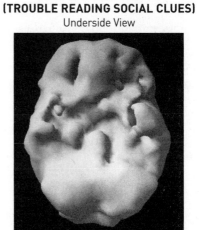

Low prefrontal cortex activity and left temporal lobe damage: learning problems

Low left and right temporal lobe activity: behavior and learning problems

Seeing is believing. When you look inside the skull, you can see that mental health problems are actually brain health problems, and it makes sense that healing the brain is the key to ending mental illness. *Looking at the brain changes everything for the better for our patients.* Our brain imaging work does the following:

- Decreases stigma, shame, and guilt (people see their problems as medical and not moral).
- Increases compliance (people want better brains).
- When taken together with patients' symptoms, helps our doctors devise personalized treatment programs specially targeted to individual brains.
- Gives a different perspective on the notions of "good" and "evil." It is easy to judge people as bad. Our brain imaging work has caused us to take a step back and ask why.
- Helps to prevent mistakes, such as stimulating an overactive brain or calming one that is underactive.
- Shows that illnesses, such as Alzheimer's disease, start decades before people have any symptoms. Imaging is an excellent early screening tool to assess your vulnerabilities.
- Shows that no two brains are the same. Treatment needs to be targeted to your brain, not a cluster of symptoms.

Looking at the brain changes everything.

Our imaging work has provided us with a greater understanding of the amazing organ between our ears, leading us to identify 12 simple principles about the brain and behavior. In the following chapter, you will discover these fundamental truths and see how they can help you begin to live the life you want.

CHAPTER 3

12 GUIDING PRINCIPLES TO CHANGE YOUR LIFE

*To expect a personality to survive the disintegration of the brain is like
expecting a cricket club to survive when all of its members are dead.*
BERTRAND RUSSELL

Our clinical and brain imaging work has led us to 12 simple principles that
underlie all we do. I've written about these principles in depth in several of
my books, including *Change Your Brain, Change Your Life*.[1] If you embrace
them, they will set a foundation for brain health—and start to change everything in your life.

1. **Your brain is involved in everything you do.** How you think, how
   you feel, how you act, and how well you get along with other people
   has to do with the moment-by-moment functioning of your brain.
   Your brain is involved in every decision you make.

2. **When your brain works right, you work right.** When your brain is
   troubled, you have trouble in your life. When your brain is healthy,
   you tend to be effective, thoughtful, creative, and energetic. When
   your brain is troubled—for whatever reason—you are much more
   likely to have problems in your life, including issues with depression, anxiety, impulsivity, anger, inflexibility, and memory. Brain
   dysfunction, even when subtle, gets in the way of your ability to be
   successful in your relationships, your work, and even your finances.

3. **Your brain is the most complicated organ in the universe.** With
   about 100 billion neurons (nerve cells) and about another 100 billion support cells, your brain has more connections than there are
   stars in the universe. Your brain accounts for only 2 percent of your

body's weight, yet it uses 20 to 30 percent of the calories you consume and 20 percent of the oxygen and blood flow in your body.

4. **Your brain has needs that must be met in order to work at optimal efficiency.** The requirements for optimal brain function include:

- Healthy blood flow (to deliver oxygen, vitamins, and essential minerals to the brain)
- Proper hydration
- Physical and mental exercise
- Stimulation (new learning)
- Fuel (aka food)
- Hormones
- A strong (but not too strong) immune system
- An efficient waste management system
- Adequate sleep
- Meaning and purpose in your life
- Being socially connected to other brains

5. **Your brain is soft, and it is housed in a very hard skull.** Your brain is about the consistency of soft butter, and it floats inside your head in a bath of cerebrospinal fluid. Inside your skull, there are sharp bony ridges that can easily damage your brain. You must protect it.

6. **Many things can hurt the brain.** It is critical for you to know what hurts the brain (the BRIGHT MINDS risk factors will be discussed in part 2). A colored version of the poster on the right hangs in more than 100,000 schools, prisons, and therapist's offices around the world as a reminder of this principle.

7. **Many things can help the brain.** It is critical for you to know what enhances the brain (see the BRIGHT MINDS interventions in part 2).

BRIGHT MINDS TIP

Many things both hurt and help the brain. It is critical for you to know the BRIGHT MINDS risk factors and interventions.

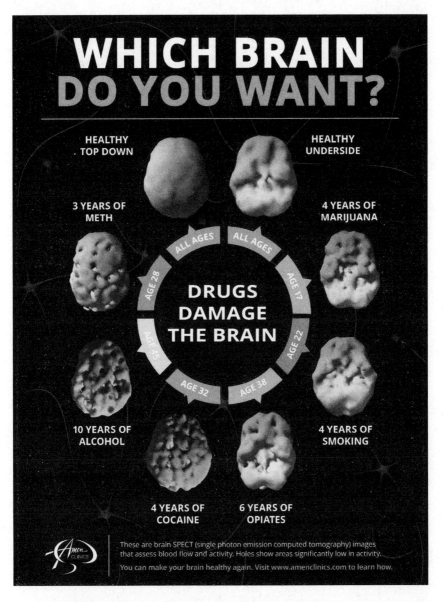

8. Like an orchestra, all parts of your brain need to be working well together to make you the best that you can be. Certain brain systems tend to do specific things. For example:

- Prefrontal cortex (PFC)—language, focus, forethought, judgment, empathy, impulse control, and learning from mistakes. This is called the executive brain because it is like the boss at work and helps you plan and make good decisions.

- Temporal lobes—visual and auditory processing, memory, learning, mood stability, and emotional reactiveness

  - On the inside of the temporal lobes are two critically important structures: the hippocampus, involved with mood and memory; and the amygdala, involved with signaling fear, emotional reactions, and anxiety.
  - The hippocampus is one of the few parts of your brain that continues to make new neurons every day. If you put it in a healing environment, it can grow bigger. If it comes under toxic attack or sustained stress, it can be easily damaged.

- Parietal lobes—direction sense, math, and constructing

- Occipital lobes—visual processing

- Cerebellum—physical, emotional, and cognitive coordination and processing speed. It houses half of the brain's neurons, even though it makes up only 10 percent of the brain's volume. It is one of the most underrated parts of the brain. I call it the "Rodney Dangerfield" part of the brain, because it gets little respect.

- Anterior cingulate cortex—shifting attention and error detection

- Basal ganglia—pleasure, motivation and adjusting movements

- Deep limbic system—sensory gating and emotional processing

None of these areas of your brain work in isolation.

9. **Understanding your brain helps you identify specific problems and which part of your brain may need help. Problems in certain brain systems tend to be associated with specific issues, such as:**

- PFC—language problems, short attention span, distractibility, a lack of planning and forethought, poor judgment, low empathy, poor impulse control, and not learning from mistakes

- Temporal lobes—visual and auditory abnormalities, poor memory, learning disabilities, mood instability, and temper issues

- Parietal lobes—poor direction sense and trouble with math

- Occipital lobes—visual processing issues

- Cerebellum—problems with physical, emotional, and thought coordination and processing speed

- Anterior cingulate cortex—trouble shifting attention, worry, holding grudges, obsessions, and excessive error detection

- Basal ganglia—addictions, tremors, and low motivation

- Deep limbic system—sensory overload, sadness, and negativity

YOUR BRAIN: A BRIEF PRIMER

Outside View of the Brain

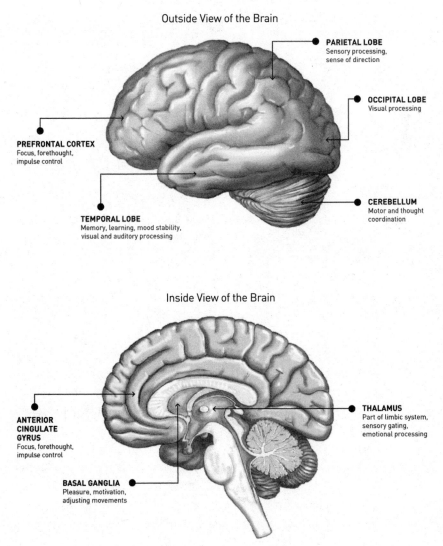

PARIETAL LOBE
Sensory processing,
sense of direction

OCCIPITAL LOBE
Visual processing

PREFRONTAL CORTEX
Focus, forethought,
impulse control

CEREBELLUM
Motor and thought
coordination

TEMPORAL LOBE
Memory, learning, mood stability,
visual and auditory processing

Inside View of the Brain

THALAMUS
Part of limbic system,
sensory gating,
emotional processing

ANTERIOR
CINGULATE
GYRUS
Focus, forethought,
impulse control

BASAL GANGLIA
Pleasure, motivation,
adjusting movements

10. **Psychiatric "illnesses" are not single or simple disorders; they all have multiple types that require their own treatments.** Taking a one-size-fits-all approach to treatment invites repeated failure and frustration. Depression, for example, is a symptom, *not* an illness. I've written books on:

- Seven types of anxiety and depression (*Healing Anxiety and Depression*)
- Seven types of ADD/ADHD (*Healing ADD*)
- Six types of addicts (*Unchain Your Brain*)
- Five types of overeaters (*Change Your Brain, Change Your Body*)

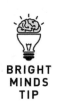

BRIGHT MINDS TIP

Psychiatric illnesses are not single or simple disorders; they all have multiple types that require their own specific treatment strategies. Taking a one-size-fits-all approach to treatment invites failure and frustration.

---

11. **The amount of "brain reserve" you have can help you handle life's stresses or make you more vulnerable to them.** Did you know that the adult brain loses an average of about 85,000 neurons a day? In early childhood, the brain is very active, sprouting new neurons and developing new connections between synapses. Older adults have significantly less activity in the brain. As we get older, our muscles tend to wither, and a similar process takes place in the brain. *What we have learned from our brain imaging work is that your day-to-day lifestyle and activities are either accelerating or slowing the brain aging process.* Just as you can train your muscles to retain a more youthful tone, you can use strategies to keep your brain functioning more optimally. Ultimately, brain aging is optional if you consistently use the right strategies.

When I talk to my patients about brain aging, I find it helpful to introduce them to the concept of "brain reserve." That's the extra cushion of brain function you have to help you deal with the stresses life throws at you. In general, the more brain reserve you have, the more resilient you are and the better your brain can handle the aging process to keep "mental health" disorders at bay. To illustrate this point to my patients, I typically show them the following "brain reserve" drawing. It shows the intersection of brain activity and age and habits. As you can see, at a certain point along the line in the graph, you cross a threshold indicating that your reserve is gone. This is when symptoms like anxiety, depression, memory problems, or temper flare-ups can appear.

Today marks one year since our first visit at Amen Clinics. My husband and I are forever grateful for you. My shame has been lifted and my mind renewed! I cannot imagine taking on this new position a year ago, thankful for how far I've come!

MEL E.

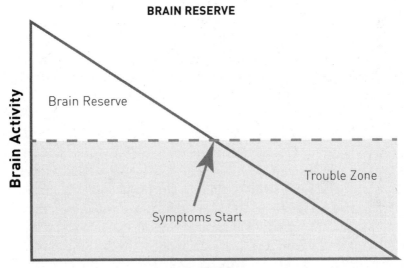

BRAIN RESERVE

Let's backtrack a bit to explain why some people have more brain reserve than others. A growing body of science is showing that even before you were conceived, your parents' lifestyle habits were laying the foundation for your overall wellbeing and physical and mental health.[2] At conception, your brain had a certain potential for reserve. However, if your mom smoked (or got second-hand smoke from your dad), drank too much alcohol, ate junk food, was chronically stressed, or had infections during the pregnancy, it depleted your reserve—even before you were born. If, on the other hand, your mom (and dad) didn't smoke, and she was healthy, ate nutritious meals, took prenatal vitamins, and was not overly stressed, it was contributing to a boost in your reserve.

After your grand entrance to the world, this increase or depletion in your brain reserve continues for the rest of your life. For example, if you were exposed to chronic stress or you witnessed domestic abuse at home, it decreased your reserve. If you fell off your bike and hit your head when you were in grade school, it lowered your reserve, even if you didn't have any symptoms. If you started smoking marijuana as a teenager, it further depleted your reserve. Then if you played tackle football or hit a lot of soccer balls with your head, it took an additional toll on your reserve. Despite all of these knocks on your reserve, you may not have developed any symptoms . . . yet.

Here's an example I like to use with my patients. Imagine two soldiers in a war-torn region. They are both in the same tank and exposed to the same blast injury at the same angles. They both survive the blast without physical injuries, yet one of them is subsequently racked by post-traumatic stress disorder (PTSD) and depression, while the other one experiences no residual mental health problems. Why? Luck? Probably not. It is far more likely that the two soldiers had different levels of brain reserve going into the accident. One soldier had more reserve because he took good care of his brain, he had lots of educational opportunities, his parents fed him well, and they didn't let him play football. The other soldier had less reserve due to an unstable home environment, three previous concussions from playing football, a junk-food diet, and drug use as a teenager. They were both effective at their jobs, but they started at different places in terms of reserve. And even though the blast diminished both of their reserves, the one with more reserve avoided any mental health consequences while the one with less reserve crossed that threshold I mentioned earlier where the reserve is gone, making him vulnerable to brain health/mental health problems like PTSD and depression.

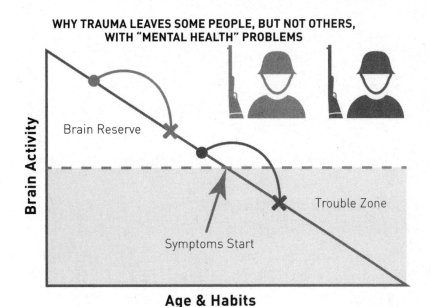

At Amen Clinics, most of the people we see are already symptomatic, which means they have crossed the brain reserve threshold (the dotted line in the previous two illustrations). Getting well is not just about eliminating the symptoms of "mental illness"; it's also about increasing brain reserve to get it back above the line. To boost your brain reserve, you need to follow three simple strategies:

- Love your brain (you have to really care about your brain).
- Avoid the things that hurt your brain.
- Do the things that help your brain.

The decisions you make and the habits you engage in on a daily basis are either boosting or stealing your brain's reserve and are either accelerating the aging process or rejuvenating your brain. When you grasp this concept, you realize that you have a lot of influence on the health and age of your brain, as well as on your own mental health and ability to end "mental illness."

12. **The most important lesson from imaging is that you are not stuck with the brain you have. You can make it better, and we can prove it.** This is perhaps the most exciting and hopeful lesson we've learned. We all need to work hard to improve how our brains function because, with a better brain, a better life and better mental health always come.

The most exciting lesson learned from nearly 160,000 brain SPECT scans is that you can change your brain, change your life, and change your mental health . . . and I can prove it.

THE 12 GUIDING PRINCIPLES AND "MENTAL ILLNESS"

When you grasp the concepts of the 12 guiding principles, it becomes increasingly clear that mental health problems are, in fact, brain health problems. And it makes even more sense that eliminating brain health/mental health disorders involves optimizing brain function and boosting brain reserve. You'll discover the interventions to help you do it in the rest of the book. I understand that you may be in a hurry to start putting these strategies into practice in your own life, but I urge you not to skip ahead. It's very important to understand why you need to take a comprehensive approach to healing. Then you'll have a stronger foundation to make the strategies in part 2 even more effective for you.

CHAPTER 4

GET YOUR BRAIN RIGHT AND YOUR MIND WILL FOLLOW

IT STARTS WITH FOUR CIRCLES AND PREVENTING OR TREATING 11 RISK FACTORS

*She will be a star if you surround her with stars. She will go
to jail if you surround her with people who go to jail.*

MY COMMENT TO THE MOTHER OF ONE OF MY TEENAGE PATIENTS

To get your mind right, you must first have a healthy brain. Imagine going to a psychotherapist for depression, anxiety, bipolar disorder, or an addiction with a brain that has been physically traumatized; a brain that is inflamed, poisoned, infected, or low in neurohormones; or a brain that works too hard or not hard enough. You spend the time, invest the money, make the effort, and open up your emotional vulnerability trying to get the help you need, but it doesn't work because you cannot focus, remember, or process the information. You are likely to quit therapy and feel demoralized and "less than others" who you assume are benefitting from similar techniques. You wonder why therapy seems to work for them but not for you. When this is the case, therapy can actually do more harm than good because of the failed expectations and wasted resources. Here is an example:

 DAVE AND BONNIE

Dave and Bonnie were struggling in their marriage. Dave had a bad temper and many negative thoughts, and Bonnie was having a hard time dealing with his behavior. They decided to go to a psychologist for marital therapy and stuck with it for three years. But it was a frustrating endeavor. Try as they might to get closer, nothing seemed to work. The therapy sessions were filled with blaming, bickering, frequent explosions, and a general sense of unhappiness. The therapist, who was very experienced, tried and tried. She had diagnosed Dave with mixed personality disorder with narcissistic and antisocial features, along with intermittent explosive disorder, but none of the usual treatments, strategies, or relationship tools helped them make any progress. After considerable thought, the doctor decided to give the couple an F in marital therapy. She told Dave and Bonnie that, in her opinion, it was time for divorce. After spending years of effort and more than $25,000 trying to heal their marriage, the couple protested, and the therapist said there was one more option. She told them about Amen Clinics, where some of her most difficult clients had found help.

After an evaluation, our team performed brain SPECT scans on the couple. Bonnie's scan was healthy. But Dave's brain scan looked shriveled and full of holes, the same pattern that we see in drug or alcohol abusers. This was odd because Dave said he didn't drink and never used drugs. To make sure, in front of Bonnie, I asked Dave if he was drinking heavily or using drugs, and he denied it.

I turned to Bonnie for more information, knowing that alcoholics are often in denial and drug abusers often lie. She said, "He's right. He doesn't drink and, as far as I know, has never used drugs. That is not his problem, Dr. Amen. He's just a jerk." As an aside, his therapist's diagnosis of mixed personality disorder with narcissistic and antisocial features was her way of calling him a jerk, but "jerk" is not a billable diagnosis.

DAVE'S TOXIC SPECT SCAN

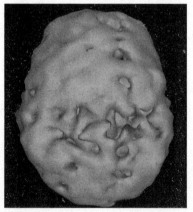

Notice shriveled appearance and huge "holes" of decreased activity

I chuckled at Bonnie's comment. But if Dave was really not a drinker or drug abuser, my mind started immediately looking for alternatives about why he had such a toxic-looking brain. My psychiatrist friend Harold Bursztajn, former codirector of the program in psychiatry and law at Harvard, often says that scans don't always give you the answer; they teach you to ask better questions. I went through the different potential medical causes in my head—brain infections, a near-drowning episode, hypothyroidism, anemia, environmental toxins. My next question to Dave was, "Where do you work?"

He replied, "I work in a furniture factory."

"What do you do there?" I asked.

"Finish furniture."

"Is there good ventilation in the room?"

"No," Dave said. "It's often hot and reeks with fumes."

Oh my goodness, I thought. *Dave has a drug-affected brain from the solvents he is using at work.* Even though he had never willfully used drugs, the chemicals were eating away at his brain. Dave thought he was going to work to support his family, but he was really being poisoned.

"Do you wear a mask?" I asked.

"No. They tell me I should, but I don't think it's important."

"Ouch," I said. "You really should." My next question was to Bonnie: "When did he start becoming a jerk?"

She thought for a moment. "We weren't always unhappy. We've been married for 15 years. It just seems that the last eight were hard. The first years were great. He was so different." Then a look of "Aha" washed over Bonnie's face. "Dave started to work at the furniture factory eight years ago. Do you think his personality change can be from his job?"

"You bet," I answered. "Something is damaging his brain and damaging his ability to be the kind, thoughtful, empathic, and loving man you married."

I urged Dave to take a six-month medical leave of absence and would only allow him to return to a nontoxic job at the plant. After seeing Dave's brain scans, Bonnie developed empathy for her husband. She went from thinking he was a jerk to seeing him as someone who was in need of help and understanding. When a person's behavior changes dramatically or does not make sense, like Dave's, it is important to consider brain health issues as a potential cause of the trouble.

It was clear to me that Dave's problem was not just psychiatric; it was *biological.* Numerous studies have shown that exposure to chemicals and solvents has negative effects on brain health, including mood, memory, and attention.[1] No amount of therapy and no amount of effort on Dave's part was going to heal the damaging effects the solvents had on his brain. The problem is virtually no marital therapists, psychologists, or psychiatrists start by mapping the brain, so they have no idea if it is healthy or unhealthy and in need of repair. And most don't look into a patient's biology that might be contributing to the problem. We can and must do better.

AMEN CLINICS FOUR CIRCLES BRIGHT MINDS PROGRAM

To end mental illness in people like Dave—as well as in my nieces, Alizé and Amelie, whom I told you about at the beginning of the book—we need to stop looking at psychiatric problems through a singular lens as just a cluster of symptoms and start assessing and treating the whole person. The Amen Clinics Four Circles BRIGHT MINDS Program was developed to help you and your loved ones achieve long-term brain health/mental health. This program has three main components:

1. Optimize the four circles of a whole life—biological, psychological, social, and spiritual (covered in this chapter).
2. Prevent or treat the 11 major risk factors that damage the brain and steal your mind (covered in part 2).
3. Target treatment to your specific needs, such as ADD/ADHD, anxiety, depression, psychosis, or insomnia (covered in part 3).

THE FOUR CIRCLES

When I started medical school in 1978, our dean, Dr. Sid Garrett, gave us one of our first lectures on how to help people of any age for any problem. He told us, "Always think of people as whole beings, never just as their symptoms." He insisted that whenever we evaluated and treated anyone, we should take into consideration the four circles of health and illness:

 Biological: how your physical body and brain function (body)

 Psychological: developmental issues and how you think (mind)

 Social: social support and interactions, and your current life situation (connections)

 Spiritual: your connection to God, the planet, and past and future generations; and your deepest sense of meaning and purpose (spirit)[2]

At Amen Clinics, we use these four circles as part of a balanced, comprehensive approach to assessment and healing. I wrote about them in *Change*

Your Brain, Change Your Life. Each of these four circles interacts with the 11 BRIGHT MINDS risk factors you will read about in part 2. The interplay of these four circles and 11 risk factors is our guide for alleviating mental illness. When you ignore the four circles, it allows your risk factors to get out of control, and they can then conspire against you to create mental illnesses. On the other hand, when you care for the four circles, it minimizes your risk factors. They begin to work in concert to help prevent or treat mental illness not only in yourself but also in the next generation, whether nieces (like Alizé and Amelie), nephews, children, or grandchildren.

In this chapter, you will see how each of the four circles affects brain health/mental health. You will also discover how modern society is attacking the four circles and contributing to the rise of mental health/brain health problems. To offset these attacks, I'll offer simple strategies to optimize each of the four circles. It starts by knowing and caring about them, avoiding anything that hurts them, and engaging in simple habits to optimize them.

FOUR CIRCLES BRIGHT MINDS PROGRAM

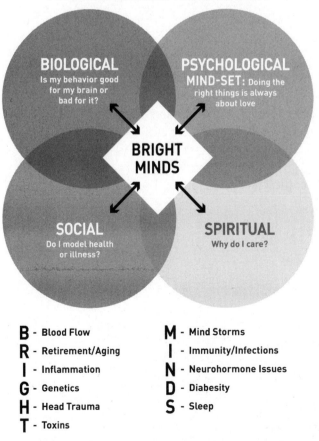

B - Blood Flow

R - Retirement/Aging

I - Inflammation

G - Genetics

H - Head Trauma

T - Toxins

M - Mind Storms

I - Immunity/Infections

N - Neurohormone Issues

D - Diabesity

S - Sleep

I want you to imagine two rulers in rival kingdoms. One is an evil ruler whose top priority is to create and perpetuate mental illness as a way to diminish and control the kingdom's subjects. How would he or she do it? The evil ruler would turn the four circles against us, creating policies and promoting behaviors guaranteed to increase the BRIGHT MINDS risk factors (part 2). The other one is a benevolent ruler, who is passionate about ending mental illness in order to create more effective, happier humans. What would he or she do to end mental illness? The good ruler would encourage people to use the four circles to enhance brain health and to advocate policies and behaviors that would help minimize their risk factors.

Throughout this chapter, you'll find charts for each of the four circles, detailing the societal influences and the steps that will contribute to either creating mental illness and making future generations (like my nieces, Alizé and Amelie) suffer or to ending mental illness and keeping future generations healthy.

B *Biological Circle*

The first circle of a whole life and a healthy brain is biology—how the physical aspects of your brain and body function together. In order for your biology to operate at peak efficiency, its machinery (cells, connections, chemicals, energy, blood flow, and waste processing) needs to work right. The brain is like a supercomputer, with both hardware and software. Think of the biological circle as the hardware. Within it are the BRIGHT MINDS factors (which will each be explored in subsequent chapters):

Blood Flow

Retirement/Aging

Inflammation

Genetics

Head Trauma

Toxins

Mind Storms (abnormal brain electrical activity)

Immunity/Infections

Neurohormone Issues

Diabesity

Sleep

When the brain's biology is healthy, all these factors work together in a positive way to maximize your success and sense of well-being. When any of the BRIGHT MINDS risk factors are troubled, you are more likely to suffer with a wide variety of symptoms.

Ⓑ BIOLOGICAL CIRCLE

THE EVIL RULER WOULD . . .	THE BENEVOLENT RULER WOULD . . .
Perpetuate the biological warfare in America by keeping 88 percent of the population metabolically unhealthy. (More biological evildoings in the BRIGHT MINDS chapters.)	Counteract the biological warfare waged on society by creating a nationwide program that would help people fall in love with their brains. It would start in schools and go into churches, businesses, and senior centers—anywhere people gather.

Unfortunately, America's population is being assaulted by biological warfare. Only 12 percent of the population is metabolically healthy.[3] According to a 2018 study, researchers reported that 88 percent of the population did not meet the following criteria for optimal health:

- Waist circumference—less than 45/35 inches for men/women
- Fasting glucose—less than 100 mg/dL and hemoglobin A1c less than 5.7 percent
- Blood pressure—systolic less than 120 and diastolic less than 80 mmHg
- Triglycerides—less than 150 mg/dL
- High-density lipoprotein (HDL) cholesterol greater than 40/50 mg/dL for men/women
- Not taking any related medication[4]

No wonder there is a high incidence of mental illness. Your brain is an organ linked to the rest of your body. When your body is unhealthy, so too is your brain. Singer Demi Lovato, who has talked openly about having bipolar disorder, has been publicly urging people to look at the biology behind mental disorders. In 2015, she told *People* magazine, "The problem with mental illness is people don't look at it as a physical illness. When you think about it, the brain is actually the most complex organ in your body. We need to treat it like a physical illness and take it seriously."[5]

BRIGHT MINDS TIP

In the biological circle, each one of the BRIGHT MINDS risk factors can create a mental illness.

Ⓑ BIOLOGICAL CIRCLE

STEPS TO CREATE MENTAL ILLNESS ... AND MAKE MY NIECES, ALIZÉ AND AMELIE, SUFFER	STEPS TO END MENTAL ILLNESS ... AND KEEP MY NIECES, ALIZÉ AND AMELIE, HEALTHY
1. Don't care about your brain.	1. Love your brain.
2. Engage in habits that hurt your brain and promote the BRIGHT MINDS risk factors (see part 2).	2. Avoid anything that hurts your brain (such as the BRIGHT MINDS risk factors, see part 2).
3. Avoid regular brain-healthy habits.	3. Engage in regular brain-healthy habits (explored throughout the rest of the book).

Here is my favorite tiny habit that relates not only to the biological circle but to all four circles.

TINY HABITS

When you come to a decision point in your day, ask, "Is the decision I'm about to make good for my brain or bad for it?" It takes three seconds, and if you consistently make good decisions, your brain and mental health will begin to improve immediately.

Ⓟ *Psychological Circle*

The psychological circle includes how we think and talk to ourselves—the running dialogue in our minds—as well as our self-concept, body image, past emotional traumas, upbringing, and significant developmental events.[6] This circle helps us decide if we are enough—good enough, smart enough, pretty enough, strong enough, rich enough, and so on. When we feel as if we are enough, we are happier and more successful in our relationships and work. When we feel less than enough, it drives a sense of sadness, anxiety, and failure.

I keep fighting voices in my head that say I'm not enough.

LAUREN DAIGLE, "YOU SAY"

Growing up in a reasonably happy home, receiving positive messages, and feeling confident and comfortable with our abilities and our bodies all contribute to good psychological health and the feeling of being enough. When we struggle in any of these areas, we are less likely to be "psychologically healthy." If we perceive ourselves as unattractive or somehow inferior to our peers, trouble starts to accumulate. If our thoughts are excessively harsh or critical—I call these automatic negative thoughts (ANTs)—it will have a negative impact on our moods, anxiety levels, and ultimately on our biology.

Developmental issues, such as adoption, neglect or abuse, or surviving a significant loss or trauma as a child, are also important. Children often believe that they are the center of the universe and if something bad happens, such as a child's dad having a heart attack, the child may think it's his fault and be racked with guilt. Successes and failures, hope, a sense of worth, and personal power or control are a part of the psychological circle.

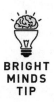

BRIGHT MINDS TIP

In the psychological circle, past emotional trauma, undisciplined thinking, ANTs, excessive social media and screen time, and shame can create a mental illness.

Ⓟ PSYCHOLOGICAL CIRCLE

THE EVIL RULER WOULD . . .	THE BENEVOLENT RULER WOULD . . .
1. Use *psychological warfare* to hurt subjects. This includes ignoring past emotional trauma created by alcoholic or drug-abusing parents and not addressing current or past traumas from earthquakes, fires, floods, immigration, and criminal behaviors. 2. Model undisciplined, negative thinking patterns and never teach people how to eliminate the ANTs that infest their minds. 3. Perpetuate shame, one of the most powerful psychological weapons. Shame is a painful emotion that results from negatively comparing yourself to others or not living up to your own standards. Social media outlets are masterful at creating shame as they invite nonstop comparisons to other people who may or may not even be real. Because of this, the evil ruler would use social media to shame others and would give people free rein to spout hateful ideas without consequences.	1. Make psychotherapy readily available for those who want or need it, especially if they've had past emotional trauma, after they have worked to optimize their brains. 2. Teach subjects how to deal with current or past emotional traumas. 3. Make rational thinking skills (eliminating the ANTs) part of the educational curriculum, along with ways to help people self-regulate their bodies and emotions with guided imagery, meditation, and hypnosis. 4. Limit social media so people cannot endlessly compare themselves to others, never feeling enough. 5. Require all therapists to have brain health modules as part of their education programs. 6. Incorporate more green space into urban planning to promote better moods and reduce the incidence of mental illness.[7]

I find Eckhart Tolle's concept of the "painbody" to be a very helpful psychological concept. He writes, "There is such a thing as old emotional pain living inside you. It is an accumulation of painful life experience that was not fully faced and accepted in the moment it arose. It leaves behind an energy form of emotional pain. It comes together with other energy forms from other instances, and so after some years you have a 'painbody,' an energy entity consisting of old emotion."[8] When your painbody bumps up against the painbodies of others, it can cause intense relational disturbances, where each painbody feeds off the others. Tolle teaches us:

Recognize the painbody when it shifts from dormant to active, when something triggers a very strong emotional reaction. At that moment, when it does take over your mind, the internal dialogue, which is dysfunctional at the best of times, now becomes the voice of the painbody talking to you internally. Everything it says is deeply colored by the old, painful emotion of the painbody. Every interpretation, everything it says, every judgment about your life, about other people, about a situation you are in, will be totally distorted by the old emotional pain.[9]

If you are present by being "in the moment," the painbody cannot feed anymore on your thoughts or on other people's reactions. The antidote to the painbody is to recognize it by asking, "Could this be my painbody talking? Am I reacting from the present moment or from pain in the past?" Tolle writes, "You can simply observe it, and be the witness, be the space for it. Then gradually, its energy will decrease."[10]

To optimize your psychological circle, it is important to train your mind to help you rather than hurt you. In a recent public television special, my 16-year-old daughter, Chloe, shared some of her own anxieties about school, the way she looked, and her future. She knows these are common worries for teens, but that doesn't mean they're not painful. For many years, she thought she was the only person who felt that way. Many adults still carry the ANTs they collected during adolescence . . . which can continue to infest them for the rest of their lives unless they learn how to eliminate them.

**BRIGHT
MINDS
TIP**

To optimize the psychological circle, it is critical to train your mind to help you by eliminating the ANTs and soothing any painbodies.

You can train your mind to help you, but left undisciplined it can spin out of control. Unfortunately, most people are never taught how to train their minds. Chloe shared the following examples of the thoughts that used to torture her.

- *I'm not good enough.*
- *I'm not smart enough.*
- *Why do I have to work harder than other people?*
- *Why am I the only person who feels this way?*
- *I don't fit in.*

I taught Chloe the following principles to train her mind:

1. Whenever you have a sad thought, a mad thought, or a hopeless thought, such as "I don't fit in," your brain releases chemicals that make you feel bad. Your hands get colder, they start to sweat, your breathing changes, your muscles tense, you can't think, and these changes happen immediately. But the opposite is also true.

2. Every time you have a happy thought, a hopeful thought, or an empowering thought, such as "I don't fit in, which may be a good thing," your brain releases a different set of chemicals that make you feel good . . . immediately. Your hands become warmer and drier, your breathing rate slows down, your muscles become more relaxed, and you feel happier.

3. Thoughts are powerful, and they can help you feel wonderful or miserable.

4. Thoughts are automatic; they just happen.

5. Unfortunately, thoughts lie. They lie a lot, and it is these bad thoughts that steal our happiness. We call them ANTs, but you can learn to kill the ANTs and be happier.

6. To kill ANTs, write down what you're thinking whenever you feel mad, sad, nervous, or out of control. Then ask yourself if the thoughts are factually true or whether you are jumping to a conclusion or making an assumption. Often ANTs are simply interpretations that you cannot prove as true. Can you absolutely know if they're true? Challenging the ANTs helps to take away their power. (For a more in-depth look at how to kill the ANTs, see my book *Feel Better Fast and Make It Last*.)

Many of my patients wear rubber bands around their wrists and snap them whenever they notice bad thoughts to remind themselves to eliminate the ANTs. You don't have to believe every thought you have. Killing the ANTs made a big difference for Chloe, and normally it only takes a few minutes. Plus, the more you do it, the easier it gets. If teenagers can do it, I think you can do it too.

Also, it is critical to program your mind to look for what is right, rather than just thinking about what is wrong. Where you bring your attention determines how you feel. I start every day with the phrase, "Today is going to be a great day." It's a simple way to begin training your brain to look for what's right rather than what's wrong, and it sets a positive tone for the rest of the day. Ending each day by journaling or meditating on what went well that day sets up your dreams to be much more positive. This simple technique will take about three minutes and can decrease depression in just 30 days. Do this as a household or family. Start every day by saying to each other, "Today is going to be a great day." End each day by asking "What went well today?" It will completely change your relational dynamics in just a few days.

Practicing gratitude is also incredibly powerful. It increases happiness, self-esteem, self-control, you live longer, and your relationships are better. Gratitude should be written at the top of every prescription your doctor gives you, and journaling gratitude doesn't have to take more than three minutes a day. It really helped Sarah, a 16-year-old who came to our clinic in Chicago in search of help for crushing depression.

Sarah Discovers the Power of Gratitude Journaling

February 2017 is when my story of mental illness began. What started out as frequent feelings of sadness slowly intensified into a numb depression. As time went on, the depression overcame and muted any feelings of happiness I had, making it seemingly impossible for me to enjoy the things I once loved. Thankfully, I hadn't lost hope yet, and I found the strength to reach out and get professional help.

In the beginning, I tried therapy. I went to many appointments with several therapists, but I left each one feeling no better than when I went in. To me, it was simple. I didn't have anything wrong with my life; I didn't have anything to talk about or "fix." When therapy didn't help, I tried medication. I spent month after month trying what seemed like randomly selected cocktails of medications. Unfortunately, this was a dead end as well. Each time a medication didn't help, I lost a little more hope.

Throughout these months my depression only continued to consume me, and anxiety decided to join the party. After tirelessly trying to feel better for months with my symptoms only declining, I settled at my lowest point yet. I had lost all hope of recovering, there was no more light to hold on to, and I felt as if there was no reason to keep trying. I gave up.

It was at this point that my grandma discovered Amen Clinics. Instead of randomly selecting medications to put me on, they would use brain scans to see exactly what I needed, my grandma explained to me. Seeing how much hope my mom and my grandma had in this, I went along with it.

In February 2018 my mom, my grandma, and I drove to the Chicago location of Amen Clinics. The first two days I was there I got both my brain scans done and completed a computer test. On the third day, I got my evaluation. From the test results, Dr. Michelle Flowers determined what the best treatment option would be for me. First, I would begin taking deliberately selected vitamins and supplements. I would also continue on the medication I was still on from my last doctor because with the help of these new supplements my body could use the medication to its full advantage. Secondly, I would begin trying a new type of therapy, and unlike the form [of] therapy I previously tried, this new therapy would be used to retrain my brain, not pick at it. And the third major piece of the puzzle was gratitude journaling.

In the beginning, it was challenging to think of pleasant moments to write about, but over time my brain learned to find these moments without thought. Before long, my brain was noticing moments to be grateful for all throughout the day.

I left knowing we had physical evidence and facts to back up the treatment plan. We had a plan that we knew would help. It wasn't just some doctor telling me it would be okay, it was a doctor show- ing me what was wrong and how we could fix it. I still have a way to go in my recovery, but I have exactly what I need to keep growing, healing, and taking on what life throws at me.

—Sarah, 16

It is important to recognize the psychological warfare being perpetuated by our society with the excessive use of social media, where teenagers and young adults are endlessly comparing themselves to others, never feeling enough. I talk about this with my nieces, Alizé and Amelie, on a regular basis to help them maintain a healthy perspective about social media. In a study of more than a million teens since 1991, researchers found that when the teens limited social media, spent time with their friends in person, exercised, played sports, attended religious services, read, and even did homework, they were happier than those who spent time on the internet and social media, playing computer games, texting, using video chat, or watching TV.[11]

Ⓟ PSYCHOLOGICAL CIRCLE

STEPS TO CREATE MENTAL ILLNESS . . . AND MAKE MY NIECES, ALIZÉ AND AMELIE, SUFFER	STEPS TO END MENTAL ILLNESS . . . AND KEEP MY NIECES, ALIZÉ AND AMELIE, HEALTHY
1. Don't think or care about your psychological health. 2. Engage in habits that hurt your mind, including: • Comparing yourself to others (the seeds of shame) • Telling yourself you are not enough • Believing the ANTs • Not recognizing the painbody or getting help for your past emotional traumas • Focusing primarily on what's wrong with you and others 3. Avoid any education or habits on how to help your mind.	1. Care deeply about your psychological health. 2. Engage in regular healthy psychological habits, including: • Telling yourself you are enough • Challenging and eliminating the ANTs • Noticing what's right about yourself more than what is wrong • Saying, "Today is going to be a great day." • At the end of the day, journaling what went well that day • Practicing gratitude • Recognizing a painbody and focusing on being present to calm it down • Seeking brain-informed psychotherapy, when needed 3. Avoid excessive social media use and bad psychological habits, such as believing every thought you have or not dealing with past emotional trauma.

Here are three of my favorite psychological circle tiny habits.

- Whenever you feel sad, mad, nervous, or out of control, write down your ANTs and ask yourself if they are assumptions, conclusions, interpretations, or truth. Can you absolutely know if they are true? Questioning your thoughts helps to take away their power.

- Every day when your feet hit the floor in the morning, say to yourself, "Today is going to be a great day!" That way your subconscious mind will find why it will be a great day. This helps to train your mind to look for what is right rather than what is wrong.

- Every night before bed, write down what went well that day. Research suggests it can improve your happiness after just one month.[12]

Ⓢ *Social Circle*

In a computer analogy, the biological circle is the hardware, the psychological circle is the software, and the social circle is the network connections. The social circle includes the quality of your relationships and any current stresses—think problems with your spouse or kids, crazy deadlines at work, a family member's health crisis, or mounting credit card debt. When we have great relationships, healthy families, a job we love, and enough money, our brains tend to do much better than when any of these areas are troubled. Dealing with difficult life circumstances—such as a divorce, moving, a job change, or the death of a close family member—elevates stress hormone levels and makes us more vulnerable to many illnesses, including depression, anxiety disorders, and more.

BRIGHT MINDS TIP

You become like the people with whom you spend the most time. Relationship health is critical to the health of your brain and mind.

Stress occurs when a person perceives excessive demands on his or her emotional or physical resources. Stress increases to toxic levels when we feel things are out of control. In 1967, US psychiatrists Thomas Holmes and Richard Rahe studied the effects of stress on health, surveying more than 5,000 medical patients. They asked them to say whether they had any of a series of life events in the previous two years. The more events someone had, the more likely they were to become physically or emotionally sick.[13] Toxic stress has been associated with obesity, heart disease, cancer, ADD/ADHD, learning disabilities, social anxiety, depression, alcohol and drug abuse, PTSD, being arrested, and an unhealthy "fight or flight" aggressive tendency in the brain. Decreasing everyday stress (relationships, work, finances, and health) lowers inflammation and improves immune system function.[14]

Ⓢ SOCIAL CIRCLE

THE EVIL RULER WOULD . . .	THE BENEVOLENT RULER WOULD . . .
1. Cause strife among the people, subjecting them to chronic stress that separates them from each other, so that the ruler could retain more power.	1. Make job training, healthcare, parent training, and financial assistance readily available to those who need it.
2. Bombard people with negative news cycles, creating an us-versus-them mentality and pitting political, racial, and other groups against each other.	2. Advocate for stress-management classes in schools and businesses.
3. Create a society where recreational marijuana dispensaries are on every corner and alcohol is promoted as a health food. (In an example of evil-ruler entrepreneurial genius, Girl Scouts are now setting up outside marijuana dispensaries. In 2014, a 13-year-old Girl Scout sold 177 boxes of Samoas, Tagalongs, and Thin Mints outside a San Francisco pot dispensary. After being there just a short time, she had to call for help to be restocked. In 2018, a nine-year-old Girl Scout sold 300 boxes of the tasty treats outside a San Diego pot dispensary in about six hours.[15] Smarter still, inside the pot dispensaries they are offering cookies with THC in them and a strain of marijuana called Girl Scout Cookies.)	3. Provide classes on decision-making skills so people would make better life decisions and be less stressed. Decisions are better when you have clear goals, sleep more than seven hours, avoid low-blood-sugar states (have protein and healthy fat at every meal), and eliminate the ANTs when they attack.
4. Increase the social pressure to stay connected to your phone and social media for work and relationships, not allowing enough time for sleep and self-care.	

Social warfare—that's when our society wages an attack on our well-being—is one of the most common causes of mental illness. Negative news cycles create an us-versus-them mentality, pitting political, racial, and other groups against each other. Just 14 minutes of negative news has been found to increase both anxious and sad moods.[16] Such chronic stress and relational separation damages brains. In addition, bad relationships, health problems, and financial stress all contribute to the social causes of mental illnesses. That's why all four circles of health matter so much.

Loneliness is also a concern in the social circle. Baby boomers are aging alone more than any generation in US history. About 10 percent of Americans who are 50 and older do not have a spouse, partner, or living child. This group has the highest rate of suicide and an increasing problem of drug addiction.[17] Loneliness is a recognized risk factor for Alzheimer's disease.[18]

We're increasingly spending more time on the internet, with social media rapidly replacing in-person connections. But social media doesn't provide us with the same benefits as socializing face-to-face. In fact, in a new study, there was a clear, causal link between Facebook, Snapchat, and Instagram and depression and loneliness, especially in teenage girls.[19] These sites also made vulnerable people feel worse about their bodies.[20] In addition, new research shows that using screens for long periods changes children's brains in a negative way. Researchers at the National Institutes of Health performed brain scans of 4,500 children. Those who had daily screen time usage of more than seven hours showed premature thinning of the cortex, the outermost brain layer responsible for processing information from the physical world.[21]

Even more frightening is the reported emergence of seemingly innocent online videos directed at children that encourage them to engage in challenges involving self-harm. For example, reports have surfaced of deadly suicide games aimed at teens called the "Momo" (a scary-looking doll-like figure) challenge and the Blue Whale challenge.[22] Even if these games don't actually exist, the social media buzz surrounding them can spread quickly among vulnerable children and teens who *think* they are real and who may act on them.

In addition, the health habits of the people with whom you spend time have a dramatic impact on your own health and habits. If you spend time with unhealthy people, you are much more likely to be unhealthy yourself. Brazilian supermodel Gisele Bündchen discovered this in her twenties when, despite her multimillion-dollar career and romantic involvement with Hollywood heartthrob Leonardo DiCaprio, she sank into depression and began to experience panic attacks. Not surprisingly, a doctor suggested she take Xanax. But the supermodel chose to make some lifestyle changes instead. The jet setter who had basically been living on wine, coffee, and cigarettes cut back on those bad habits, reduced her work schedule, and integrated yoga, meditation, and family time into her daily life.

"I've learned that our thoughts, words, and actions are all connected, and why we need to be careful with them. I began nourishing my body, mind, and spirit through meditation, healing foods, and a positive outlook, and as a result was able to experience a deeper clarity and greater sense of purpose," she wrote in her book *Lessons: My Path to a Meaningful Life.*[23] That's when she came to realize her boyfriend was not quite right for her, and the pair split. Getting healthy means avoiding people who encourage habits that contribute to illness and, instead, surrounding yourself with those who support brain-healthy choices.

Social connections are also essential to mental health. German Emperor Frederick II conducted a barbaric 13th-century experiment because he wanted to know what language and words children would speak if they were raised without hearing any words at all. He took a number of infants from their homes and put them with people who fed them but had strict instructions not to touch, cuddle, or talk to them. The babies never spoke a word. They all died before they could speak. Salimbene, a historian of the time, wrote of the experiment in 1248, "They could not live without petting."[24] This powerful finding has been rediscovered over and over. In the early 1990s, thousands of Romanian infants were orphaned and warehoused without touch sometimes for years at a time. PET studies (similar to SPECT studies) of a number of these deprived children have shown marked overall decreased activity across the whole brain.[25]

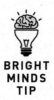

BRIGHT MINDS TIP

In the social circle, an us-versus-them mentality, chronic stress, social pressure that encourages bad habits and illness, loneliness, and a lack of affection and touch can create a mental illness.

Ⓢ SOCIAL CIRCLE

STEPS TO CREATE MENTAL ILLNESS ... AND MAKE MY NIECES, ALIZÉ AND AMELIE, SUFFER	STEPS TO END MENTAL ILLNESS ... AND KEEP MY NIECES, ALIZÉ AND AMELIE, HEALTHY
1. Don't think about your social connections or how you manage stress.	1. Care about your social connections and how you manage stress.
2. Engage in things that damage your social connections and generate stress, including:	2. Avoid anything that hurts your relationships or increases stress, such as:
• Loneliness, social isolation	• Unhealthy people
• Poor or disconnected relationships	• Us-versus-them mentality
• Us-versus-them mentality, pitting social or political groups against each other	• Negative news cycles
• Excessive health, school, job, financial, relational, or legal stress	• Unnecessary stress
• Toxic societal stress; constant negative news cycles	• Excessive screen time and social media
• Associating with people with negative health habits	3. Engage in habits that strengthen your relationships and lower unnecessary stress, such as:
• Being in easy proximity to illness temptations, such as fast food restaurants, marijuana dispensaries, happy hour, decadent holiday parties, etc.	• Positive relationship habits (responsibility, empathy, time, listening, assertiveness, noticing what you like more than what you don't, forgiveness)
• Staying connected to your phone and other devices at all times	• Volunteering to help others in need
• Choosing social media connections over in-person relationships	• Looking for ways to bring your social connections together
3. Avoid any education or habits on how to strengthen your social connections or lower stress.	• Cultivating stress management and decision-making skills
	• Surrounding yourself with positive, healthy people—the fastest way to get healthy is to find the healthiest people you can stand and spend as much time around them as possible.
	• Keeping your distance from fast food restaurants, marijuana dispensaries, happy hour, decadent holiday parties, etc.

Here are three of my favorite social circle tiny habits.

- After I've had a fight with a loved one, I will take responsibility for my part and quickly apologize.

- When I feel overwhelmed or stressed, I will take five deep breaths, taking twice as long to exhale to settle and center myself.

- If I have children, I'll spend at least 20 minutes a day fully present with them, doing something they want to do. I will make no commands, ask no questions, and give no directions. It is just a time to be together. (This dramatically improves bonding.)

SP *Spiritual Circle*

Beyond the biological, psychological, and social aspects of our lives, we are also spiritual beings. To fully heal and be your best, it is important to recognize that we are more than just our cells, thoughts, and connections. We are all spiritual beings created with divine purpose, whether or not we believe in God. Having a sense of purpose and a moral code, as well as connections to God, the planet, past generations (my grandfather, as an example: I was named after him, and he was my best friend growing up), and future generations (my grandchildren and great-grandchildren) reminds us that our lives matter; we have a role to play and a calling to fulfill. Without this spiritual connection, many people experience a sense of despair or meaninglessness, which can lead to depression.

SP SPIRITUAL CIRCLE

THE EVIL RULER WOULD . . .	THE BENEVOLENT RULER WOULD . . .
1. Lead people to live meaningless lives, devoid of values and connection to a life beyond themselves.	1. Model a purposeful life and encourage everyone else to do the same.
2. Model an amoral life, making it seem normal, even desirable.	2. Encourage spiritual beliefs and practices without dictating them, such as prayer, meditation, worship, and service.
	3. Foster a deep connection to the past, the future, and the planet.

Purposeful people, defined as having "the psychological tendency to derive meaning from life's experiences and to possess a sense of intentionality and goal directedness that guides behavior," live longer and are healthier overall.[26] In a large study, purposeful people were found to have better mental health, less depression, greater happiness and satisfaction, more personal growth and self-acceptance, and better sleep. Over time, higher scores on this scale were also associated with a reduced risk of Alzheimer's disease, less cognitive impairment, and a slower rate of cognitive decline in old age.[27]

Research shows that having a strong "purpose in life" also reduces the chances that your self-esteem will fluctuate with the number of likes you get on social media.[28] Ultimately, feeling as if your life matters and living purposefully helps protect you from the social warfare you now understand is behind so much mental illness. On the flip side, a lack of purpose has been linked to higher levels of the stress hormone cortisol, more abdominal fat, and other negative health markers. It's easy to see how increased stress, a bigger belly, and poorer health can contribute to negative feelings that, when combined with low brain reserve, can create mental illness. Think of how easily that can be passed on to younger people, such as my nieces, who are vulnerable.

In our society, the media constantly highlights people—such as politicians, religious and business leaders, and celebrities—who model amoral lives. In addition, on a day-to-day basis, we often come into contact with people—including our own parents, teachers, or bosses—whose lives are devoid of meaning and purpose. With so much confusion about the spiritual circle in our society, how can we find our purpose in life?

Dr. Viktor Frankl, a psychiatrist, World War II concentration camp survivor, and author of *Man's Search for Meaning*, believed there were three ways to create meaning:

1. Purposeful work or being productive—asking questions such as, "Why is the world a better place because I am here?" or "What do I contribute?"
2. Love for the people who are central to our lives.
3. Courage in the face of difficulty—shouldering whatever difficult fate we have and helping others shoulder theirs.

I suggest engaging in spiritual practices, such as prayer, meditation, worship, and service. I stay connected to God and my Christian faith through daily prayers, meditation, and attending church with my family. Think of your church or other places of worship, as well as any nurturing environment, as a space that fosters all four circles of health. I also have my patients ask themselves:

- What does your life mean?
- What is your purpose?
- Why are you here?
- What are your values?
- Do you believe in God or a higher power?
- How does that affect your life?
- What is your connection to past generations, future generations, and the planet?[29]

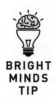

BRIGHT MINDS TIP

In the spiritual circle, a lack of purpose or connections to something larger than yourself and not living up to your own moral code can create a mental illness.

Here are two of my favorite spiritual circle tiny habits.

- In the morning, I will ask myself, *What one purposeful thing will I do today?*

- When I start getting upset about something happening in my day, I'll ask myself, *Does this have eternal value?*

SP SPIRITUAL CIRCLE

STEPS TO CREATE MENTAL ILLNESS . . . AND MAKE MY NIECES, ALIZÉ AND AMELIE, SUFFER	STEPS TO END MENTAL ILLNESS . . . AND KEEP MY NIECES, ALIZÉ AND AMELIE, HEALTHY
1. Don't care or think about your spiritual well-being or purpose in life.	1. Care about your deepest sense of meaning and purpose. You are more than just your cells, thoughts, and connections.
2. Live a meaningless existence, focused solely on yourself and the pleasures of the moment.	2. Stop engaging in habits that hurt your spiritual circle.
3. Behave in opposition to a moral code (anger, gluttony, addictions, affairs, pornography, etc.).	3. Live by a moral code.
4. Look up to people who live amoral lives.	4. Engage in regular positive spiritual habits, including:
5. Avoid a sense of passion or purpose.	• Living with intentionality, being goal oriented toward a higher purpose.
6. Avoid connections to the past, future, and planet.	• Building or rediscovering connections with God, the church, the past, the future, and/or the planet.
7. Avoid role models who are living spiritual lives.	• Engaging in meaningful work, such as volunteering at your church or place of worship.
	• Engaging in meaningful relationships with people who share your values and faith.
	• Having courage and faith in the face of challenges.
	• Living with the end in mind— what does God want you to accomplish while you are alive?

THE POWER OF PURPOSE AND THE SPIRITUAL CIRCLE

I met Byron Katie in 2005, and we immediately became friends. She is the author of one of my favorite books *Loving What Is* and was helpful to me personally during a difficult time of grief. She worked with people I loved to help discipline their minds, and I worked with people she loved to help balance their brains. Eventually, I scanned Katie's brain. It was not healthy and looked like the scan of someone who was suffering. Yet she was at peace. Her spiritual practice overrode her brain issues.

Likewise, a number of years ago, I scanned Sam, who had been practicing loving-kindness meditation for 20 years. Of note, his SPECT scan looked quite terrible, with decreased activity to his left frontal and temporal lobes. He told me he'd had a motorcycle accident 20 years earlier, and he started the meditation practice to deal with the depression he experienced after the trauma. In the last 15 years, he had started his own chiropractic office, had been very successful, and had not experienced any more depression, although he admitted he was quite disorganized and relied on his wonderful wife and practice manager to keep him on track.

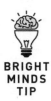

BRIGHT MINDS TIP

Psychological health, positive social connections, and spiritual practices can help stabilize troubled brains.

Both Byron Katie's story and Sam's story point to how psychological health, positive social connections, and spiritual practices can help override brains that are in trouble. Getting and staying well involves all four circles. In part 2, you'll see how the four circles intersect with and influence the 11 BRIGHT MINDS risk factors. And I'll introduce you to some simple strategies using each of the four circles that you can use to prevent or heal those risk factors to enhance your brain health and end mental illness.

HOW TO CREATE OR ELIMINATE MENTAL ILLNESS: A BRIGHT MINDS APPROACH

To keep your brain and mind healthy, or to rescue it if it is headed for trouble, you have to prevent or treat the 11 major BRIGHT MINDS risk factors that steal your mind. In *Memory Rescue*, I wrote extensively about these risk factors in relation to memory and cognitive decline. But these risk factors also have huge implications on other areas of brain health/mental health. Addressing them can help you prevent or reverse "mental illness," and your memory will also benefit in the long run.

The following chapters will help you determine which of the risk factors you may have and how to prevent and treat them, including specific strategies and nutraceuticals when appropriate. Foods to support each risk factor will be discussed in chapter 18.

CHAPTER 5

<u>B</u> IS FOR BLOOD FLOW

OPTIMIZE THE FOUNDATION OF LIFE

One way to get high blood pressure is to go mountain climbing over molehills.
EARL WILSON

 DANIEL

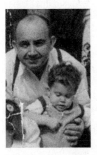 Daniel Ara was the kindest person I've ever known. He was my grandfather. I was named after him, and he was my best friend growing up. Being the third of seven children, I did not have much individual time with my parents, but when I was at his home, it felt like I was the most special person in the world. Plus, he was a professional candy maker. It doesn't get any better than that for a child. My earliest memories were of standing by the white stove in his kitchen, learning how to make fudge and pralines. Yum.

Yet all the sugar took a toll on him, and he had his first heart attack at age 69. Before that, I can't remember a single time when Grandpa was irritable or upset, even being married to my grandmother, which could be stressful. He was happy, always smiling, and positive. But after his heart attack, he changed. He cried easily, had trouble sleeping, and lost his joy. He was clinically diagnosed with major depression and put on antidepressant medication. I was in college and medical school during that time and learned firsthand about the connection between cardiovascular disease and depression. His funeral was the saddest day of my life. He was one of the main reasons why I fell in love with helping people who are suffering from brain health/mental health issues.

I wish I had known then what I know now about sugar, blood flow, heart disease, and depression. Blood flow is critical for life. It transports nutrients, including oxygen, to every cell in your body and flushes away toxins. Even though your brain, which weighs about three pounds, makes up only 2 percent of your body's weight, it uses 20 percent of the oxygen and blood flow in your body. Anything that damages your blood vessels or impairs blood flow hurts your brain. This means that taking care of your heart and blood vessels to ensure healthy blood flow to your brain is not just important for your physical health, but it is also essential for your mental well-being. And this relationship goes both ways.

People with depression, anxiety, bipolar disorder, and schizophrenia are more likely to develop cardiovascular disease, even at young ages; and people with cardiovascular disease are more likely to suffer from depression and dementia.[1] Exciting new research dispels the long-held belief that our brain cells age quickly; rather, it is the blood vessels that feed our neurons that are aging faster.[2] If you want to keep your brain healthy, your mind sharp, and your mental health strong for as long as possible, you need to protect your blood vessels.

SPECT measures the brain's blood flow and activity. Low blood flow on SPECT has been seen with depression, suicide, bipolar disorder, schizophrenia, attention deficit disorder/attention deficit hyperactivity disorder (ADD/ADHD), traumatic brain injury (TBI), hoarding, murder, substance abuse, seizure activity, and more. Low blood flow is the number one brain imaging predictor that a person will develop Alzheimer's disease.[3]

Low blood flow on SPECT has been seen with depression, suicide, bipolar disorder, schizophrenia, ADD/ADHD, substance abuse, hoarding, murder, seizure activity, head trauma, and more.

This is why I was so concerned when I scanned my niece Alizé's brain when she was 13 and discovered that it showed lower overall blood flow. To end mental illness with Alizé and her sister, Amelie, I would have to teach her how to boost blood flow, and she would have to get serious about caring for her brain. As any parent knows, getting a teen to adopt new habits can be a challenge. But showing Alizé a healthy brain scan and putting it next to her own scan helped her see that her brain needed help and motivated her to get on board with the Four Circles BRIGHT MINDS program.

ALIZÉ'S SPECT STUDY

Before   After

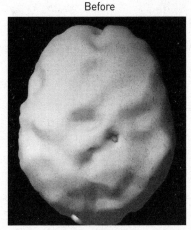

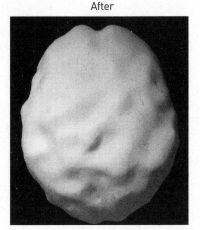

Low overall blood flow,   Improved overall
especially for her age

Less than a year later, we rescanned Alizé's brain, and it showed marked improvement in overall blood flow after taking supplements and doing hyperbaric oxygen therapy (HBOT). Seeing the improvement helped her know she was on the right track and gave her encouragement to stick with the program.

My niece Alizé and my grandfather are prime examples of how much the four circles can come into play in blood flow.

- **B** • **Biological:** Having compromised blood flow like Alizé, or a heart attack like my grandfather, is linked with a higher risk for brain health/mental health issues.

- **P** • **Psychological:** In my grandfather's case, he didn't know at the time that he could take action to improve his blood flow and minimize his depression. But, as Alizé is already learning, when you believe you have the power to change your brain and change your life, you can improve blood flow to the brain and reduce symptoms of mental illness.

- **S** • **Social:** Alizé grew up in an environment that was contributing to lower blood flow in the brain. When she came to live with me and my wife, however, we surrounded her with people who live brain-healthy lives. It has inspired her to start adopting healthier habits that are boosting blood flow to her brain.

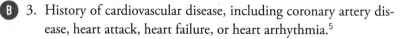

SP • **Spiritual:** For many people, like my grandfather, taking care of others takes precedence over taking care of themselves. Making your own health a priority may feel selfish, but making sure you are happy, healthy, and energetic is the key to being there for your family and friends.

Our brain imaging research has taught us that the number one strategy to support your brain and mental health is to protect, nurture, and optimize your heart and blood vessels. Anything that damages your blood vessels damages your mind. Do you have any of the following risk factors for low blood flow to the brain?

Blood Flow Risk Factors
(and the Four Circles They Represent)

B 1. History of a stroke,[4] which indicates blood vessels are already damaged or vulnerable to trouble.

B S 2. More than two cups of caffeinated drinks a day, which constricts blood flow to the brain (social circle if you're drinking it with friends or coworkers).

B 3. History of cardiovascular disease, including coronary artery disease, heart attack, heart failure, or heart arrhythmia.[5]

B S 4. High low-density lipoprotein (LDL) cholesterol in the blood, particularly with a high content of small LDL particles (social circle if, when eating with friends or family, you eat foods that negatively impact LDL cholesterol). One caveat, which over-enthusiastic cardiologists will rarely tell you, is that lowering total cholesterol levels below 160 mg/dL can *increase* the risk of depression and aggression. The body actually needs cholesterol for certain vital functions, so don't go too low.[6]

B P 5. Prehypertension or hypertension in midlife,[7] which decreases blood flow to the brain (psychological circle if chronic stress is contributing to high blood pressure). Low blood pressure in later life[8] also lessens blood flow.

B 6. Erectile dysfunction.[9] If you have blood flow problems anywhere, it likely means they are everywhere.

B 7. Sedentary lifestyle and limited exercise, less than twice a week.[10] More than 90 percent of teenagers do not get the CDC's recommended level of exercise, which could be one of the major reasons brain health/mental health issues among teens have skyrocketed in the last 30 years.[11]

B 8. Prediabetes or diabetes (see chapter 14, "<u>D</u> Is for Diabesity"). High blood sugar levels cause blood vessels to become brittle and more likely to break, delaying healing and causing disease complications.

B **S** 9. Smoking or ingesting nicotine (see chapter 10, "<u>T</u> Is for Toxins"), which constricts blood flow to the brain (social circle if you smoke with friends).

B **S** 10. Excessive alcohol use (see chapter 10, "<u>T</u> Is for Toxins"), which lowers overall blood flow to the brain (social circle if you drink in social situations).

B 11. Sleep apnea (see chapter 15, "<u>S</u> Is for Sleep"), which lowers overall blood flow to the brain, but especially in the areas that die first in Alzheimer's disease.

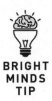

BRIGHT MINDS TIP

The number one strategy to keep your brain and mind healthy is to protect, nurture, and optimize your heart and blood vessels. Anything that damages them damages your mind.

Take a look at how the evil and benevolent rulers would influence blood flow to increase or decrease mental illness.

BLOOD FLOW

THE EVIL RULER WOULD . . .	THE BENEVOLENT RULER WOULD . . .

1. Tell people they must not exercise, which decreases blood vessel flexibility and hurt brain health.
 	
2. Pass out video game consoles and online streaming services to all subjects, stealing their time and attention so they can't find the time to exercise.
 	
3. Encourage schools to cut physical-education programs from the curriculum.
 	
4. Encourage a higher incidence of hypertension and heart diseases, such as heart attacks (depression risk is significantly elevated after a heart attack[12]), and hardening of the arteries by
 	
  • Making cigarettes and marijuana widely available for a low price (both decrease blood flow[13]).
  • Putting fast food restaurants on every street corner, allowing subjects to supersize meals for just a few pennies, withholding calorie counts on menus so people have no idea how much they are consuming, and giving away free desserts with every meal—*because the population deserves it!*
  • Making coffee shops plentiful (caffeine constricts blood flow to the brain)
	1. Encourage exercise in schools, churches, and the workplace.
	
	2. Limit video games and screen time, so children and adults will spend more time outdoors exercising.
	
	3. Advocate annual screening for any vascular issues and enthusiastically treat them early when signs of trouble arise.
	
	4. Make brain health education mandatory at schools and businesses on the blood flow effects of caffeine, including energy drinks, nicotine, and marijuana.

PRESCRIPTIONS FOR REDUCING YOUR BLOOD FLOW RISK FACTORS
(AND THE FOUR CIRCLES THEY REPRESENT)

The Strategies

Here are the primary strategies that can help support your overall blood flow and blood pressure.

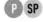 1. **Care about your blood vessels.** They are important to every other part of your body.

2. **Avoid anything that decreases brain blood flow.** Examples include a sedentary lifestyle, obesity,[14] more than one serving of caffeine a day,[15] ingesting nicotine,[16] smoking marijuana,[17] and dehydration.[18] When people stop smoking, anxiety, depression, and stress levels are lower, quality of life and mood improves, and even the dosages of some medications used to treat psychiatric issues can be reduced.[19] Video gaming is also related to decreased blood flow in the prefrontal cortex in both children and adults,[20] and playing violent video games leads to lower perfusion to the anterior cingulate cortex.[21]

3. **Get medical help for anything that damages your blood flow.** Don't ignore or delay treating health problems you know you have, such as coronary artery disease, heart arrhythmias, prediabetes and diabetes, prehypertension and hypertension, insomnia, sleep apnea, erectile dysfunction, and drug and alcohol abuse.

4. **Practice natural strategies to support healthy blood pressure.** In addition to the other strategies on this list, these will help keep your blood pressure healthy.

   - Hydrate better! If you drink at least five glasses of water a day, you could decrease your risk of hypertension.[22]
   - Eat mostly plants.
   - Limit salt intake.
   - Eat more foods high in magnesium, such as avocados, nuts, and seeds, and potassium, such as spinach and sweet potatoes.
   - Incorporate foods that lower blood pressure, such as beet juice, broccoli, celery, garlic, chickpeas, and mushrooms.

- Limit alcohol, caffeine, fruit juices, and sodas (including diet sodas).
- Sleep seven to eight hours a night, and if you have sleep apnea, get it assessed and treated.

(B) 5. **Take medication if you need it.** I prefer a natural approach to health problems, but high blood pressure or excessively high cholesterol must be managed properly. The thoughtful use of medicines, when combined with the above lifestyle strategies, can be very helpful.

(B) (P) (S) (SP) 6. **Engage regularly in behaviors that enhance blood flow.**

(SP) • **Spend 10 to 20 minutes a day in prayer or meditation.**[23] Both prayer and meditation have been shown to improve blood flow to the prefrontal cortex, decrease anxiety, and improve mood. They are also both effective stress-management tools.

(B) (S) • **Build regular physical exercise into your lifestyle** (social circle if you exercise with friends). In a review of research on more than 10,000 people, exercise was found to be similar in effectiveness to antihypertensive medication.[24] The benefits of exercise for brain health are lasting and impressive. Just ask Lena Dunham, the creator of the hit HBO series *Girls*. She wrote on Instagram, "Promised myself I would not let exercise be the first thing to go by the wayside when I got busy with *Girls* Season 5 and here is why: It has helped with my anxiety in ways I never dreamed possible. To those struggling with anxiety, OCD, depression: I know it's mad annoying when people tell you to exercise, and it took me about 16 medicated years to listen. I'm glad I did."

Dunham is right. Just 100 minutes a week of exercise (that's just 20 minutes a day, five times a week), together with a healthy diet, decreased brain age by nearly 10 years.[25] Plus, regular physical exercise does the following:

- Lowers the risk of developing depression (and that's by jogging for just 15 minutes a day).[26]
- Improves mood, anxiety, and even cognitive health in patients with depression and schizophrenia.[27]

- Reduces depression and anxiety in prisoners[28] and methamphetamine abusers.[29]
- Improves anxiety, depression, and insomnia in postmenopausal women[30] and breast cancer survivors.[31]
- Increases the size of the hippocampus,[32] one of the brain's major memory and mood centers.
- Protects the hippocampus from stress-related hormones, like cortisol,[33] which normally shrink it. Even leisurely walking has been shown to increase the size of the hippocampus in women.[34]
- Stimulates the production of growth factors, such as BDNF (brain-derived neurotrophic factors), which improves neuroplasticity (brain adaptability).[35]
- Stimulates "neurogenesis," the ability of the brain to generate new neurons. In exercising laboratory rats, research shows that they generate new neurons in the frontal lobe and hippocampus, which survive for about four weeks and then die off unless they are stimulated.[36] If you stimulate these new neurons through mental or social interaction, they can then connect to other neurons and become integrated into brain circuits that help maintain their functions throughout your life. This is why people who go to the library or take music lessons after a workout are smarter than those who work out and then veg out.
- Improves cognitive flexibility[37] and is an effective treatment for obsessive-compulsive disorder (OCD)[38] and post-traumatic stress disorder (PTSD).[39]
- Improves the heart's ability to pump blood throughout the body and brain, which increases oxygen and nutrient delivery.
- Boosts nitric oxide production and the flexibility of blood vessels, which decreases the risk for high blood pressure, stroke, and heart disease.
- Enhances insulin's ability to lower high blood sugar levels, reducing the risk of diabetes.
- Helps you maintain coordination, agility, and speed.
- Allows for greater detoxification through sweat.
- Improves the quality of sleep.

The following four types of exercise are great for your brain. Of course, you should check with your physician before starting any new exercise routines.

- **Burst training.** This involves 30- to 60-second bursts at go-for-broke intensity followed by a few minutes of lower-intensity exertion. Short burst training also helps raise endorphins, lift your mood, and make you feel more energized.
- **Strength training.** Strength training decreases anxiety and increases energy and mood.[40] I recommend two 30- to 45-minute weight-lifting sessions a week, one or two days apart—one for the lower body, the other for the upper body.
- **Coordination activities.** Dancing, pickleball, table tennis (the world's best brain sport), and similar exercises that require coordination boost the activity in the cerebellum. The cerebellum contains 50 percent of the brain's neurons and controls your physical and thought coordination. In a study from Taiwan,[41] table tennis was found to improve social behaviors and executive function in children who have ADD/ADHD.
- **Mindful exercise.** Exercises such as yoga, Pilates, and tai chi help anxiety and depression and increase focus and energy, boosting your brain health.

B 7. **Undergo hyperbaric oxygen therapy (HBOT).** HBOT is a simple, noninvasive, painless treatment with minimal side effects that uses the power of oxygen to enhance the healing process and reduce inflammation. My introduction to HBOT, which has been used for decades, came in the 1990s courtesy of Michael Uszler, MD, a nuclear medicine physician, who gave a lecture on it at UCLA. One of the original pioneers in using brain SPECT imaging in the 1980s, Michael showed before-and-after SPECT scans of his patients who had undergone HBOT. The scans revealed remarkable improvement in blood flow and inspired me to introduce this therapy into my own practice. Many of my patients who underwent HBOT, especially those with low blood flow, experienced similar improvement.

How does HBOT work? HBOT provides people with concentrated oxygen in a special pressurized chamber. This increased pressure allows the lungs to take in more oxygen than usual, which is beneficial because oxygen is critical to the healing process. As more oxygen enters the blood vessels and tissues, it can boost production of growth factors and stem cells that promote healing.

Typically, it is only red blood cells that shuttle oxygen throughout the body. With HBOT, oxygen dissolves into other bodily fluids, such as plasma, cerebral spinal fluid, and lymph, which can then transport it to areas where circulation is low or impaired. For example, in strokes, vascular problems, and non-healing wounds, adequate amounts of oxygen are unable to reach the troubled areas, diminishing the body's ability to heal. When extra oxygen is able to penetrate these damaged regions, it speeds the recovery process.

Researchers have found that increased oxygen can promote healing after mild TBIs. A 2013 study on 56 mild TBI patients with postconcussion syndrome showed that HBOT improved cognitive and emotional functioning and quality of life.[42] Other research has concluded that HBOT enhances brain repair after TBI.[43]

In 2011, Paul Harch, MD, colleagues, and I published a study on 16 soldiers who had experienced blast-induced TBIs and subsequent PTSD.[44] They were studied with brain SPECT imaging and neuropsychological testing before and after 40 sessions of HBOT. After treatment, our patients demonstrated significant improvement in their symptoms; full-scale IQ (a term for complete cognitive capacity; up 14.8 points); delayed and working memory scores; tests of impulsivity, mood, anxiety; and quality-of-life scores. Their SPECT scans showed remarkable overall improvement in blood flow.

Many of the NFL and NHL players we have treated with HBOT at Amen Clinics also experienced benefits.

HBOT has been found beneficial for many other conditions as well. For example, a 2016 study showed HBOT improved both blood flow to the brain and neuropsychiatric function in patients who had significant neuropsychological issues caused by carbon monoxide poisoning.[45] Research suggests HBOT can also be helpful for:

- Stroke[46]
- Fibromyalgia[47]
- Lyme disease (as a helpful add-on treatment)[48]
- Burns[49]
- Diabetic ulcers and complications[50]
- Wound healing[51]
- Multiple sclerosis[52]
- Irritable bowel disease[53]
- Post-surgical healing[54]
- Autism[55]
- Cerebral palsy[56]

B   8. **Take supplements with research-based evidence to help maintain healthy blood pressure[57] and increase blood flow.** A nutraceutical is a vitamin, mineral, other nutrient, or standardized herbal extract that has shown health benefits in well-controlled human clinical trials.

- **Ginkgo biloba:** In controlled studies, this supplement has helped cerebral blood flow,[58] memory,[59] and neuropsychiatric symptoms,[60] including depression[61] and anxiety.[62]
  Dose suggestion: 60–120 milligrams (mg) twice a day. I recommend starting at the lower dose for several weeks and then increasing to the higher dose to see which is best for you.

- **Cocoa flavanols**[63] improve blood flow, support healthy blood pressure,[64] and improve brain functions,[65] even in those who haven't had enough sleep.[66] Being the grandson of a candy maker, this finding made me happy.
  Dose suggestion: I recommend one piece of sugar-free, dairy-free dark chocolate every day.

- **Omega-3 fatty acids** can improve blood flow,[67] brain function,[68] memory,[69] and mood;[70] as well as reduce inflammation[71] and brain shrinkage from aging.[72] There are two active compounds in omega-3s: EPA (eicosapentaenoic acid) and DHA (docosahexaenoic acid). You need both.
  Dose suggestion: For most of our patients, I prefer 1,400 mg or more with a ratio of approximately 60/40 EPA-to-DHA. (Check out information on the Omega-3 Index in chapter 7, which will let you know if you're on the right track toward Omega-3 protection.)

- **Green tea catechins** (GTCs) are good for blood flow,[73] blood vessels, and blood pressure.[74] GTCs also improve cholesterol[75] and help regulate blood sugar.[76] Research shows that taking GTCs on a daily basis improves depression[77] and reduces the risk of cognitive decline, especially in women and people with a genetic risk for Alzheimer's disease.[78]
  Dose suggestion: I recommend keeping the daily dosage to less than 720 mg.

- **Resveratrol** boosts blood flow.[79]
  Dose suggestion: Research shows that a daily dose of 75 mg is effective.

In chapter 16, you'll find additional recommendations and dosages for supplements that help the BRIGHT MINDS risk factors and brain health/mental health problems.

Here are scans of a 40-year-old woman, Brooke, with ADHD. She had significantly low blood flow to the front part of her brain. She did not want to take medication, so she tried nutraceuticals, including the ones listed above plus a multiple vitamin and fish oil. She felt remarkably better, and you can see the improvement in her scans a month later.

BROOKE'S SPECT STUDY

Before   After One Month on Nutraceuticals

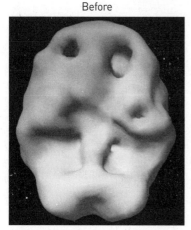 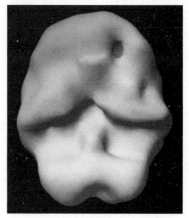

Low blood flow to frontal lobes   Improved overall

BRIGHT MINDS: BLOOD FLOW

STEPS TO CREATE MENTAL ILLNESS . . . AND MAKE MY NIECES, ALIZÉ AND AMELIE, SUFFER	STEPS TO END MENTAL ILLNESS . . . AND KEEP MY NIECES, ALIZÉ AND AMELIE, HEALTHY
1. Don't care about your blood flow.	1. Care about your blood flow.
2. Engage in habits that damage your blood vessels and impair blood flow. • Limit exercise. • Play video games and use streaming services to distract you from exercising. • Use cigarettes and marijuana.	2. Avoid anything that damages your blood vessels or hurts your blood flow, such as nicotine, caffeine, and marijuana.
3. Avoid the strategies that enhance blood flow.	3. Engage regularly in healthy habits that boost blood flow. • Exercise at least 100 minutes each week. • Take a walk every day. • Limit video games and screen time. • Screen for any vascular issues on a yearly basis and treat them early when signs of trouble arise. • Take nutraceuticals that increase blood flow. • Drink plenty of water.

Let's go back to my grandfather. If I could travel back in time, I would encourage him to limit candy because sugar (as you'll see in chapter 14) damages blood vessels and contributes to heart disease. Knowing that heart disease is associated with depression, I would have scanned his brain to see what was going on and started him on a comprehensive treatment plan using the BRIGHT MINDS strategies and nutraceuticals to boost his blood flow. I think it would have helped him continue to be the happy, loving man he had been before his heart attack. And ultimately, he might have lived longer. Sadly, it's too late for me to help my grandfather, but he is one of the main reasons why I am so passionate about ending mental illness so my nieces, Alizé and Amelie, won't have to suffer.

Pick One BRIGHT MINDS Blood Flow Tiny Habit to Start Today

TINY
HABITS

1. I'll focus on drinking more water—and remember that my brain and other bodily organs are mostly water.

2. I'll avoid caffeine and nicotine.

3. I'll take up a racquet sport.

4. For a treat, I'll enjoy a small piece of sugar-free dark chocolate.

5. As one of my supplements, I'll take ginkgo biloba standardized extract. (The healthiest SPECT scans I see often belong to people who are taking a standardized extract of this Chinese herb.)

6. When eating, I'll consume more foods that enhance blood flow. (You'll find many listed in chapter 18.)

CHAPTER 6

<u>R</u> IS FOR RETIREMENT AND AGING

WHEN YOU STOP LEARNING, YOUR BRAIN STARTS DYING

We don't stop playing because we grow old.
We grow old because we stop playing.
GEORGE BERNARD SHAW

 BETTY

Betty was 94 when she first came to see me. I had seen three generations of people in her family for attention deficit hyperactivity disorder (ADHD): her son, grandson, and great-granddaughter. When I asked her why she wanted to be evaluated, she said that she wanted to be able to finish reading the paper in the morning, something she had never been able to do. When Betty came back for her first follow-up visit after a month on our program, she told me she had read her first book! It was a joyous appointment. Several months later, she wondered aloud how her life would have been different if she had addressed her attention and impulse-control issues earlier in her life, yet she was grateful her children, grandchildren, and great-grandchildren would not have to suffer as she had.

Too often, elderly (let's say those over 70) people are dismissed with brain health/mental health issues—such as ADD/ADHD, depression, anxiety or memory issues—because they are older; but research has found that no matter what your age, your brain can be better if you put it in a healing environment. Brain imaging work at the Amen Clinics has also clearly shown the gravity of age. As your skin starts to sag and wrinkle and show other signs of aging, the same type of process occurs in the brain. Following are three typical scans at 35, 55, and 85.

TYPICAL AGING BRAIN SPECT SCANS

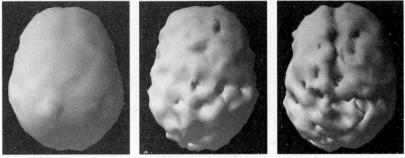

| 35 years old | 55 years old | 85 years old |

Yet your brain doesn't have to deteriorate with age if you remain diligent about your health for as long as you want to have a clear and happy mind! Here is a scan of my grandmother Margaret when she was a 92-year-old, and she was cognitively sharp until the day she died at age 98. One of her secrets of brain health was that she knitted her whole adult life, which is an exercise that works out the cerebellum.

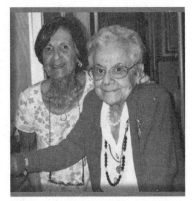

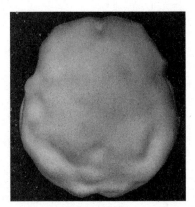

Grandmother　　　　　　　　　　Scan at 92

In a study the Amen Clinics and others published in the *Journal of Alzheimer's Disease* in 2018 on 62,454 SPECT scans, we presented the overall pattern of brain aging and factors that accelerated it.[1] For example, we showed that children have very active brains that tend to settle down in activity around their mid-20s. From the mid-20s, brain activity then tends to stay relatively stable until the 60s, when it begins to decline, often due to poor vascular health and the other BRIGHT MINDS risk factors. But this doesn't have to happen—there's nothing inevitable about it. We have scanned many elderly patients and found really healthy scans, mostly because they were serious about taking care of themselves. Look at a typical aging pattern for the posterior cingulate gyrus, an area critical to memory and mood, in the graph below.

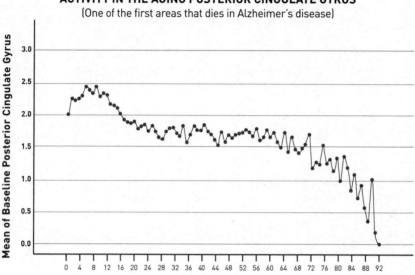

ACTIVITY IN THE AGING POSTERIOR CINGULATE GYRUS
(One of the first areas that dies in Alzheimer's disease)

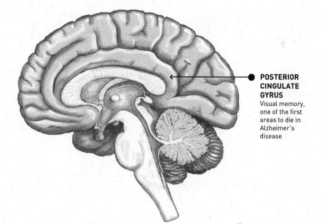

POSTERIOR CINGULATE GYRUS
Visual memory, one of the first areas to die in Alzheimer's disease

These were the factors that accelerated aging the most in our study in order of importance: schizophrenia, marijuana abuse, bipolar disorder, and ADD/ADHD, along with alcohol abuse, and smoking. Other studies show that high iron levels in your blood[2] and red meat consumption[3] are also associated with premature aging.

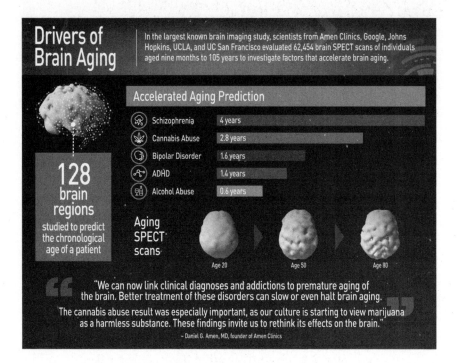

Drivers of Brain Aging

In the largest known brain imaging study, scientists from Amen Clinics, Google, Johns Hopkins, UCLA, and UC San Francisco evaluated 62,454 brain SPECT scans of individuals aged nine months to 105 years to investigate factors that accelerate brain aging.

128 brain regions studied to predict the chronological age of a patient

Accelerated Aging Prediction

Schizophrenia	4 years	
Cannabis Abuse	2.8 years	
Bipolar Disorder	1.6 years	
ADHD	1.4 years	
Alcohol Abuse	0.6 years	

Aging SPECT scans

Age 20   Age 50   Age 80

"We can now link clinical diagnoses and addictions to premature aging of the brain. Better treatment of these disorders can slow or even halt brain aging. The cannabis abuse result was especially important, as our culture is starting to view marijuana as a harmless substance. These findings invite us to rethink its effects on the brain."

~ Daniel G. Amen, MD, founder of Amen Clinics

The world's population is on average becoming older, and age is the biggest risk factor for Alzheimer's disease and other forms of dementia.[4] According to the World Health Organization, between 2015 and 2050 the percentage of people over 60 years will nearly double, from 12 percent to 22 percent.[5] This is really challenging for individuals as well as governments because as many as 10 percent of all people 65 years of age and older have serious memory problems, and up to 50 percent of all people 85 and older will be diagnosed with dementia. That means that if you are fortunate enough to live to 85, you have a one in two chance of losing your mind. Plus, the really bad news is that our research and the scientific findings of others have shown that Alzheimer's disease and other forms of dementia actually start in the brain decades before people have any symptoms. For too many people, the golden years are anything but golden. The older you get, the more serious you need to be about the health of your brain.

Other brain health/mental health issues also worsen with age. The older you get, the more likely you are to struggle with your memory, social isolation, hearing problems, and overall cognitive function. As the brain deteriorates with age, it leads to a greater risk of mood problems, anxiety, irritability, temper flare-ups, and irrational behavior. Combine the lowered brain activity with detrimental changes to the four circles—biological, psychological, social, and spiritual—and it can accelerate brain health/mental health issues. Let's look at how the four circles can contribute to brain health/mental health issues in the aging brain:

- **B** • **Biological:** If you're racked by pain and stiffness (especially if you played football in high school like yours truly), it can make you feel cranky and depressed. (Try fish oil, s-adenosyl methionine [SAMe], and curcumins as I do to help pain.) If you have a medical condition, such as cancer, it can sap the joy from your life. If you have failing eyesight (*Where did I put my glasses?*), you may have a hard time enjoying your favorite hobbies, like reading or knitting. If you're experiencing hearing issues ("What?" is the most common word I seem to say), you may begin feeling disconnected from your loved ones. As you'll learn in chapter 18, what you put into your body (i.e., food) also matters. For example, consuming charred meats—think about those burgers or steaks on the grill at summer barbecues—creates toxic chemicals called glycotoxins that have been linked to memory problems and other cognitive problems.[6]

- **P** • **Psychological:** You may become increasingly worried about being either financially or physically dependent on others. You may find that your thoughts are more focused on what's wrong with you than on what's right.

- **S** • **Social:** The death of parents, siblings, or friends can increase a sense of loneliness, which can have a major impact on your mental well-being. Unfortunately, one-third of seniors between the ages of 50 and 80 say they feel a lack of companionship, and 25 percent of them feel socially isolated, according to a 2018 University of Michigan poll.[7]

- **SP** • **Spiritual:** Retiring from work may leave you feeling as if you have no purpose in life. When you lack passion, purpose, social contribution, faith, or a connection to God or something greater than yourself, you are at a higher risk for developing brain health/mental health issues. Depression is more common after retirement, especially when retirees don't find a new source of purpose. In fact, following an initial boost in health, retirement increases your risk of clinical depression by 40 percent while raising your chances of being diagnosed with a physical illness by 60 percent.[8]

I saw some of these changes happening to one of my uncles. As he aged, his behavior became downright embarrassing whenever we went to dinner together. He had always been a bit impulsive, but later in life he was rude to servers and often made inappropriate comments. I could see his brain deteriorating before my eyes. Also, when depression strikes in the elderly, it may well be one of the first signs of dementia. Ultimately, when you stop learning, your brain starts dying.

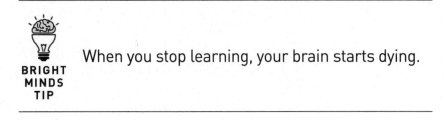

When you stop learning, your brain starts dying.

BRIGHT MINDS TIP

YOU DON'T HAVE TO BE OLDER TO HAVE THESE ISSUES

Anyone who is in a job that does not require ongoing learning is at a higher risk of memory problems and brain health/mental health issues. Numerous studies show that people who struggled in school, who learned to hate learning, or who dropped out of school early also have a higher incidence of cognitive problems and mental health challenges.

If you want to create a mental illness, never fully support children with ADD/ADHD or learning disabilities. Every day of their lives that they feel they are failing or that someone is disappointed in them ratchets up chronic stress, which shrinks the hippocampus, a critically important brain structure involved in memory, mood, and learning. My nieces were at great risk for this because of their home situation before their mother got help for her brain. Likewise, if you want to create a mental illness, start your children in school too early. Research shows that younger children in school are more likely to be diagnosed with ADD/ADHD and treated with stimulant medication.[9]

Research also shows that purpose and social contribution across the lifespan have a surprising pattern: They tend to peak when people are young (late adolescence/young adulthood), then begin to wane during middle age and decline sharply through late adulthood.[10] When purpose is absent or low, it increases the risk of mental illnesses, particularly depression, and decreases self-acceptance.[11]

Likewise, you are more likely to develop a mental illness if you have an "old mind-set," where you find yourself saying things such as:

I'm too old for that.
I don't have the energy for that.
I just want to be left alone.
I'm going to die soon, so why bother changing my habits?
This is how I've done things for years, so why should I change now?
I can't give up . . . candy, muffins, wine, chips . . . you name it. I'd rather deal with anxiety or get Alzheimer's disease.

Retirement/Aging Risk Factors
(and the Four Circles They Represent)

(B) 1. Increasing age, especially over 65.

(B)(P) 2. Having a job that does not require new learning.

(S) 3. Loneliness or social isolation. Humans are social animals: Social connectivity is hardwired into our brains, and when we are lonely and/or disconnected from others, it can have negative consequences for us cognitively, emotionally, and physically.[12] More than one in eight people report having no close friends.[13] The loneliest among us experience cognitive decline 20 percent faster than people who are connected to others, and loneliness has been associated with depression, social anxiety, addictions, even hoarding.[14] Loneliness peaks at several periods in life: during the late 20s, mid-50s, and late 80s.[15] Loneliness does not mean being alone or not having friends. It is subjective distress, meaning the discrepancy between the social relationships you have and the ones you want. The physical damage associated with being lonely was found to be equivalent to 15 cigarettes a day.

(SP) 4. Retired without new learning endeavors or passion or purpose.

(B) 5. Too much or too little iron (blood test)—ferritin measures iron stores in the blood. Get yours checked. Levels between 50 and 100 nanograms/mL are ideal. Levels below 50 ng/mL can cause problems, such as anxiety, fatigue, restless legs, and ADD/ADHD. A 2015 study among psychiatric patients found that more than 25 percent of them were also suffering from anemia, with the condition being most common in people with psychotic disorders, anxiety, obsessive-compulsive disorder (OCD), and bipolar disorder.[16] High levels (over 250 ng/mL) are associated with iron overload and increase the risk of inflammation, heart disease and neurodegenerative diseases, such as Parkinson's and Alzheimer's disease.[17]

B 6. Decline of neurotransmitters (brain chemicals), such as serotonin, dopamine, gamma-aminobutyric acid (GABA), and acetylcholine. As we age, we lose brain cells that produce these important chemicals that help our neurons communicate effectively. Low serotonin activity increases risk of depression;[18] low dopamine increases risk of Parkinson's disease and loss of motivation and pleasure;[19] low GABA increases the risk of anxiety;[20] and low acetylcholine can affect learning and memory.[21]

Take a look at how the evil and benevolent rulers would ensure that aging and retirement helped or perpetuated mental illness.

RETIREMENT/AGING

THE EVIL RULER WOULD . . .	THE BENEVOLENT RULER WOULD . . .
1. Recommend everyone retire early, stop learning new things, and watch all the television they want, especially the news that focuses on violence, natural disasters, and partisan politics that breeds anger and stress.	1. Encourage lifelong learning, purpose, and knitting.
	2. Discourage children from starting school too young.
	3. Promote cross-training in the workplace.
2. Let people watch as many scary movies as they want or play violent video games, both of which wear out the pleasure centers.	4. Limit television, social media, and scary movies to keep the pleasure centers healthy.
3. Encourage people to spend their days in meaningless activities in isolation and demand that people spend hours on social media every day, which increases the risk of depression and obesity.	5. Encourage regular blood donation for those who have high iron blood levels.
	6. Educate people about the benefits of intermittent fasting.
4. Start children in school too young.	7. Provide treatment for ADD/ADHD and learning disabilities, so people would enjoy learning.
	8. Mandate brain health education at schools and businesses, which would highlight the positive effects of lifelong learning.

Despite the dire news about aging and your brain, you don't have to give in to decline. Yes, you will age, but you can slow the process while keeping your brain sharp, focused, and clear. Imagine entering the latter part of your life with just as much mental capacity and energy as you have now, if not more. It's possible.

PRESCRIPTIONS FOR REDUCING YOUR RETIREMENT/AGING RISK FACTORS
(AND THE FOUR CIRCLES THEY REPRESENT)

P SP 1. **Care! The older you get, the more serious you need to be.** I turned 65 this year, and I'm planning to have one of the healthiest brains when I reach my 90s. I often ask myself, "Do you want an old brain or a young one?" to stay motivated when I don't feel like working out or eating well. I recently saw a world-famous boxing champ who was struggling with his memory. After looking at his brain, I used the metaphor that he was in the "fight of his life." He was going to have to break up with Colonel Sanders, one of his great loves, if he was going to keep his memory healthy. He told me he would train diligently because "you ain't got nothing without your memory."

B P S SP 2. **Avoid anything that accelerates aging**—such as no new learning, being in a job that does not require ongoing learning, high iron levels, smoking anything, alcohol or marijuana abuse, standard American diet, loneliness, and a lack of purpose.

SP 3. **Know your *why* for being healthy.** Do you believe you need to be healthy because God has a calling for you? Is it independence? I love my four children, but honestly, I never want to have to live with them. I never want to be a burden, and I do not want them telling me what to eat or what to wear or worrying about taking my driver's license from me. If that is true for you, then you need to be serious about your health.

B P 4. **Exercise your brain with new learning.** Engage in lifelong learning to keep your brain strong. Take a cue from actress Dame Judi Dench, who continues to act even though she is now in her eighties. She told the *Telegraph* in 2015 that *retired* is the rudest word in the dictionary. "I don't think age matters at all. What matters is your determination not to give up and not to stop learning new things."[22]

The best mental exercises involve acquiring new knowledge and doing things you haven't done before. Even if your daily activities are complex, such as teaching coding, interpreting brain scans, or engineering a new bridge, they won't challenge your brain as much as new learning. Whenever the brain repeats an activity over and over, it uses less and less energy each time to accomplish it. New learning, such as a new hobby or game, establishes new connections, which maintains and improves other brain areas that you use less often.

The parts of your brain that you use will grow, and the parts of your brain that you do not use will atrophy, or shrink. This provides guidance on how to exercise the brain. If you were to only play Scrabble or do the Sunday crossword puzzle, you wouldn't get the full benefits you want. That's like going to work out and only doing right bicep curls and then leaving. See the graphic below for more ideas.

BRAIN HEALTH WORKOUTS BY REGION

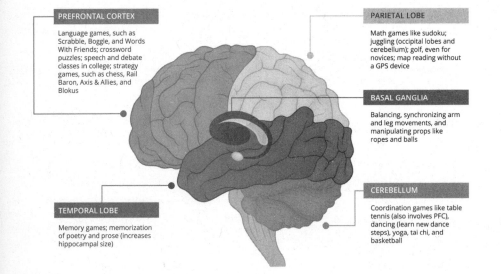

PREFRONTAL CORTEX

Language games, such as Scrabble, Boggle, and Words With Friends; crossword puzzles; speech and debate classes in college; strategy games, such as chess, Rail Baron, Axis & Allies, and Blokus

PARIETAL LOBE

Math games like sudoku; juggling (occipital lobes and cerebellum); golf, even for novices; map reading without a GPS device

BASAL GANGLIA

Balancing, synchronizing arm and leg movements, and manipulating props like ropes and balls

TEMPORAL LOBE

Memory games; memorization of poetry and prose (increases hippocampal size)

CEREBELLUM

Coordination games like table tennis (also involves PFC), dancing (learn new dance steps), yoga, tai chi, and basketball

5. **Balance your iron levels.** Causes of too much iron include regular alcohol consumption, cooking in iron pans, foods fortified with iron, well water high in iron, or vitamin or mineral supplements with extra iron. Some people are genetically predisposed to absorb too much iron from food. Donating blood can help you lower iron levels. Green tea, rosemary[23], and curcumin may also help.[24]

    If you are low in iron, supplement with iron but never take iron in combination with other vitamins because it can make them toxic, and always take the iron supplement a couple of hours away from other supplements.

 6. **Fast intermittently.** Fasting helps your brain stay healthy because it cleans out the buildup of toxic proteins that damage neurons, reducing inflammation and slowing down aging. A simple way to do a nightly 12- to 16-hour fast is to eat dinner at 7 p.m., for example, and not eat again until 7 a.m. (or 11 a.m. for a longer fast). Even longer fasts of 24 hours can also be helpful.

 7. **Get connected.** To reduce the risk of loneliness and isolation, invest time with your family, church, or other groups. Sign up for a class or meet new people, anything to stay connected and build relationships. Research shows that caring for others increases your life expectancy.[25] Grandparents who care for their grandchildren, for example, live longer, on average, than grandparents who do not. In one study, older people who volunteered over two years actually increased the size of their hippocampus (involved in mood and memory).[26]

8. **Take nutraceuticals that are most useful to slow aging.**

    • **N-acetylcysteine (NAC).** NAC has shown promising results in people with bipolar disorder, schizophrenia, OCD, and addictions.[27] It can also decrease inflammation[28] and may help delay brain atrophy in Alzheimer's disease.[29]
Dose suggestion: The typical adult dose is 600–2,400 mg a day; more than 1,800 mg/day can upset your stomach. I usually start patients at 600 mg twice a day.

    • **Huperzine A.** This remarkable compound, studied in China for nearly 20 years, improves the cognitive impairment that is often seen in people with depression[30] or schizophrenia,[31] as well as with several types of dementia.[32] It can have adverse side effects such as gastrointestinal issues, headaches, dizziness, and increased urination, as well as side effects with certain medications. Caution: Huperzine A should only be used with a doctor's supervision.

Dose suggestion: The typical adult dose is 50–100 micrograms (mcg) twice a day.

- **Saffron.** Recent clinical trials have found that it helps for depression,[33] bipolar disorder, and anxiety. As a potent antioxidant[34] and nerve protector,[35] saffron enhances memory,[36] protects the hippocampus, boosts blood flow[37] and acetylcholine,[38] and fights toxic buildup of the proteins thought to cause dementia.[39]

  Dose suggestion: The typical dose of saffron in trial is 30 mg a day of standardized concentrates. The dose of the patented preparation of saffron called Satiereal is 176.5 mg a day, and its potency is comparable to that of 30 mg per day of other saffron concentrates.

- **Sage.** In the 17th century, herbalist Nicholas Culpeper wrote that the herb sage could "heal" the memory while "warming and quickening the senses." Centuries later, research shows the brain-enhancing effects of sage extracts[40] including potential relief from depression.[41]

  Dose suggestion: The typical dose is 300–600 mg of dried sage leaf in capsules or essential oil in doses of 25–50 microliters (mcL). **Caution:** *Those who have high blood pressure or seizure disorders should only use it under the direction of their physicians.*

- **Phosphatidylserine (PS).** Clinical trials show that PS improves attention, learning, memory and verbal skills in aging people with cognitive decline, and it is the best documented nutraceutical for memory. Even people with Alzheimer's have been found to benefit from taking PS. PS may also be effective in controlling stress, as it has been found to reduce cortisol levels,[42] and may reduce symptoms of ADD/ADHD in children.[43] You can get PS from egg yolks, muscle meats, and organ meats.

  Dose suggestion: The typical adult dose is 100–300 mg a day.

BRIGHT MINDS: RETIREMENT/AGING

STEPS TO CREATE MENTAL ILLNESS ... AND MAKE MY NIECES, ALIZÉ AND AMELIE, SUFFER	STEPS TO END MENTAL ILLNESS ... AND KEEP MY NIECES, ALIZÉ AND AMELIE, HEALTHY

1. Don't care about your aging brain.
 	
2. Engage in habits that accelerate brain aging.
 	
  • Don't treat ADD/ADHD or learning disabilities so children learn to hate learning.
  • Have a job that requires no new learning.
  • Retire early without a new hobby, passion, or purpose in life.
  • Don't think about *why* you want to have a healthy brain.
  • Live alone and isolate yourself from friends and family.
  • Don't check your iron level or treat abnormal levels.
  • Focus on all your aches and pains and other reasons why your life isn't as good as it used to be.
  • Adopt an "old mind-set."
  • Watch a lot of TV, especially news that focuses on violence, natural disasters, and partisan politics that breeds anger.
  • Spend hours on social media, which increases the risk of depression and obesity.
 	
3. Avoid the strategies that slow the brain aging process.
	1. Care about your brain at all ages.
	
	2. Avoid anything that prematurely ages your brain.
	
	3. Engage regularly in healthy habits that slow the aging process.
	
	  • Focus on learning new things to keep your mind active, and engage in a variety of exercises that work different brain regions.
	  • Cross-train at work to learn new skills.
	  • At retirement age, continue working or volunteering, or find a new passion.
	  • Know *why* you want to keep your brain healthy as you age.
	  • Consider intermittent fasting to help clear the brain of toxic proteins that damage neurons.
	  • Stay connected to family and friends, and engage in church or other group activities to form bonds with others.
	  • Check your iron level and treat it if it is abnormal.
	  • Maintain a youthful outlook on life.
	  • Avoid watching too much distressing TV news.
	  • Limit the amount of time you spend on social media.
	  • Get treatment for ADD/ADHD or other learning disabilities so you will enjoy learning.
	  • Consider nutraceuticals to optimize your brain health.

Pick One BRIGHT MINDS Retirement/Aging Tiny Habit to Start Today

---

TINY HABITS

1. I'll limit charred meats.

2. I'll ask my doctor to check my ferritin (iron) levels.

3. If my iron is too high, I'll donate blood.

4. I'll try a daily fast for 12–16 hours.

5. In my diet, I'll include potent antioxidants such as blueberries, other berries, green tea, and cloves.

6. To obtain the basic nutrients my brain needs to generate energy and use it to power its functions, I'll take a multiple vitamin-mineral supplement and concentrated fish oil.

7. I'll add acetylcholine-rich foods, such as shrimp.

8. I'll stay connected to others and volunteer to avoid loneliness and isolation.

9. I'll start or continue music training.[44]

10. Today, I'll start a daily habit of new learning.

CHAPTER 7

I IS FOR INFLAMMATION

QUENCHING THE FIRE WITHIN

Reduce inflammation to treat the root of many issues. If your
gut isn't working right it can cause so many other issues.

JAY WOODMAN

 LYNN

Lynn, 53, was looking forward to marrying the love of her life when her fiancé, Will, had a heart attack one evening and died in her arms. She was devastated and suffered with intense grief that would not go away. It eventually drove her to come to see me. She complained of depression, panic attacks, shortness of breath, insomnia, and crushing chest pain, which her primary doctor said was a well-known sign of grief and a "broken heart." Lynn was referred to me by her sister, Debbie, who had seen me years earlier for an anxiety disorder. I had also seen Debbie's daughter and son-in-law.

When I saw Lynn, the grief was palpable. I could see why it was easy to assume it was just "normal" grief, but we put her through our usual process. I ordered a SPECT scan, which showed overall decreased blood flow to her brain and premature aging. She was also obese, and her screening lab tests showed that her blood marker for inflammation, C-reactive protein (CRP), was dramatically elevated at 78 mg/L (normal is less than 1.0 mg/L), and that she had low thyroid, low testosterone, and a high fasting blood sugar level. I immediately sent her to a cardiologist, who told us she had a 95 percent blockage in three of her coronary arteries. She underwent coronary artery bypass surgery the next week, which helped alleviate her chest pain. Then, together, we worked to eliminate all of her BRIGHT MINDS risk factors. Within six months, her mood brightened, the grief lessened, her inflammation markers went back into the normal range, she was down 30 pounds, and her follow-up scan was improved.

LYNN'S SCAN BEFORE TREATMENT **AFTER TREATMENT**

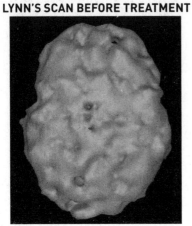

Overall low activity (common with Overall improved blood flow and activity
heart disease and inflammation)

The word *inflammation* comes from the Latin *inflammare*, meaning "to set on fire." Inflammation is your body's natural way of coping with an injury or foreign invader, such as a splinter, virus, or bacterial infection.

When you are injured or develop an infection, your body's natural defense mechanism jumps into action: Blood vessels dilate so blood can rush to the troubled area, and your immune system's army of white blood cells (plus substances they produce) hurry to the scene to handle the situation—like firefighters to a fire. The affected area becomes swollen, warm, red, and painful as your immune system launches an assault to destroy foreign substances and initiate the healing process. Usually, after a few hours or a few days, the immune response downshifts back to neutral, and the inflammation subsides. This critically important bodily process is intended to help keep you healthy. You would never want to completely eliminate inflammation because it would leave you vulnerable to infections and unable to heal from injuries.

In some people, however, the inflammatory response gets stuck on "high" mode and doesn't subside. Or it mistakes healthy tissue for a foreign invader and begins attacking it (like "friendly fire"). When inflammation becomes chronic, it is like having a constant, low-level fire in your body that damages your organs and tissue. Persistent inflammation, as in Lynn's case, has been linked to a host of physical ailments, including heart disease, cancer, arthritis, pain syndromes, and gastrointestinal disorders. In fact, chronic degenerative conditions like these represent the number one health threat worldwide, according to the World Health Organization. And inflammation is often one of the main causes of disease.

BRIGHT MINDS TIP If you have been treated for a brain health/mental health issue without success, it may be time to look at inflammation as a possible root cause.

What does chronic inflammation have to do with brain health/mental health issues? Just as it can ravage your body, it can also damage your brain and mind. It has been associated with a wide range of neurological and psychiatric illnesses, including depression, bipolar disorder, obsessive-compulsive disorder (OCD), schizophrenia, personality disorders, Alzheimer's disease, and Parkinson's disease.[1] High levels of inflammation have also been associated with decreased motivation[2] and suicidal behavior,[3] along with activation of parts of the brain that feel social rejection, fear, and threats.[4] If you have been treated for a brain health/mental health issue without success, it may be time to look at inflammation as a possible root cause.[5]

For example, did you know that depression is a primary side effect of drugs that purposefully increase inflammation, such as vaccinations or interferon, which is used to treat hepatitis or certain types of cancer? On the flip side, some anti-inflammatory medications, such as aspirin and ibuprofen,[6] and nutraceuticals, such as omega-3 fatty acids and curcumin, have been found to decrease depression in people who have evidence of persistent inflammation.

> *Depression is a primary side effect of drugs that increase inflammation; and anti-inflammatory supplements, such as curcumin and omega-3 fatty acids, decrease depression.*

Because of the link between inflammation and brain health/mental health issues, it's important to be aware of the many risk factors that may trigger or promote inflammation—*injury and infection aren't the only ones!* Here are ways to know if you likely have persistent inflammation as a risk factor.

Inflammation Risk Factors
(and the Four Circles They Represent)

B 1. High C-reactive protein (blood test): A healthy range is between 0.0 and 1.0 mg/L.

B 2. High homocysteine (blood test): Associated with inflammation, hardening and narrowing of the arteries, and an increased risk of heart attacks, strokes, blood clots, and possibly Alzheimer's disease. The level should be less than 8 micromoles/liter.

B 3. Low levels of vitamin D

B 4. Environmental toxins

B P S SP 5. Smoking (biological because it damages the body, psychological because you may smoke to self-medicate, social because you may smoke in social situations, and spiritual because you need to find the *why* to quit)

B P S SP 6. Excessive alcohol (psychological because you may drink to self-medicate, social because you may drink in social situations, and spiritual because you need to find the *why* to limit your intake)

B P S SP 7. Chronic stress

P 8. Childhood trauma[7]

B 9. Gum disease

B P S SP 10. Obesity, especially belly fat (biological because poor food choices and obesity are pro-inflammatory, psychological because you may eat to self-medicate, social because you may overeat or make bad food choices in social situations, and spiritual because you need to find the *why* to take control of your eating)

B 11. Prediabetes or diabetes

B P 12. Insomnia, especially in shift workers (psychological circle if stressful thoughts keep you up at night)

B P S 13. Excessive exercise (psychological circle if you exercise obsessively, plus social circle if you over-exercise because your friends do)

B **P** **S** **SP** 14. Proinflammatory foods

- Sugar
- High-glycemic, low-fiber foods that quickly turn to sugar (bread, pasta, potatoes, and rice)
- Trans fats
- Excessive omega-6 fatty acids from corn, soy, and vegetable oils
- Artificial sweeteners
- Gluten

B 15. Low Omega-3 Index (a drop of blood): measures the total amount of omega-3 fatty acids EPA and DHA in red blood cells, which, as it turns out, directly reflects their levels in the brain. A low Omega-3 Index increases the risk of cognitive decline by as much as 77 percent.[8] Aim for an Omega-3 Index level above 8 percent.

B 16. Leaky gut and/or unhealthy microbiome

The remainder of this chapter will focus primarily on two of the most common causes of inflammation: leaky gut and/or an unhealthy microbiome and a low Omega-3 Index.

THE GUT-INFLAMMATION-BRAIN CONNECTION

The gut—your gastrointestinal tract (GI)—is often called the second brain because it is lined with about 100 million neurons. That's more neurons than you have in your spinal cord or in your peripheral nervous system. This nerve tissue is in direct communication with the brain inside your skull, which is why you get butterflies before a big job interview or feel queasy when you're upset. Emotional and psychological pain—anxiety, depression, stress, and grief—are often also expressed with gut distress.

You have about 30 feet of tubing (including your stomach) that goes from your mouth to the other end. It is lined with a single layer of cells with tight junctions that protects it from foreign invaders and allows you to digest food in an efficient way. Big trouble happens when the cell junctions widen and the lining becomes excessively porous, a condition known as leaky gut.

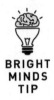

BRIGHT
MINDS
TIP

The gut lining is only a single cell layer thick. Anything that causes the cell junctions to widen or become porous allows toxins into your body that can cause inflammation.

Leaky gut is associated with brain problems, including mood and anxiety disorders,[9] attention deficit disorder/attention deficit hyperactivity disorder (ADD/ADHD),[10] Parkinson's, and Alzheimer's.[11] Leaky gut is also linked to chronic inflammation, along with a host of other issues from autoimmune diseases[12] (such as lupus, rheumatoid arthritis, Hashimoto's thyroiditis, and multiple sclerosis) and digestive issues (gas, bloating, constipation, and diarrhea) to seasonal allergies and skin problems (acne and rosacea).[13]

LEAKY GUT SYNDROME

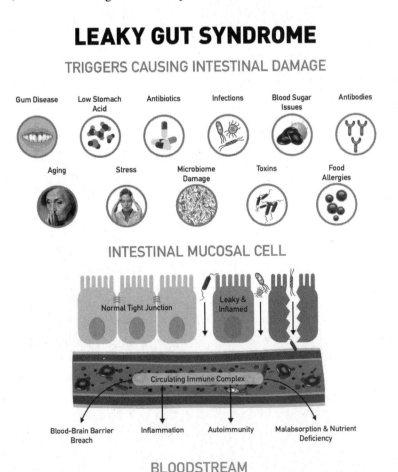

INSIDE YOUR GUT: GOOD BUGS VERSUS BAD BUGS

Considering all the neurons in your GI tract and the direct communication it has with the brain, the health of your gut is tightly linked to the health of your brain and mind. In large part, the health of your gut depends on bugs. That's right, your GI tract is host to an estimated 100 trillion micro-organisms (bacteria, yeast, and others), about 10 times the total number of cells in the rest of the human body. This community of "bugs" is collectively known as the *microbiome.*

Some of these bugs are beneficial to your health and well-being while others are harmful. And in a classic good guys versus bad guys scenario, they are all trying to wrestle for control of your microbiome. When the ratio of good bugs to bad bugs is about 85 percent good guys to 15 percent trouble-makers, it creates a healthy gut. When the ratio is tipped the other way, the bad bugs cause trouble that can lead to a leaky gut, as well as physical and mental problems. *Keeping your gut microbiome in proper balance is essential to your mental health.*[14]

The microbiome plays a vital role in protecting your gut lining, digestion, nutrient absorption, and the synthesis of vitamins (K, B12) and neurotransmitters, such as serotonin. Your microbiome is involved in detoxification and helps manage inflammation, immunity, appetite, and blood sugar levels. There is evidence that friendly gut bacteria deter invading troublemakers, such as E-coli bacteria, and help you withstand stress.[15]

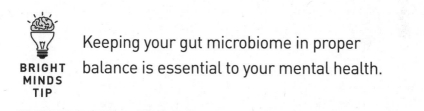

BRIGHT MINDS TIP

Keeping your gut microbiome in proper balance is essential to your mental health.

However, if the good bugs are deficient—whether it's due to a poor diet, such as consuming too much sugar, which feeds yeast overgrowth (bad bugs); excessive use of antibiotics (even as far back as childhood) that killed good bacteria; or being born by cesarean section and missing out on being swathed in all the good bugs in the birth canal—you are more likely to feel anxious, stressed, depressed, and tired.

What Decreases the Good Bugs?

- Medications (antibiotics, oral contraceptives, proton pump inhibitors, steroids, NSAIDS)
- Low levels of omega-3 fatty acids
- Stress
- Sugar and high fructose corn syrup
- Artificial sweeteners
- Gluten
- Allergies to the environment or food
- Insomnia (especially among soldiers and those involved in shift work)
- Toxins (antimicrobial chemicals in soaps; pesticides; heavy metals)
- Intestinal infections (H. pylori, parasites, Candida)
- Low levels of vitamin D
- Radiation/chemotherapy
- Excessive high-intensity exercise
- Excessive alcohol[16]

Let's take a closer look at how medications, and in particular antibiotics, can affect the bugs in your gut. Antibiotics are intended to kill the harmful bacteria that make you sick, but at the same time, they also harm some of the good bacteria in your gut. In some people, overuse of antibiotics can deplete the population of good bugs and tip the ratio in favor of the bad bugs. In a 2016 study,[17] mice that were given antibiotics showed decreased gut bacteria, which lowered the number of white blood cells that communicate among the gut, brain, and immune system. Surprisingly, the antibiotics stopped the growth of new cells in the hippocampus and impaired memory. Remember, the hippocampus is also involved in mood regulation. Probiotics and exercise reversed the trouble in the hippocampus.

> **BRIGHT MINDS TIP**
>
> Antibiotics stop the growth of new cells in the hippocampus and impair memory. The hippocampus is involved in mood regulation. Chronic use of antibiotics in childhood can affect the rest of your life. Probiotics and exercise reverse the trouble in the hippocampus.

What may surprise you is that the greatest danger from antibiotics does not come from those prescribed by your doctor but, rather, from the foods you eat. An estimated 70 percent of the antibiotics used in the United States are given to livestock, and the prevalence of these drugs in conventionally raised meats and dairy has the potential to throw off the balance of good to bad bacteria in the gut. This is why it is critical to eat antibiotic- and hormone-free meats whenever possible. In short, you need to take care of your gut, or your brain could be in big trouble.

OMEGA-3 FATTY ACIDS: LOWER INFLAMMATION AND BOOST BRAIN HEALTH/MENTAL HEALTH

Having low levels of the omega-3 fatty acids EPA and DHA in your bloodstream is associated with inflammation.[18] It's also one of the leading preventable causes of death, according to researchers at the Harvard School of Public Health.[19] Low levels of EPA and DHA are also linked to

- Depression and bipolar disorder[20]
- Suicidal behavior[21]
- ADD/ADHD[22]
- Cognitive impairment and dementia[23]
- Obesity[24]
- Heart disease[25]

Did you know that most people are low in the omega-3 fatty acids EPA and DHA? Chances are you are too, unless you make it a point to eat fatty fish (which can be high in mercury and other toxins) on a regular basis or you take a high-quality omega-3 fatty acid EPA plus DHA supplement. At Amen

Clinics in 2016, we tested the omega-3 fatty acids levels of 50 consecutive patients who were not taking fish oil (the most commonly used source of EPA and DHA) and found that 49 had suboptimal levels. In another study,[26] our research team correlated the SPECT scans of 130 patients with their EPA and DHA levels and found those with the lowest levels had lower blood flow (the number one predictor of future brain problems) in the right hippocampus and posterior cingulate (one of the first areas to die in Alzheimer's disease), among other areas. On cognitive testing, we also found low omega-3s correlated with decreased scores in mood.[27]

Increasing scientific evidence points to a connection between cognitive function, mental health, and the omega-3 fatty acids EPA and DHA, and taking fish oil rich in EPA and DHA may help ease symptoms of depression.[28] One 20-year study involving 3,317 men and women found that people— especially women—with the highest consumption of EPA and DHA were less likely to have symptoms of depression.[29] And some experts suggest these effects are thanks to the anti-inflammatory properties of omega-3s.[30]

Additional brain health/mental health benefits of omega-3 EPA and DHA include increased attention in people with ADD/ADHD,[31] reduced stress, and a lower risk for psychosis.[32] And at Amen Clinics, when we put a group of retired football players on highly concentrated fish oil supplements, many of them were able to decrease or completely eliminate their pain medications.

Take a look at how the evil and benevolent rulers would promote or prevent inflammation throughout society.

BRIGHT MINDS TIP

Low fish intake, processed foods, and a leaky gut can increase inflammation and brain health/mental health challenges.

INFLAMMATION

THE EVIL RULER WOULD . . .	THE BENEVOLENT RULER WOULD . . .
1. Increase availability and marketing of processed foods loaded with corn and soy products and refined oils (high in omega-6 fatty acids that promote inflammation).	1. Regularly test subjects for CRP, homocysteine, and the Omega-3 index.
2. Increase chronic stress by encouraging subjects to watch hateful political talk shows for hours a day, where the negative news and conflicts dominate headlines.	2. Limit unnecessary antibiotic therapy, pesticides, processed foods, and sugar.
3. Promote inflammation by limiting availability of sustainable fatty fish.	3. Promote diets loaded with organic colorful vegetables and prebiotic and probiotic foods.
4. Increase use of pesticides and spray crops with potentially dangerous glyphosates.	4. Encourage healthy stress management and rest.
5. Fool population into thinking alcohol is a health food and dictate everyone must drink two glasses of wine a day.	5. Make probiotic (live bacteria of the good gut variety) or prebiotic (dietary fiber that feeds the good bugs) nutraceuticals available to everyone.
6. Promote the belief that being busy is a valid substitute for a deeper sense of purpose.	6. Encourage healthy fish consumption (see www.seafoodwatch.org) and pass out high-quality omega-3 nutraceuticals.
7. Ban flossing.	7. Teach about inflammation in schools, especially how important flossing and gum health are to the brain.
8. Prohibit probiotic and prebiotic foods, and discourage anything that supports the good bugs in the gut.	
9. Mandate antibiotics at the first sign of sniffles or coughs for children and adults, killing off beneficial gut bacteria.	
10. Increase sugar-laden foods (proinflammatory) and encourage food manufacturers to add hidden sugars into their products to wipe out good bugs in the gut.	

PRESCRIPTIONS FOR REDUCING YOUR INFLAMMATION RISK
(AND THE FOUR CIRCLES THEY REPRESENT)

The Strategies

B **SP** 1. **Care about your level of inflammation and ask your doctor to test for it on a regular basis** with CRP, homocysteine, and the Omega-3 Index. CRP levels are important for other reasons too. Exciting research points to CRP levels as a way to help determine which antidepressant medication will be most effective in people with major depression.[33]

B 2. **Avoid anything that increases inflammation**, such as leaky gut, low omega-3 fatty acid levels, excessive omega-6 intake, and gum disease.

3. **Engage regularly in habits that lower inflammation.**

B **S** • **Consumer prebiotics (dietary fiber that promotes good bugs).** These include apples, beans, cabbage, psyllium, artichokes, onions, leeks, asparagus, squash, and root veggies, such as sweet potatoes, yams, jicama, beets, carrots, and turnips (social circle because your friends and family influence what you eat).

B • **Add probiotics with either probiotic supplements** (see below) or fermented foods that contain live bacteria: kefir, kombucha, and unsweetened yogurt (goat or coconut); kimchi, pickled fruits and vegetables, and sauerkraut.

B • **Be cautious about taking antibiotics.** If you have had a number of antibiotics in the past, then probiotics and a healthy diet are essential to maintaining brain health.

B • **Reduce homocysteine.** B vitamins—especially B6, B12, and folate—reduce high levels of homocysteine. They also support brain health and can reduce the amount of brain shrinkage by up to 90 percent.[34]

B • **Take care of your gums.** This is an easy one. Avoid periodontal (gum) disease, which is a risk factor for depression and dementia,[35] by brushing your teeth twice a day, flossing daily, and getting regular dental cleanings.

4. **Take nutraceuticals that lower inflammation** (social circle because your friends and family influence what you eat). Rarely do I meet patients who do not need to lower inflammation. It is a risk factor for nearly everyone. The following supplements help lower your inflammation and rebuild your microbiome:

- **Probiotics:** These have been shown in clinical studies to decrease homocysteine and inflammation.[36] They were found to be even more effective when given with prebiotics.[37] Prebiotics support and promote the growth of probiotics. Look for products that contain both Lactobacillus and Bifidobacterium strains. The number of probiotics in a supplement is less important than the quality of the strains.
  Dose suggestion: The probiotic I often recommend was found to be effective at 3 billion live organisms a day.

- **Folate, vitamin B6, vitamin B12, and betaine:** I recommend that my patients with high homocysteine levels take these supplements.

- **Folate**
  Dose suggestion: 800 micrograms (mcg) a day as methyl folate, which is the body's naturally most active form as opposed to folic acid, which is synthetic

- **Vitamin B6**
  Dose suggestion: 20 mg a day as pyridoxine hydrochloride or as pyridoxal-5-phosphate (both are well absorbed and utilized)

- **Vitamin B12**
  Dose suggestion: 500 mcg a day as methyl cobalamin; hydroxocobalamin is also safe. Both are preferable to cyanocobalamin, a widely sold form that contains potentially toxic cyanide.

- **Betaine (trimethylglycine)**
  Dose suggestion: 1,000–3,000 mg a day; this substance is naturally present in our cells and very useful as a methyl backup.

- **Curcumin:** This is a collective name for the three active "curcuminoids" from turmeric root (used in making curries), which have potent anti-inflammatory effects. More than 7,000 published articles have revealed the benefits of curcumin, including powerful anti-inflammatory properties, as well as antioxidant, blood sugar regulation, and anti-cancer activities.[38] However, be aware that curcuminoids are very poorly absorbed when taken by themselves. Look for preparations that are more absorbable, such as the one made by Longvida, which is proven to have high absorption. *Dose suggestion: I recommend 500–2,000 mg a day of a highly bioavailable curcumin supplement.*

- **Omega-3:** The omega-3 fatty acids EPA and DHA can reduce inflammation,[39] anxiety,[40] and depression;[41] increase blood flow;[42] mood,[43] working memory,[44] and executive function;[45] and slow brain atrophy.[46]

  Your body has very limited capacity to produce EPA and DHA, meaning you have to get most of your supply from foods or supplements. Plants make a type of omega-3 fatty acid called alpha-linolenic acid (ALA) that your body can convert into EPA and DHA, but it isn't very efficient. The best dietary source of EPA and DHA is cold-water fish, including salmon, sardines, trout, tuna, mackerel, herring, and halibut. However, it's important to choose fish that won't poison you with mercury, PCBs, or dioxins. Choose wild rather than farm-raised fish, and do your best to ensure it is free of toxic contamination. The safest and most efficient way to increase your Omega-3 Index is to take highly concentrated, high-quality fish oil supplements that provide at least 1,000 mg of EPA and DHA per day.

BRIGHT MINDS: INFLAMMATION

STEPS TO CREATE MENTAL ILLNESS ... AND MAKE MY NIECES, ALIZÉ AND AMELIE, SUFFER	STEPS TO END MENTAL ILLNESS ... AND KEEP MY NIECES, ALIZÉ AND AMELIE, HEALTHY
1. Don't care about inflammation.	1. Care about inflammation.
2. Engage in habits that promote inflammation. • Eat processed foods and those filled with trans fats. • Choose produce that's been sprayed with pesticides. • Opt for meat, eggs, and other foods that come from animals treated with hormones and antibiotics. • Eat sugar or artificial sweeteners at every meal. • Drink two or more glasses of alcohol a day. • Let stress dominate your days. • Neglect your dental health and floss infrequently or not at all. • Don't check your CRP, homocysteine, or Omega-3 Index levels. 3. Avoid the strategies that calm inflammation.	2. Avoid anything that increases inflammation. 3. Engage regularly in healthy habits that turn down the fire within. • Avoid processed foods and trans fats. • Choose organic produce. • Eat foods that are hormone- and antibiotic-free. • Limit sugar and artificial sweeteners in your diet. • Limit alcohol consumption. • Practice stress management. • Floss your teeth daily, and visit your dentist for regular check-ups. • Ask your doctor to test your CRP, homocysteine, and Omega-3 Index levels. • Take vitamins and supplements that have anti-inflammatory properties.

Pick One BRIGHT MINDS Inflammation Tiny Habit to Start Today

1. When I finish brushing my teeth before bed, I will floss.

2. When I make dinner, I will put more green leafy vegetables on my plate.

3. When I go to the doctor for my annual checkup, I will ask to have my CRP, homocysteine, and Omega-3 Index levels checked.

4. When I go to the grocery store, I will shop on the outside of the aisles to avoid processed foods.

5. When I eat, I will limit omega-6 rich foods (corn, soy, refined oils, and processed foods).

6. When I plan my menus, I will include more omega-3 rich foods (fish, avocados, walnuts).

7. When I take my supplements each day, I will include an omega-3 supplement, vitamins B6 and B12, and methylfolate.

8. When I make my shopping list, I will put prebiotic foods at the top of the list so I don't forget them.

9. When I eat breakfast, I will include probiotic foods and/or supplements.

CHAPTER 8

<u>G</u> IS FOR GENETICS

KNOW YOUR VULNERABILITIES,
BUT YOUR HISTORY IS NOT YOUR DESTINY

The individual nature of a single cell can be compared to that of a manuscript. Each cell inherits the same first draft. Over time, words are scratched out and others are added; genes are silenced or activated. Different qualities or phrases are emphasized; and a unique novel is born from an otherwise standard script. Humans derive their individuality from epigenomes, which are triggered by chance events, like injuries, smells, infections, or falling in love.

SIDDHARTHA MUKHERJEE, *THE GENE: AN INTIMATE HISTORY*

 EMMY

Emmy, our nine-year-old granddaughter, started having intense seizures when she was just five months old. In one day, she had 160 of them. I was lecturing in Boston when my daughter texted me videos of the seizures where it looked as if Emmy was being electrocuted. Emmy was diagnosed with infantile spasms (later shown to be caused by a very rare genetic disorder, Koolen-de Vries Syndrome), which is associated with seizures, heart disease, and developmental delays. The neurologist gave us the grim news that Emmy might never walk and had a 30 percent chance of dying before the age of three. He wanted to put her on a medicine that was $26,000 a dose and loaded with side effects, including wiping out her immune system.

I asked about trying the ketogenic diet, which has been found to be helpful for many children with seizure disorders. Her doctor laughed at me and told me it didn't have any science supporting its use. My wife, Tana, later told me she knew the relationship had gone sour when I asked the doctor if he knew how to read. "You're kidding me," I said. "It has more than 75 studies showing it decreases seizure frequency in children, with some children becoming seizure free. The studies were done at a little place in Baltimore called Johns Hopkins. You've heard of Johns Hopkins?" I was frustrated.

The doctor said if we wanted to try the ketogenic diet, he would not be Emmy's doctor. "You're fired," I replied. "How did you get through medical school without learning about informed consent? You're supposed to give us reasonable options, and we decide what to do, remember?"

I then called the ketogenic clinic at Oregon Health & Science University and talked to their director, who told us the diet was an option for Emmy. Within three months on the diet, her seizures subsided, and by age three, Emmy was walking to preschool.[1] It was through Emmy and many children like her I learned that although genes may increase your risk for brain health/mental health illness they can often be modified by smart, targeted interventions.

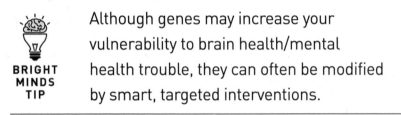

BRIGHT MINDS TIP

Although genes may increase your vulnerability to brain health/mental health trouble, they can often be modified by smart, targeted interventions.

If you have family members with brain health/mental health challenges, such as anxiety disorders, obsessive-compulsive disorder (OCD), depression, bipolar disorder, schizophrenia, addictions, attention deficit disorder/ attention deficit hyperactivity disorder (ADD/ADHD), Alzheimer's disease, or Parkinson's, you have a higher risk of having them too. Studies on identical twins and within families have shown the high genetic nature of many brain health/mental health issues.

FAMILIAL RISK OF PSYCHIATRIC ILLNESS[2]

	Identical Twins	Siblings	General Population
Autism	69%	6%	0.6%
Schizophrenia	50%	9%	0.9%
Bipolar Disorder	40%	5%	1%
Depression	44%	20%	6%
Anxiety Disorder	40%	25%	6%
ADHD	66%	36%	5–15%

Yet having a genetic risk is not a death sentence; it should be a wake-up call for you to know your vulnerabilities and get serious about taking care of your brain. As you can see in the chart above, identical twins, who have identical genes, are just as likely *not* to develop the same conditions as their twin when it comes to schizophrenia, bipolar disorder, depression, and anxiety disorders. Genes load the gun; your behavior and environment pull the trigger.

BRIGHT MINDS TIP

Genes load the gun; your behavior and environment pull the trigger.

The Lincoln Legacy

Abraham Lincoln's family tree is loaded with brain health/mental health issues. His mother, Nancy Lincoln, was described as sad, and his father often got the "blues" with strange spells where he wanted to be alone. His paternal great uncle told a court he had a "deranged mind." His uncle Mordecai Lincoln had severe mood swings, which got worse with heavy drinking. Mordecai's three sons struggled with depression, and one of them swung between depression and mania. One of Abraham Lincoln's first cousins had a daughter, Mary Jane Lincoln, who was committed to the Illinois State Hospital for the Insane. During her trial, the jury concluded, "The disease is with her hereditary," meaning that mental illness ran in her family.[3] It is clear that Abraham Lincoln suffered with periods of depression, even voicing suicidal thoughts. Yet, at the same time, in many ways, he was the epitome of mental health and was able to keep the United States together during its darkest days. His genes were not his destiny.

GENETICS AND THE FOUR CIRCLES

You may think that genetics are purely biological, but they can impact all four circles and, likewise, all four circles can influence your genes, as well as those of your children, grandchildren, and beyond—just as my nieces, Alizé and Amelie, were at risk because of their family history.

- **(B)** • **Biological:** Humans are made up of 23 pairs of chromosomes—one set from each parent—that are found in their DNA in the nuclei of their cells. All humans share 99.99 percent of their genetic code with other humans (so much for feeling special). We share about 98 percent with chimpanzees, about 60 percent with bananas, and about 33 percent with yeast. A gene is a very small part of a chromosome that codes for making different proteins, which in turn make up your cells and, ultimately, you. A lucky person has just the right number of chromosomes and genes. When the number of chromosomes is wrong, when there are extra or defective genes, or when there are certain gene variants, you become more susceptible to issues. For example, heart disease and obesity run in my family, but I do not have either because I don't give in to the behaviors that make them more likely.

- **(P)** • **Psychological:** Too many people believe the false notion that they are condemned to have diabetes, obesity, hypertension, bipolar disorder, depression, or Alzheimer's disease because of their genetic family history. This leads them to develop a defeatist attitude and bad habits that make it likely to be so.

- **(S)** • **Social:** Many people adopt their families' unhealthy behaviors, which increases their risk of developing the brain/mental illnesses for which they have a genetic predisposition.

- **(SP)** • **Spiritual:** If you don't have a strong purpose in life, you are less likely to know *why* you want to turn off those genetic vulnerabilities.

HOW PSYCHIATRIC ISSUES IN YOUR FAMILY MAKE YOU MORE SUSCEPTIBLE TO TROUBLE

- **(B)** 1. You have the genetic vulnerability.

- **(B)(P)** 2. You are more likely to have experienced lasting stress because of the psychiatric challenges in your family. For example, children who grow up with stress or abuse from a parent or relative are significantly more likely to experience lasting anxiety or depression.

B 3. The stress of the illnesses in prior generations changed your genes to become more vulnerable to trouble. Stress, poor diets, environmental toxins, and prenatal nutrition in earlier generations actually changed their genes (epigenetics) to be more likely to express trouble.

S 4. If your family members self-medicate with bad habits, you are likely to pick up those same behaviors, which increases your risk of brain health/mental health issues.

SP 5. If your family doesn't care enough about their own health or about your well-being to change their behavior, it can be harder for you to learn to love yourself enough to adopt a healthier lifestyle.

The more of these factors you have, the higher your risk. Think of it this way: When my daughters, Breanne, Kaitlyn, and Chloe, and granddaughters, Emmy and Haven, were born, they were born with all of the eggs in their ovaries they will ever have. They were all influenced by their mother's habits and my habits. In turn, their habits will turn on or off certain genes that will make illness more or less likely in them and, subsequently, in their babies and grandbabies. Similarly, my nieces, Alizé and Amelie, were born with genes that were influenced by the habits of their parents and grandparents. To end mental illness in Alizé and Amelie and their future children and grandchildren, they need to focus on brain health in an attempt to turn off any of those genes that increased their vulnerability to psychiatric issues.

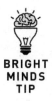

BRIGHT MINDS TIP

Genes are not a death sentence; they should be a wake-up call for you to know your risks and work hard to prevent them.

YOUR ANXIETY MAY BE FROM ANOTHER TIME

In fascinating but disturbing research, fear has been shown to be passed down through generations. You may be afraid of something and have absolutely no idea why. Researchers Brian Dias and Kerry Ressler from Emory University made mice afraid of a cherry blossom scent by shocking them whenever the smell was in the air.[4] In scientific circles, this is called classical fear conditioning, and this result came as no surprise. What was startling, however, was the fact that the rodents' offspring and even the following generation were also afraid of the scent of cherry blossoms, even though they were never exposed to the shocks. The fear was actually transmitted epigenetically.

The implications of this research are wide-reaching. Emotions like fear, anxiety, and perhaps even hatred may have ancestral origins. If you are afraid of something and have no idea why, go back through your genealogy and look for any clues that the fear may actually have nothing to do with your own experience. Prior-generation stress has also been associated with depression, antisocial behaviors, and memory impairment. Fortunately, it seems that stress in your ancestors can go both ways; another study suggested prior-generation stress can help animals learn to better cope with stress.[5]

GENETIC RISKS FOR BRAIN HEALTH ISSUES

- Family history of neurological illnesses
- Family history of psychiatric illnesses, including addictions
- Not being serious about health, despite family history
- Epigenetic factors, such as poor diet, environmental toxins, unresolved emotional trauma, and so on

Would it be any surprise how an evil or benevolent ruler would use your genetics against you or to help you?

GENETICS

THE EVIL RULER WOULD . . .	THE BENEVOLENT RULER WOULD . . .
1. Tell people who have a family history of brain health/mental health illnesses not to worry about taking care of their health because there is nothing they can do about it.	1. Inform the population that genes are not everything and learn from the misguided eugenics movement of the 19th and 20th centuries.
2. Adopt "Live It Up While You Can" as the nation's public health slogan.	2. Educate the population to know their genetic risks and vulnerabilities by having families tell accurate stories of their ancestors and be serious about prevention as soon as possible.
3. Tell subjects there's no point in dealing with their emotional baggage because once they are dead, they are finished.	3. Encourage people to be serious about healthy BRIGHT MINDS lifestyle habits and develop public service programs to let people know about epigenetics.
	4. Remind people that their behavior is not just about them; it is about generations of them.

SOME GUIDING GENETIC PRINCIPLES

1. Genes do not cause illnesses. They make proteins, which have specific functions. The translation process from gene to functional protein is controlled and regulated by other genes and by the availability of nutrients that come from the diet.

2. Few medical illnesses are caused by a malfunction of a single gene.

3. Very rarely is any brain health/mental health disorder caused by a single gene. More often, multiple genes are involved.

4. Even though we are born with all the genes we'll ever have; their expression is influenced by all of the four circles (biological, psychological, social, and spiritual) and BRIGHT MINDS risk factors. This process is called epigenetics. It is rarely your genes by themselves that cause trouble. Nature and nurture always work together to create who we are and how we feel.

5. Small genetic abnormalities are more common in those with autism, schizophrenia, bipolar disorder, and nicotine dependence than in healthy people.[6]

6. Genetic testing is still in its infancy but will likely play an important role in the future of brain health/mental health. For now, genetic testing cannot give a brain health/mental health diagnosis, but it may give clues about vulnerabilities, which medications or supplements may help, and how you metabolize certain medications. For example, if you are of Asian ancestry and your doctor is considering the mood stabilizer carbamazepine (Tegretol), the genetic marker HLA-B*1502 should be tested because it substantially increases the risk of developing serious side effects.[7]

   Genetic testing is beyond the scope of this book, but I want to give you a sense of a few of the genes researchers believe may have some practical application to brain health. There is not a consensus about these findings among scientists, so be cautious in how you interpret this information.

   Some terminology can help:

   - Every person has two copies of each gene, one from their mother and one from their father.
   - *Genotype* is the array of genes an individual has.
   - A *nonideal variant* contains one or two copies of affected genes, also called alleles. Alleles are the variations of any one specific gene.
   - The genetic markers below are simply markers of genetic predisposition. Dietary, environmental, and epigenetic factors often modify the influence of these markers on a person's health. Having a positive marker does not necessarily mean that an action needs to be taken.

PRESCRIPTIONS FOR REDUCING YOUR GENETIC RISK FACTORS
(AND THE FOUR CIRCLES THEY REPRESENT)

The Strategies

B **SP** 1. **Care about your genes and know your vulnerability.** If you have genetic risk factors or a family history of brain health/

mental health issues, get an early screening for the genes listed above. Genomind (www.genomind.com) and Genesight (www .genesight.com) are two companies our clinicians use at Amen Clinics. Questionnaires to screen for brain health/mental health issues, cognitive testing, and possibly brain SPECT imaging may be helpful.

B **S** 2. **Avoid any risk factors that accelerate disease for your genetics** (social circle if you do these activities with friends). Here's an example: Any child who wants to play a contact sport with a likelihood of concussions (football, soccer, hockey, horseback riding, etc.) should be screened for the *APOE* e4 gene. Its presence increases the risk of cognitive decline and dementia later in life tenfold![8] If they have an *APOE* e4 gene, they should consider noncontact sports, such as golf, tennis, table tennis, cross-country running, track, and dance.

B **P** **S** **SP** 3. **Engage in regular healthy habits to decrease the expression of problem-promoting genes.** Be serious about prevention as soon as possible and attack all 11 of the BRIGHT MINDS risk factors. If you have brain health/mental health issues in your family, you should want to be vigilant about brain health. It could make all the difference for you and your family. Studies have shown a lower risk of dementia in people with one or two of the *APOE* e4 genes if they had higher education levels and participated in leisure activities like sports or hobbies that involved new learning.[9] They also did better if their blood flow and vascular risk factors, such as hypertension, smoking, or heart problems, were low.

B 4. **Take nutraceuticals related to any genetic variants you may have.** Refer to the chart in appendix B, and work with an integrative practitioner to determine your risks.

DO YOU WANT A BETTER BRAIN 11 YEARS FROM NOW?

One of my all-time favorite stories involves my friend Leeza Gibbons. Leeza has been a television personality for decades, having appeared as a correspondent and cohost of *Entertainment Tonight* for 16 years and then hosting her own daytime talk show, where we met. Her grandmother and mother died with Alzheimer's disease, and she was terrified she would get it as well. During a stressful time, she came to one of our clinics when she was 51, and her scan was not healthy, which, given her family history, was very concerning. But Leeza didn't allow the news to depress her; rather, it motivated her to follow the strategies in this book to enhance her brain. When I scanned her 11 years later, it was remarkably better. You are not stuck with the brain you have; you can make it better, even 11 years later.

LEEZA AND DR. AMEN

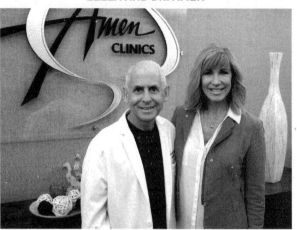

Leeza, Age 51 SPECT Scan

Age 62

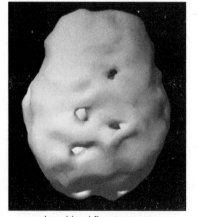

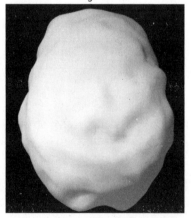

Low blood flow to areas
vulnerable to Alzheimer's

Improved overall

BRIGHT MINDS: GENETICS

STEPS TO CREATE MENTAL ILLNESS ... AND MAKE MY NIECES, ALIZÉ AND AMELIE, SUFFER	STEPS TO END MENTAL ILLNESS ... AND KEEP MY NIECES, ALIZÉ AND AMELIE, HEALTHY

1. Believe your genes are your destiny.
 	
2. Engage in habits that turn on genetic vulnerabilities.
 	
   • Adopt your family's poor eating habits.
   • Self-medicate with substances like alcohol, cigarettes, and sugar.
   • Ignore stress management techniques.
   • Don't deal with the emotional trauma from living with family members with psychiatric illness.
   • Don't seek to understand how your genetics may make you more vulnerable to brain health/mental health issues.
   • Think that your behaviors affect no one but yourself.
 	
3. Avoid the strategies that turn off genetic vulnerabilities.
	1. Believe your behavior can turn on or turn off the genes that increase your vulnerability for brain health/mental health issues.
	
	2. Avoid anything that turns on genetic vulnerabilities.
	
	3. Engage regularly in healthy habits that turn off genetic vulnerabilities.
	
	   • Consume a BRIGHT MINDS diet.
	   • Address all your BRIGHT MINDS risk factors to deal with any brain health/mental health issues.
	   • Practice prayer, meditation, or other ways to cope with stress.
	   • Work on addressing past emotional trauma so you do not have to spread it to future generations. If you already did, help those generations get help.
	   • Consider genetic testing to identify any vulnerabilities.
	   • Remember that your behavior is not just about you; it's about generations of you.

Pick One BRIGHT MINDS Genetics Tiny Habit to Start Today

1. If there are brain health/mental health issues in my family, I will consider early screening.

2. If there is a family history of psychiatric problems in my family, I will remember that my behavior and environment can turn on or off the genes that increase my chances for brain/mental illness.

3. When I suspect I may have a brain health/mental health issue, I will consider testing my genetic vulnerabilities.

4. If I have the APO E4 gene, I will avoid contact sports and other head trauma risks.

5. When I make lifestyle choices, I will remember that my choices affect not only me, but also my children, my grandchildren, and future generations.

CHAPTER 9

<u>H</u> IS FOR HEAD TRAUMA

THE SILENT EPIDEMIC THAT UNDERLIES
MANY MENTAL ILLNESSES

*After at least five concussions, SPECT and hyperbaric
oxygen therapy helped my brain get back to normal.*

HALL-OF-FAME NFL QUARTERBACK JOE NAMATH[1]

 GARY

On December 4, 1988, Gary Busey was involved in a near-fatal motorcycle accident, striking his head on a curb. The Academy Award-nominated actor, who had been appearing on screen since 1971, was not wearing a helmet and suffered massive head injuries. Surgeons opened up his scalp, drilled holes through his skull, and scraped the temporal side of his brain. The brain surgery was deemed a success, the scars on his scalp sealed over, and he underwent occupational and speech therapy. Gary thought he was healed, but for 30 years, the traumatic brain injury (TBI) inside his skull went untreated. After the accident, the rising star tumbled into freefall. He suffered explosive outbursts (many of them caught on camera in reality TV shows), was arrested on battery charges, overdosed on cocaine, and went to rehab.

In 2008, he met his future wife, Steffanie Sampson. At first, she found him charismatic. "Sometimes he's ultimately charming and appears caring," she said "and then sometimes he's just in your face like a bull in a china shop. It's weird." Over the years, she became so worn out she felt like she couldn't put up with his erratic behavior anymore and threatened to leave if he didn't do something about it. In order to save his relationship, Gary agreed to get help, and that's when he came to see me. When we scanned his brain, it showed very low activity in parts of the prefrontal cortex (PFC) and temporal lobes—areas involved in judgment, forethought, empathy, impulse control, and anger management. When Gary and Steffanie saw the scans, they were stunned. Gary had thought he had fully recovered from the accident.

In taking Gary's history, we learned that the motorcycle accident was only one of many things affecting his brain. He likely had attention deficit hyperactivity disorder (ADHD) as a child; he played tackle football in high school and college; he smoked cigars; he abused cocaine and smoked marijuana; and when he had cancer of the sinuses, he had radiation that affected the brain. All of this chipped away at his brain reserve, leading to a breaking point.

Now we're fixing Gary's brain (see the chart below). In the first few months of treatment with our BRIGHT MINDS program, he has cut out marijuana, cigars, and sodas. He has increased his water intake; he is eating healthy, organic, nutrient-dense foods; he's having hyperbaric oxygen therapy (HBOT) treatments and is taking supplements. He's even lost weight. I'm excited to see how much more of a change it will make in Gary's life. I know you are not stuck with the brain you have. You can make it better, and Gary and I are proving it.

BRIGHT MINDS	GARY'S RISK FACTORS	INTERVENTIONS
Blood Flow	Low blood flow on SPECT	Exercise, BRIGHT MINDS diet, omega-3 EPA and DHA, ginkgo
Retirement/Aging	Age 75	New learning
Inflammation	High CRP, low Omega-3 Index	BRIGHT MINDS diet
Genetics		
Head Trauma	Motorcycle accident, playing tackle football	HBOT, neurofeedback, nutraceuticals
Toxins	Drug use, cigar smoking	Stop using drugs, stop smoking
Mind Storms	Temper flares	Stress management tools
Immunity/Infections	Low vitamin D level	Vitamin D
Neurohormone Issues	Low testosterone	Testosterone replacement
Diabesity	High blood-sugar levels	Eliminate sugar and sodas, BRIGHT MINDS diet, exercise, targeted nutraceuticals
Sleep	Insomnia	Sleep strategies

GARY'S SPECT SCAN BEFORE

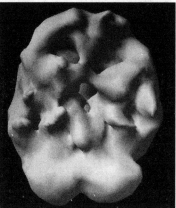

Overall low activity, especially to frontal and temporal lobes

As you have seen throughout this book, your brain is at the heart of what makes you who you are. When it works right, you work right; and when it is troubled for whatever reason, you are much more likely to have trouble in your life. Many people think the brain is rubbery and fixed within the skull, but it isn't. As I've taught for decades, your brain is soft, about the consistency of soft butter, tofu, or custard—somewhere between egg whites and gelatin. It floats in cerebrospinal fluid and is housed in a very hard skull that has many sharp bony ridges (see next page). As such, it is easily damaged.

In this chapter, we are focusing on physical trauma to the brain (biological circle). Whiplash, jarring motions (think shaken baby syndrome), blast injuries, and blows to the head can cause the brain to slosh around, slamming into the hard ridges inside the skull. Here is what happens in the brain after physical trauma:

- Bruising
- Broken blood vessels and bleeding
- Increased pressure
- Lack of oxygen
- Damage to nerve cell connections
- Ripping open of brain cells that spill out proteins like "tau" that cause inflammatory reactions

On top of that, your pituitary gland (which regulates your hormones) sits in a vulnerable part of your skull, so it is often hurt in head injuries, causing major hormonal imbalances.

A LOOK INSIDE THE SKULL

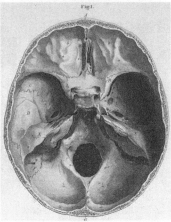

Looking down from the top, you can see the protective bony ridges,
which can damage your soft brain in an accident or injury.

According to the CDC,[2] more than 2 million new head injuries occur in
the United States every year. That means over the last 40 years, more than
80 million people have sustained head injuries. And the number of concussions is also rising, especially among children. From 2010 to 2015, concussion diagnoses jumped 43 percent among the general population. For young
people from 10 to 19 years of age, however, concussion diagnoses skyrocketed
71 percent.[3] We have to do a much better job of preventing TBIs as well as
repairing the brain whenever they occur.

Common causes of head injuries include:

- Falls—falling out of bed, slipping in the bath or shower, falling down
  steps, or falling off ladders
- Motor vehicle–related collisions—involving cars, motorcycles, or
  bicycles; also, accidents where pedestrians are involved.
- Violence—caused by gunshot wounds, assaults, domestic violence,
  or child abuse
- Sports injuries—besides football, they are common in soccer, boxing,
  baseball, lacrosse, skateboarding, hockey, cycling, basketball, and
  other high-impact or extreme sports
- Explosive blasts and other combat injuries[4]

At Amen Clinics, we see patients with head injuries from all of these
causes. In particular, we have been studying the association between football

and brain injuries for several years. When I first started looking at scans, I saw Pop Warner and high school players between the ages of 8 and 18 with clear evidence of TBIs. I was horrified. And then I saw college players whose brains showed even more damage. In the past decade, I've met with many active and former NFL players whose scans were even worse. I was heartened when President Barack Obama and LeBron James both said they would not let their children play tackle football. I took it as a sign that this principle is beginning to become part of our cultural fabric. However, this message isn't hitting the population equally. A 2019 article in the *Atlantic* reported that white boys in upper-income communities are ditching football for other sports while black boys in lower-income neighborhoods are still flocking to football. In a study of 50,000 students from 8th grade to 12th grade, 44 percent of black boys reported playing tackle football compared with 29 percent of white boys.[5] We need to do a better job of getting the message out to all parents and young people that tackle football and other contact sports can have devastating lasting effects on their lives.

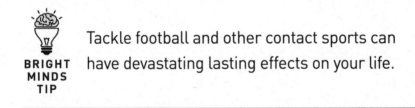

BRIGHT MINDS TIP — Tackle football and other contact sports can have devastating lasting effects on your life.

Since 2000, more than 350,000 military veterans have had TBIs.[6] Those injuries mean the Iraq and Afghanistan wars will likely have consequences for the next 70 years because these veterans will have an increased risk for brain health/mental health issues. And as you have seen, the impact of those TBIs will spread beyond the veterans themselves and affect their children and the generations after that. To put an end to this, they need our BRIGHT MINDS approach more than ever and to stand against the cultural norms that dismiss head trauma as a serious issue.

HEAD TRAUMA

THE EVIL RULER WOULD...	THE BENEVOLENT RULER WOULD...
1. Allow children to hit soccer balls with their heads; play tackle football; ski or ride bicycles without helmets; ride large horses; play hockey; and engage in other high-risk behaviors. 2. Encourage players on a team (especially the better ones) to go back into the game as quickly as possible after suffering a concussion. 3. Put fluorescent lights in all classrooms and workspaces to increase symptoms of anxiety, irritability, depression, or decreased concentration related to Irlen syndrome.	1. Encourage the population to love their brains and the brains of their children and protect them at all costs. 2. Ban children and teenagers from hitting soccer balls with their head or engaging in high-risk activities. Children and teens cannot give informed consent admitting they know and accept the risks of head injuries. Often parents approve of behaviors where they are unaware of the risks. 3. Consider delaying teens getting their driver's licenses by a year to help cut down on motor vehicle accidents and head injuries.

HEAD INJURY AND MENTAL ILLNESS

Research shows that head injuries increase the risk of:

- Depression[7]
- Anxiety and panic disorders[8]
- Psychosis[9]
- Post-traumatic stress disorder (PTSD)[10]
- Suicide[11]
- Drug and alcohol abuse[12]
- ADD/ADHD[13]
- Learning problems[14]
- Borderline and antisocial personality disorders[15]
- Dementia[16]
- Aggression[17]
- Homelessness[18]
- Victimization[19]
- Loss of or changes in sense of smell or taste[20]

Head trauma may also increase the risk of incarceration.[21] In the United States, 25 to 87 percent of inmates say they have suffered a TBI compared with 10 to 38 percent of the general population.[22] And the latest statistics from the Bureau of Justice Statistics show that 181,500 veterans are incarcerated.[23]

In our database of tens of thousands of patients, 40 percent had a significant brain injury before they came to see us. When people ask me what the single most important lesson I've learned from looking at more than 170,000 brain scans is, I reply, "Mild traumatic brain injury is a major cause of psychiatric problems, and very few people know it."

I hate the terms *mild traumatic brain injury* and *mild concussions* because they imply these injuries don't cause lasting damage, which is often not the case at all. Anyone who has played a contact sport likely has experienced many subconcussive blows, which jostled the brain but did not cause immediate symptoms. The famous boxer Joe Louis (1914–1981) is quoted as saying, "It's not the big hits that cause dementia, but rather it is the thousands of little hits."

Head trauma is a major cause of psychiatric illness, and very few people know it because most mental health professionals never look at the brains of their patients, nor do they check the hormones of the brain.

It is important to note that many people forget they've had a significant head injury in the past. At Amen Clinics, we routinely ask patients several times whether they have had a head injury. Our intake paperwork asks the question "Have you ever had a head injury?" The historian, who gathers patients' histories before they see the physician, asks them again about head injuries. The computer testing we have patients complete asks a third time about head injuries. If I see no, no, no as answers, I ask again. If I get a fourth no, I will then say, "Are you sure? Have you ever fallen out of a tree, fallen off a fence, or dived into a shallow pool? Did you play contact sports? Have you ever been in a car accident?"

I'm constantly amazed at how many people think their head injuries were too insignificant to mention. For others, they simply do not remember the incident because amnesia is a common occurrence in head traumas. When asked the question for the fifth time, one patient put his hand on his forehead and said, "Oh, yeah! When I was five years old, I fell out of a second-story window." Likewise, I have had other patients forget they went through windshields, fell out of moving vehicles, or were knocked unconscious when they fell off their bicycles.

Consider YouTube superstar Logan Paul. The controversial internet personality, who is known for his wild, risk-taking pranks and dangerous stunts, has gained more than 15 million followers. But he has also amassed some harsh critics and was named one of the most hated celebrities of 2018. Some people demanded he be banned from YouTube after he posted an insensitive video of a corpse hanging in a Japanese forest where people go to die by suicide. Logan came to see me to find out why he makes so many bad decisions, why he lacks empathy, and why he is incapable of maintaining a committed relationship. "I want to figure out why I think and act the way I do," he said in a video about his visit to Amen Clinics. "I'm a bit of a hooligan, a troublemaker."

As I do with all our patients, I asked him if he had ever experienced head trauma. He told me about a trampoline accident that had fractured his skull when he was in seventh grade. I asked him if there was any other trauma, and he said no. But a few hours later, he revealed something else. Logan shared that he had also been a linebacker and running back on his high school football team. "I was always getting hit in the head," he admitted. He didn't think of that as "trauma," though.

Logan's brain SPECT scan showed low blood flow and abnormal activity in key areas of his PFC. His history of repetitive head trauma from football combined with the trampoline accident was the main reason behind his bad decisions, lack of empathy, and trouble with relationships.

One of the saddest professional encounters I had was with a mother after I wrote a column on head trauma in the *Daily Republic*, the local newspaper where I lived in Northern California during the 1990s. A week or so after it appeared, a mother came to see me. She told me that her 20-year-old daughter had killed herself several months earlier, and she was grief stricken over the unbelievable turn of events in her life. "She was the most ideal child a mother could have," she said. "She did great in school. She was polite, cooperative, and a joy to have around. Then it all changed. Two years ago, she had a bicycle accident. She accidentally hit a branch in the street and was flipped over the handlebars, landing on the left side of her face. She was unconscious when an onlooker got to her, but shortly thereafter she came to. Nothing was the same after that. She was moody, angry, easily set off. She started to complain of 'bad thoughts' in her head. I took her to see a therapist, but it didn't seem to help. One evening, I heard a loud noise out front. She had shot and killed herself on our front lawn."

Head Trauma Risk Factors
(and the Four Circles They Represent)

B 1. One or more head injuries

B **S** 2. Contact sports with concussions

B **S** 3. Contact sports with subconcussive blows

B 4. Irlen syndrome

Unrecognized Irlen Syndrome
Leads to Mental Illness

Irlen syndrome is a visual processing problem, where certain colors of the light spectrum irritate the brain. It runs in families and is common after TBIs. Anyone experiencing symptoms of anxiety, irritability, depression, or decreased concentration should be screened for it. Common symptoms include

- light sensitivity; being bothered by glare, sunlight, headlights, or streetlights
- strain or fatigue with computer use
- fatigue, headaches, mood changes, restlessness, or an inability to stay focused with bright or fluorescent lights
- trouble reading words that are on white, glossy paper
- words or letters shifting, shaking, blurring, moving, running together, disappearing, or becoming difficult to perceive while reading
- difficulty reading music
- feeling tense, tired, sleepy, or even getting headaches with reading
- problems judging distance and difficulty with such things as escalators, stairs, ball sports, driving, or coordination
- migraine headaches
    You can learn more about Irlen syndrome at www.irlen.com.

PRESCRIPTIONS FOR REDUCING YOUR HEAD TRAUMA RISK FACTORS
(AND THE FOUR CIRCLES THEY REPRESENT)

The Strategies

(P) (SP) 1. **Love your brain, and find out if you have had a concussion or head injury** (psychological circle because you need to recognize what constitutes head trauma).
Think back (or ask your mom). Did you ever . . .

- Fall out of a tree or down stairs?
- Fall off a horse or roof?
- Dive into a shallow pool?
- Fall off a fence head first?
- Have a car accident (as a driver or passenger)?
- Have a whiplash accident?
- Have a work-related head injury?
- Hit your head on a ball, the ground, or someone else's helmet in sports?
- Suffer a concussion playing sports?[24]

(B) 2. **Avoid any future head injuries by protecting your head.** This is worth repeating over and over: Protect your head. It contains your brain, which runs everything in your life. Seems obvious, right?

Yet we let little children hit soccer balls with their heads and do dangerous gymnastic routines. Explosive new research shows that professional soccer players have a 300 to 500 percent increased risk of dementia.[25] People cheer at high school football games when the opposing quarterback is knocked out of the game with a vicious hit to his head. Many fans love the fights in hockey so much that the NHL has not yet considered eliminating them from the game.[26] I, too, was a crazy football fan. I played football in high school and for fun on weekends; I was a passionate Los Angeles Rams and Washington Redskins fan. The Redskins won the Super Bowl when I lived near Washington, DC, where I was doing my psychiatric residency at the Walter Reed Army Medical Center. Football had been part of my life, and nothing in my medical training caused me to question my devotion to it—until I started to look at the brain and could clearly see the damage it was doing to people's brains and their lives.

Only engage in high-risk activities if you don't care about the rest of your life. Other sports besides football can also be problematic, including hockey, soccer,[27] horseback riding, auto racing, skiing, and others. Wear your seat belt and, as you age, protect yourself from falls, which is one of the greatest risk factors for head injuries.

B P 3. **Actively engage in repairing any past head injuries** (psychological circle because you need to believe that you can heal your brain). If you have had a head injury, the appropriate treatment can help if you are serious about doing the right things for your brain, providing the support it needs, and attacking all of the BRIGHT MINDS risk factors. I believe the secret to our success with our patients with TBIs is that we use a BRIGHT MINDS approach in all areas, including nutraceuticals. Other treatments include neurofeedback and HBOT, which are detailed below.

   • **Neurofeedback:** Using your mind to control your physiology for better brain health/mental health. Did you know that you can control your hand temperature, heart rate, and even brain waves with your mind? Or that in doing so, you can reduce the symptoms of TBI, stress, anxiety, depression, and more? Your mind is more powerful than you know. I first began learning about therapies that involve using the mind to control our physiology back in the 1980s.

   In 1987, I took a ten-day training course in a treatment technique called biofeedback that uses technology to measure heart rate, breathing rate, brain wave patterns, hand temperature, sweat gland activity, and muscle tension. The basic concept is simple—once you know your heart rate or breathing patterns, for example, you can learn to use mental exercises and focused attention to control them. You can learn to slow your heart rate, warm your hands, decrease sweat gland activity, and so on.

   That same year, I was assigned to be the chief psychiatrist at Fort Irwin in the Mojave Desert, where army soldiers were training to fight the Russians. Among the soldiers in that isolated desert, there was a high incidence of stress, depression, anxiety disorders, drug abuse, and domestic violence. In an effort to help them, I used biofeedback to help them change their own physiology and reduce their stress. As I taught people about this method, I developed a consistent internal thought in dealing with my patients: "Teach them skills to manage their emotions and mind; don't just give them pills."

As fascinating and helpful as biofeedback was, the part of the training course I took that really changed the trajectory of my psychiatric career was a technique called neurofeedback— also called brainwave or EEG biofeedback. While many psychiatrists at that time still considered the brain to be a "black box," the professors in this course showed it was possible to look at brain wave signatures and teach patients how to manipulate them. It turned my view of treatment upside down and paved the way for me to become interested in looking at the brain with SPECT scans. It was in that series of lectures that I first got the idea that would become the signature statement of my professional life: "You are not stuck with the brain you have; you can change it! You can change your brain *and* your life."

When I introduced neurofeedback to the soldiers at Fort Irwin, I saw firsthand how it helped them decrease their impulsivity and anxiety and improve their attention, learning, and mood. Now, more than 30 years later, there are more than 1,000 scientific studies showing that neurofeedback can help a wide variety of mental health and brain-related conditions, such as

- TBI[28]
- Depression[29]
- ADD/ADHD[30]
- Obsessive-compulsive disorder (OCD)[31]
- Addiction[32]
- Memory in healthy people[33]
- Memory post-stroke[34]
- Epilepsy[35]
- Pain[36]
- Balance in Parkinson's patients[37]

BRIGHT MINDS TIP

Skills, not just pills.

Brain Wave Basics

What are brain waves? When masses of neurons communicate with each other, the electrical activity that's transmitted creates brain waves. The most common brain wave patterns are:

- *delta waves* (1–4 cycles per second)—very slow brain waves, seen mostly during sleep; high in TBI and poor memory states
- *theta waves* (5–7 cycles per second)—slow brain waves, seen during creativity, daydreaming, and twilight states; higher in ADD/ADHD, impulsivity, poor memory, and brain fog states
- *alpha waves* (8–12 cycles per second)—brain waves seen during relaxed states
- *beta waves* (13–20 cycles per second)—fast brain waves seen during focused, thinking, analytic states; higher in anxiety states
- *high beta waves* (21–40 cycles per second)—fast brain waves seen during intense concentration or anxiety
- *gamma waves* (>40 cycles per second)—very fast brain waves, often seen during meditation and creative states

Neurofeedback is a computer-based interactive therapy that uses video games to help people regulate their brain wave states. For example, at Amen Clinics, patients sit in front of a computer monitor and play a biofeedback game. If they increase the "beta" activity or decrease the "theta" activity, the game continues. However, if the player is unable to maintain the desired brain wave state, the game stops. People find the activity fun, and they gradually learn to achieve a healthier brain wave pattern. Retraining the brain to maintain a more optimal brain wave state takes time, however, and people often require 20 to 60 sessions before being able to recreate the results on their own. Many people find that the benefits are worth it.

- Hyperbaric oxygen therapy (HBOT)—see chapter 5, "B Is for Blood Flow."

B 4. **Get your hormones tested, including thyroid, DHEA, and testosterone. Remember that your pituitary gland often gets injured during head trauma.** Hormones are often low in people who have sustained head injuries. (For more information, see chapter 13, "N Is for Neurohormone Issues.")

B 5. **Consider getting a functional imaging study**, such as SPECT or QEEG, if you are struggling with your behavior or memory.

B 6. **Take nutraceuticals** that are essential to help support the brain's healing process.

- **Multivitamin/mineral complex**—a high dose supplement, with higher doses of vitamins B6, B12, folate, and D for nutrient support.

- **Omega-3 fatty acids**—highly concentrated and purified, two grams of total EPA+DHA. Dr. Michael Lewis's book *When Brains Collide* details how omega-3 fatty acids can facilitate healing after a concussion and relieve symptoms without medication.[38]

- **A combination of ginkgo** (to support blood flow), **acetyl-L-carnitine** (to support mitochondrial energy), **huperzine A** (to support acetylcholine), **N-acetylcysteine, alpha-lipoic acid** (for antioxidant support), and **phosphatidylserine** (for nerve cell membrane support).

BRIGHT MINDS: HEAD TRAUMA

STEPS TO CREATE MENTAL ILLNESS ... AND MAKE MY NIECES, ALIZÉ AND AMELIE, SUFFER	STEPS TO END MENTAL ILLNESS ... AND KEEP MY NIECES, ALIZÉ AND AMELIE, HEALTHY
1. Deny that brain injuries are likely to cause mental health issues. 2. Engage in habits that increase your risk for head trauma. • Play contact sports. • Never wear a helmet while skiing, biking, riding a motorcycle, etc. • Play soccer and head soccer balls repeatedly. • Participate in high-risk adventure activities—free climbing, bungee jumping, etc. • Climb trees and ladders and go on the roof. • Dive into the ocean or pool without knowing the depth of the water. • Don't wear a seat belt. • Drive too fast and text while driving. • Text while walking. • Don't practice balance exercises as you age. 3. Avoid the strategies that protect your brain.	1. Acknowledge that brain injuries could be causing mental health issues and actively repair past head trauma. 2. Avoid anything that increases your risk for head trauma. 3. Engage regularly in healthy habits that protect your brain. • Avoid contact sports. • Avoid high-risk activities. • Don't climb trees or ladders or go on the roof. • Don't dive headfirst into any body of water. • Always wear a seat belt in the car. • Always wear a helmet when skiing or riding a bike. • Don't text while driving or walking. • Consider neurofeedback, HBOT, and nutraceuticals. • Practice balance exercises, especially as you age.

Pick One BRIGHT MINDS Head Trauma Tiny Habit to Start Today

1. When I get in the car, I will fasten my seat belt.

2. When I go into the house, I will limit the number of packages I carry at one time to minimize the risk of falling.

3. When I go skiing or biking, I will put on a helmet.

4. When I must go up on the roof, I will make sure it is absolutely safe.

5. When I walk or drive, I will slow down and pay attention to my surroundings.

6. When I walk or drive, I will put my phone out of sight so I cannot text.

7. When I go downstairs, I will hold the handrail.

8. When (and if) I experience a head trauma, I will check my hormones and optimize any that are low.

CHAPTER 10

T IS FOR TOXINS

DETOX YOUR MIND AND BODY

Toxicity is the primary driver of disease.
DR. JOSEPH PIZZORNO, NP, *THE TOXIN SOLUTION*

 STEVEN

Steven, 32, was a firefighter who suffered from depression, brain fog, and symptoms of post-traumatic stress disorder (PTSD) when he first came to see me. I had already seen his brother for learning issues at school, his father for job-related anxiety, and his stepmother for depression. All of them had mentioned to me their concern for Steven, especially after learning about the connection between brain health and mental health. Firefighters are exposed to environmental toxins, head trauma, and emotional trauma.

Steven initially asked me, "How can I deal with the trauma? I wish I could forget what my eyes have seen, from children being burned to losing whole families in car crashes and fires." His scan showed signs of PTSD, with his emotional brain working way too hard, plus he also had evidence of toxic exposure, likely from breathing in carbon monoxide and the poisonous chemicals often released by burning furniture. This toxic look is very common among the many firefighters we have seen. Seeing his scan caused Steven to get serious about brain health. Within six months, he felt much better and his brain was healthier.

STEVEN'S SPECT SCANS BEFORE AND AFTER TREATMENT

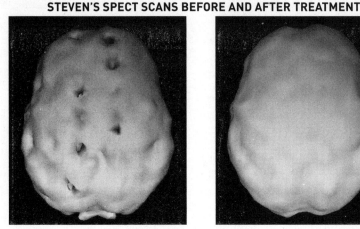

Toxic: overall low blood flow   Healthier overall

Steven isn't alone. The dangerous professions of firefighters, police officers, first responders, and other everyday heroes subject those workers to long-lasting negative impact on their brain function. They are exposed to environmental toxins such as carbon monoxide, benzene, asbestos, and diesel exhaust; head injuries; and emotional trauma. Studies show an elevated risk of PTSD, depression, heavy drinking, and suicide in first responders.[1] Unfortunately, they are less likely to seek help because of the stigma associated with having a mental illness, fearing they will be labeled as weak or unfit for duty. Their professions have convinced them that they are superheroes and nothing could or should get to them.[2]

TOXINS AND THE BRAIN

Your brain is the most metabolically active organ in your body. As such, it is vulnerable to damage from toxins. Toxins are one of the major causes of brain health/mental health issues that traditional psychiatrists almost completely ignore. During my first decade as a psychiatrist I ignored them too. But when I started our work with brain SPECT imaging, I quickly began to see toxic patterns on patients who were not substance abusers. *Uh-oh*, I thought to myself, *there is much more to my patients' problem than I have considered. I wonder, how many people with toxic exposure have I missed?*

Toxins are one of the major causes of brain health/mental health issues that traditional psychiatrists almost completely ignore.

Environmental toxins impact nearly every aspect of your body and can damage the brain, leading to a variety of physical and psychiatric symptoms. On the physical side, issues can include autoimmune diseases, diabetes, cancer, fatigue, numbness, tingling, tremors, allergies, abdominal pain, diarrhea, smelly stools, bad breath, weight issues, skin rashes, sweats, and more. From a psychiatric standpoint, exposure to toxins can increase the risk of depression, suicide, attention deficit disorder/attention deficit hyperactivity disorder (ADD/ADHD), learning problems, memory problems, brain fog, autism, temper outbursts, psychotic behavior, and dementia. Our biological systems get rid of toxins (through the gut, liver, kidneys, and skin), but when those natural detoxification processes are overwhelmed, we can experience brain fog, fatigue, and even life-threatening illnesses. And it can certainly disrupt our mental health.

TEN WAYS TOXINS POISON YOUR BRAIN AND CONTRIBUTE TO MENTAL ILLNESS

1. **Reduce cerebral blood flow**, which on SPECT scans has been associated with depression, bipolar disorder, schizophrenia, ADD/ADHD, and more. As you learned in chapter 5, low blood flow is the number one brain-imaging predictor that a person will develop Alzheimer's disease.[3]

2. **Disrupt the endocrine system**, interfering with hormone production, causing serious imbalances, and increasing the risk of depression, anxiety, and panic attacks.

3. **Impair the immune system**, increasing your risk of autoimmune disorders and cancer, as well as anxiety, depression, and even psychosis.

4. **Disrupt the gut microbiome**, resulting in leaky gut and accompanying problems, such as mood and anxiety disorders, ADD/ADHD, Parkinson's, and Alzheimer's.

5. **Increase the likelihood of developing diabetes and obesity**, since as toxic load rises, so does risk. Toxins are also called *diabesogens* and *obesogens* because they contribute to diabetes and obesity, which raise the risk for anxiety, depression, and Alzheimer's disease.

6. **Damage DNA**, which can accelerate aging of the brain and lead to problems with mood, anxiety, irritability, temper, and irrational behavior, as well as memory.

7. **Impair enzyme systems**, which disrupts many biological processes, such as the ability to produce energy and fight free radicals.

8. **Harm organs**, including the digestive tract, liver, kidneys, and brain. This damage reduces your detoxification system's ability to do its job, creating an even greater buildup of toxins.

9. **Alter gene expression**, possibly turning on harmful gene variants and/or turning off beneficial ones.

10. **Damage cell membranes** and disrupt communication between cells.

How Toxic Is Your Brain?
Toxins Exposure Quiz

Over the years, our clinic has developed a checklist to help patients determine how much contact they may have had with harmful substances. By answering the questions below, you can begin to determine your own risk—and begin taking steps to combat that exposure.

1. Do you smoke, or are you around secondhand smoke?

2. Do you smoke marijuana?

3. Do you use conventional cleaning products and inadvertently breathe the fumes?

4. Have you been exposed to carbon monoxide?

5. Do you travel on planes more than six times a year?

6. Do you pump your own gas or breathe automobile exhaust?

7. Do you live in an area with moderate to high air pollution?[4]

8. Have you lived or worked in a building that had water damage and mold in it?

9. Do you come in contact with flame-resistant clothing or carpet, or with furnishings sprayed with chemicals to prevent stains?

10. Do you spray your garden, farm, or orchard with pesticides or live near an area with pesticides?[5]

11. Do you paint indoors without ventilation?

12. Do you have more than four glasses of alcohol a week?

13. Do you regularly eat processed or fast foods?

14. Do you regularly eat conventionally raised produce, meat, or dairy, or farm-raised fish?

15. Do you eat large (i.e., mercury-contaminated) fish, such as swordfish?

16. Do you eat nonorganic fruits and vegetables on a regular basis?

17. Do you consume foods with artificial colors or sweeteners, such as diet sodas, or use artificial sweeteners, such as aspartame (NutraSweet), sucralose (Splenda), or saccharin (Sweet'N Low)?

18. Do you use more than two health and/or beauty products per day? (Most people never read the labels or understand how many chemicals are included.)

19. Do you live in a house that contains lead pipes or copper plumbing soldered with lead (built prior to 1978)?

20. Do you wear lipstick or kiss someone with lipstick made with lead? (Sixty percent of the lipstick sold in the United States has lead in it.[6])

21. Do you have mercury amalgam fillings? How many?

22. Do you work in a job where you are exposed to environmental toxins, such as firefighting, painting, welding, longshoreman?

23. Have you had general anesthesia? How many times?[7]

TOXINS

THE EVIL RULER WOULD . . .	THE BENEVOLENT RULER WOULD . . .
1. Repeal laws that ensure clean air, clean water, and safe buildings.	1. Strengthen laws that ensure clean air, clean water, and safe buildings.
2. Ignore companies that dump toxic waste.	2. Penalize companies that dump toxic waste.
3. Promote chemically laden foods.	3. Expose the dangers of chemical-laden foods.
4. Highlight research that touts the health benefits of alcohol and marijuana.	4. Highlight research that reveals how alcohol and marijuana affect brain health.
5. Encourage teens to start smoking cannabis, because it has been found to increase the risk of depression and suicide later in life. One study found that using the drug as a teen contributes to mental illness in over 500,000 people in adulthood.[8]	5. Discourage tweens and teens from smoking cannabis.
6. Disallow labeling of the ingredients in personal care products, so people wouldn't have to worry about the chemicals they are putting on their bodies.	6. Require truthful labeling of all ingredients in personal care products, so people can make an informed decision about what they are putting on their bodies.

HOW MODERN SOCIETY IS POISONING THE BRAIN AND CONTRIBUTING TO MENTAL ILLNESS

Every single day, we are exposed to a host of chemicals, pesticides, fumes, and products that poison the human brain. Common toxins in the air we breathe, the foods we eat, and the products we rub on our skin are absorbed into our bodies via our lungs, digestive system, and pores and can eventually impact the brain. The more exposure you have to these everyday toxins, the more you are putting your brain at risk and increasing your chances of brain health/mental health issues. Look at the following lists and check how many toxic substances you may have been exposed to, either currently or in the past.

You can't avoid toxins, but you can limit your exposure and boost your natural ability to detoxify. Detoxifying your world will help you and everyone in your household, including children. My nieces, Alizé and Amelie, don't need to increase their risk factors. So we do everything we can to clean up our environment.

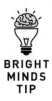

BRIGHT MINDS TIP

The more exposure you have to these everyday toxins, the more you are putting your brain at risk and increasing your chances of brain health/mental health issues.

Common Toxins . . .

THAT CAN BE INHALED[9]

- Air pollution
- Asbestos
- Automobile exhaust
- Aviation fumes
- Carbon monoxide
- Cigarette smoke, secondhand smoke, marijuana smoke
- Cleaning chemicals
- Fireplace fumes
- Fire retardant fumes
- Fire toxins (inhaled by first responders fighting fires)
- Gasoline fumes
- Mold
- Paint and solvent fumes
- Pesticide or herbicide residues near farms (also backyard applications)
- Welding, soldering fumes

THAT CAN BE INGESTED OR ABSORBED THROUGH THE SKIN[10]

- Apples sprayed with diphenylamine, which makes them shiny but breaks down into cancer-causing nitrosamines,[11] associated with Parkinson's and Alzheimer's[12]
- Artificial food dyes, preservatives, and sweeteners
- BPA (or bisphenol A; found in plastics, food and drink containers, dental sealants, and the coating of cash-register receipts)
- Chemotherapy

- General anesthesia in some patients
- Heavy metals, such as
  - Mercury: in "silver" dental fillings (50 percent mercury) and contaminated fish. (The Environmental Protection Agency recommends pregnant women eat fish no more than twice a week and avoid the big four: king mackerel, swordfish, shark, and tilefish. Also limit grouper and albacore tuna.)
  - Lead: in paint, pipes, airline fuel, and lipstick (see pages 187–188)
  - Cadmium: in cigarettes; soils treated with synthetic fertilizers; and industrial and hazardous waste sites. It is highly toxic and accumulates in the liver and kidneys and damages your ability to detoxify. It is linked to osteoporosis, heart disease, cancer and diabetes. Once it is in your body, it takes 16 years to get rid of just half of it!
- Excessive alcohol
- Foods manufactured with plastic equipment, leaking plasticizers
- Health and beauty products (see chart on pages 190–191)
- Herbicides such as glyphosate—for example, Roundup (used in genetically modified crops)—disrupt the body's endocrine or hormonal system, affecting both testosterone and estrogen,[13] and raise the risk of cancer by 41 percent.[14] Herbicides may also damage DNA, making cells age faster and increasing their susceptibility to cancer.
- Many medications, such as benzodiazepines (for anxiety, insomnia) or narcotic pain medications
- Marijuana
- MSG (monosodium glutamate)
- PCBs (polychlorinated biphenyls) (see "Gone but Not Forgotten" on page 193)
- Pesticides—such as organochlorines and organophosphates (neurotoxins)—stimulate enzymes that turn calories into fat, where toxins are stored. Those in the top 5 percent of organophosphate exposure have a 650 percent increase in dementia.[15]
- Polluted or tainted water (including lead and arsenic)
- Silicone breast implants that leaked

COMMON TOXINS AT THE ROOT OF MENTAL ILLNESS

As a psychiatrist, I have seen many patients with depression, brain fog, anxiety, poor memory and concentration, word confusion, headaches, vertigo, and cravings who all had the same thing in common: exposure to toxins. Here are eight of the most common toxic issues we see at Amen Clinics.

1. Alcohol: not a health food

Some large-scale studies have found that light-to-moderate alcohol use may benefit the heart and brain.[16] But I see alcohol from a different point of view. I worked as an ambulance driver and in emergency rooms where I witnessed the tragedy of lives lost due to drunk driving. As a psychiatrist for nearly 40 years, I have met with many patients whose lives and families have been wrecked by alcohol abuse. And as a brain imaging expert, I have seen thousands of SPECT scans of "moderate" drinkers, whose brains look terrible, and the scans of alcohol abusers that look even worse.

When it comes to the brain, alcohol is not necessarily the health food it's reported to be. Alcohol can harm your cognitive function and psychological well-being, and alcohol abuse can contribute to mental illness. For example, did you know that people who drink every day have smaller brains?[17] *When it comes to the brain, size matters!* Heavy alcohol use can alter neurotransmitter and hormonal systems that are involved in mood and anxiety disorders.[18] And did you know that compared to nondrinkers and light drinkers, moderate-to-heavy drinkers increase their risk of dementia by 57 percent—and develop it earlier?[19] Alcohol can also decrease judgment and decision-making skills and increase cravings. And because alcohol lowers blood flow to the cerebellum, an amazing part of the brain that is associated with physical movement, it can make you less coordinated. In the United States, there are 30 million children of alcoholics, and many of them suffer from PTSD as a result of growing up in an unpredictable, abusive alcoholic home. Excessive alcohol use is also a major cause of divorce, incarceration, and financial problems, which can contribute to sadness, anxiety, and despair.

Alcohol is listed as the seventh leading preventable cause of death and is related to seven different types of cancer.[20] Why do nurses rub alcohol on your skin before they give you a shot or insert an IV needle? To kill bacteria. What is the reason alcohol is used to preserve dead specimens? To kill all the cells and tissues in the specimen. This should make you wonder what alcohol is doing to your gut. If you want a better brain, less is more. For people who want to drink and who do not have a history of addiction in their families, I recommend no more than two to four normal-size drinks a week.

BRAIN SPECT SCAN OF HEAVY ALCOHOL USE

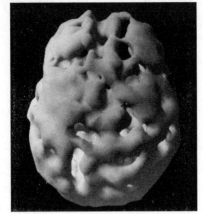

Overall low activity

2. Marijuana: reason for caution

A growing number of states are legalizing marijuana for medical and recreational use, which has boosted the interest in the drug as a potential therapy for physical and mental health issues. Some research suggests it may have some benefit for people dealing with depression, anxiety, and PTSD;[21] however, other studies have found that marijuana can have a negative impact on mental health. In 2016, we published the largest brain imaging study on marijuana users, showing the overall decreased blood flow of 982 users compared to a healthy group.[22] Blood flow was decreased the most in the right hippocampus, which is often involved with Alzheimer's disease and all types of memory loss. A 2019 review of 11 studies involving more than 23,000 people found that using cannabis as an adolescent increased the risk of developing depression and suicidal thoughts or suicide attempts in young adulthood.[23] Other research shows marijuana impairs short-term memory, contributes to learning and attention problems, reduces focus and coordination, and increases the risk for psychosis. In fact, a 2019 study in *The Lancet Psychiatry* found that potent cannabis may be associated with 10 percent of new cases of psychosis.[24]

3. Smoking/vaping: more toxic than you thought

Cigarettes are some of the most toxic substances around. According to the American Lung Association, as cigarettes burn they create about 7,000 chemicals, many of which are poisonous.

Here are just 10 of the toxins found in cigarettes:

TOXINS	ALSO FOUND IN . . .
Acetic acid	Hair dye
Ammonia	Cleaning products
Arsenic	Rat poison
Benzene	Rubber cement
Butane	Lighter fluid
Cadmium	Battery acid
Formaldehyde	Embalming fluid
Methanol	Rocket fuel
Tar	Road materials
Toluene	Paint

It's common knowledge that the tobacco industry has promoted smoking despite its serious negative health effects. But what you may not know is that it has also promoted the use of its products within psychiatric settings and has funded research suggesting people with schizophrenia can benefit from self-medicating with cigarettes.[25] Today, as many as 80 percent of people with schizophrenia smoke.[26] They aren't alone. People with brain health/mental health or substance abuse issues are more likely to smoke cigarettes than the general population. In fact, they smoke nearly 40 percent of all cigarettes, according to the CDC.[27]

Although smoking rates have been going down for years, rates of vaping e-cigarettes are on the rise. A 2018 report involving more than 40,000 teens nationwide showed that more than 20 percent of twelfth graders said they had vaped nicotine in the previous month. That's twice the number who had reported vaping in 2017. And 11 percent of eighth graders admit vaping nicotine in the past year.[28] The rate of young people vaping is rising so rapidly that in 2018, the US surgeon general called e-cigarette vaping among youth an epidemic.[29]

Cigarettes—tobacco and marijuana—as well as vaping nicotine and caffeine delivery systems cause you to inhale into your lungs a host of fine and ultrafine toxic junk that can also penetrate your brain. Does size matter? Yes! The smaller the particle you inhale, the greater its ability to cause inflammatory reactions and damage your brain.

I wanted to see what vaping caffeine does to the brain, so for an episode of *The Dr. Oz Show*, I scanned Dr. Oz before and after he vaped. The results weren't pretty. After vaping, his scans showed increased activity in the occipital lobes (the area that makes you notice someone attractive) and decreased activity in the frontal lobes (the area that puts on the brakes to prevent bad behavior). This seems like a prescription for divorce!

4. Mold: a mental illness creator

One of the first lessons I learned from our brain imaging work is that many everyday things are toxic to brain function—and one of the worst is mold. Take it from Bulletproof Coffee CEO Dave Asprey. He had been struggling with focus and memory and was barely able to pass his classes at Wharton. Then, in 2003, after reading my book *Change Your Brain, Change Your Life*, he got a brain SPECT scan. He says it changed everything in his life. It turned out that Dave had been exposed to toxic mold in his home. His health dramatically improved after following specific healing protocols, and he went on to produce *Moldy: The Toxic Mold Movie* (watch it online at https://moldymovie.com).[30]

COMMON TOXIC MOLDS

MOLD VARIETY	DESCRIPTION AND CONSEQUENCE
Ochratoxin A	Foodborne mold; causes cancer
Aflatoxins	Foodborne mold; causes cancer, can stunt growth in children
Fumonisins	Contaminant in maize as well as wheat and other cereals; implicated in neural tube defects and stunted growth[31]
Zearalenone and other Fusarium mycotoxins	Crop contaminants; disrupts hormone balance (estrogenic)[32]
Aspergillus	Found indoors and outside; especially concerning in children[33]
Tricothecene, "black mold"	Crop contaminants that can also grow in damp indoor environments; inhibits protein synthesis; extremely dangerous to skin, kidneys, liver, and more[34]

Another patient, George, 32, came to see us complaining of anxiety, brain fog, memory problems, and sleep disturbance. From the detailed history we collected, it became clear that George's symptoms began when he moved back home from college into his parents' basement apartment. Mold diagnostic testing revealed George had high levels of mold toxins in his body. Only after seeing these lab results did George remember that the basement had flooded on several occasions.[35]

We recommended that George remove himself immediately from the moldy environment, which is the first step for anyone with mold toxicity. Next, we began treatment consisting of binding agents and other medications, such as antifungals, as well as metabolic support supplements. With proper treatment and remediation of the mold problem, George's symptoms improved. He did not need psychiatric medications; he simply needed an accurate diagnosis and appropriate treatment. If no one had checked him for mold toxins, he probably would have been diagnosed with one or more mental illnesses and treated (unsuccessfully) with psychiatric medications. He could have gone years with worsening symptoms.

Six Common Symptoms of Mold Exposure

- Unexplained muscle problems
- Brain fog, memory problems
- Difficulty focusing
- Numbness or "pins and needles" feeling
- Digestive issues
- Breathing problems (chronic cough, sinus problems, wheezing)

5. Lead: a clear and present danger

Lead harms the brain, and lead exposure is associated with lower IQ, speech problems, cancer, cardiovascular problems, arthritis, seizures, headaches, anemia, kidney disease, a metallic taste, and death from all causes. Lead exposure is also related to a variety of mental health issues. In children, it has been associated with ADD/ADHD,[36] learning problems, irritability, aggression, fearfulness, anti-social behavior, and more.[37] It has also been linked to adult-onset schizophrenia.[38] In a 2010 study with nearly 2,000 young adults with low levels of lead exposure, higher blood levels of lead was associated with an increased risk of depression and panic disorder. The researchers concluded that even at levels generally considered safe, lead exposure could negatively affect mental health.[39]

The US government used to report that a "safe" level of lead in the bloodstream was less than 60 µg/dL (micrograms per deciliter). The current "safe" level is under 10 µg/dL, and in July 2012, the CDC reported that the range of 5.0–10.0 µg/dL is highly risky for children. Many scientists say that any level of lead is unsafe. Depending on your age, you may recall that the government dictated that lead be removed from gasoline and paint. Strangely, this didn't apply to small aircraft aviation fuel. At the Amen Clinics, we scanned 100 pilots and saw significant brain toxicity in two-thirds of them. We suspected it was caused by lead and other toxins that they are exposed to when they fly. In regard to paint, any house painted white before 1978 has high levels of lead, and once it chips or peels, it exposes those in the home to lead. And houses built or remodeled before 1984 likely have lead in the pipe solder.

One of the most widely used cosmetics—lipstick—still contains lead since no regulation has required that lead be removed from it. Lead was found in 60 percent of national brands.[40] In 2013, researchers at the University of California, Berkeley, found lead in 24 of 32 lip products tested. Many of the products contained high levels of eight other metals, including cadmium and chromium.[41]

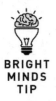

BRIGHT MINDS TIP

To avoid buying and ingesting lead-contaminated lip products, know your lipstick brands and go to www.safecosmetics.org to learn more.

---

6. General anesthesia: the risk surgeons don't warn you about[42]

I first became aware of the potentially toxic risk of general anesthesia[43] when one of my patients called me in tears after having knee surgery. She told me she felt as if she had brain fog and was afraid she was developing Alzheimer's disease. I had already done a SPECT scan on her, so I rescanned her to see if her brain had changed. On the new scan, her brain looked toxic. Her frontal and temporal lobes, which are both involved in memory and attention, looked dramatically worse. Something had negatively affected her brain after that first scan. With the BRIGHT MINDS approach in this book, she was able to clear the brain fog and regain her memory.

Some scientific studies show no lasting negative effects and others show toxic effects from general anesthesia, but two recent studies are notable. In one, children who had undergone general anesthesia before the age of four had lower IQ, diminished language comprehension, and decreased gray matter in the back of their brains.[44] Also, a before-and-after SPECT study of patients who underwent coronary artery bypass surgery showed that 68 percent had diminished blood flow, which was linked to decreased verbal and visual memory six months later.[45] As you've seen in this book, low blood flow is one of the BRIGHT MINDS risk factors that can contribute to mental illness. If you have to undergo surgery, I recommend local or spinal anesthesia whenever possible. If that is not an option, make sure you do everything you can to optimize your brain before going under the knife.

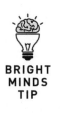

BRIGHT MINDS TIP

> If you have to undergo surgery, I recommend local or spinal anesthesia whenever possible. If that is not an option, make sure you do everything you can to optimize your brain before going under the knife.

One of my treasured assistants, Karen, who is beloved by our patients, discovered she had an aortic aneurysm. We had a prior SPECT scan, one shortly after her aneurysm surgery, and then one after she worked hard to rehabilitate her brain. No doubt, the surgery had a very negative impact on her brain and mind, but that was recoverable with the right BRIGHT MINDS program.

KAREN'S SPECT SCANS BEFORE, AFTER AORTIC ANEURYSM SURGERY, AFTER BRIGHT MINDS

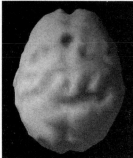 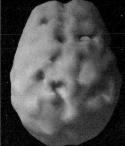 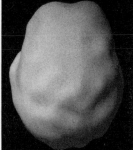

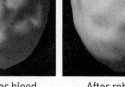

Before   Overall lower blood flow after surgery   After rehabilitation

7. Chemotherapy and heavy metals: stealing your mind

At Amen Clinics, we see many patients who have treated cancer with chemotherapy. Chemotherapy kills cancer cells, but it unfortunately can kill healthy brain cells too.[46] High exposure to heavy metals (e.g., arsenic, mercury, iron, and aluminum) can also lead to memory problems. I recommend asking your physician to screen you for heavy metals, especially if you know you've been exposed to any.

8. *Personal care products: the ugly side of health and beauty aids*

How many personal care and cosmetic products do you use each day? If you're like the average American woman, you apply about 12 products, or like the average man, about six.[47] According to Statista, the cosmetics, perfume, and other toilet preparations industry is expected to spend close to $19 billion on advertising in 2019 to encourage us to use more of these everyday items.[48] But the chemicals in these products are easily absorbed through your pores and can be transported to every organ in your body, including your brain. This means while trying to look better on the outside, you could be poisoning yourself on the inside and increasing your risk for brain health/mental health issues. The risk from these items is real. In 2016, Johnson & Johnson was ordered to pay $72 million to the family of a woman whose death from ovarian cancer was associated with the daily use of Johnson's Baby Powder among other company products.[49]

If you have symptoms associated with brain health/mental health issues, I highly recommend that you ditch personal care products with harmful ingredients to lighten your toxic load. The Environmental Working Group's Skin Deep database (http://www.ewg.org/skindeep/) can help. It offers information on many products with toxic ingredients and suggests healthier alternatives. The following chart lists chemicals commonly found in personal care products—along with a brief description of the damage they can do, and is from *The Toxin Solution*, an exceptional book by Joseph Pizzorno, ND, a founder of Bastyr University.

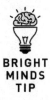

BRIGHT MINDS TIP

What goes *on* your body goes *in* your body.

COMMON CHEMICALS FOUND IN HEALTH AND BEAUTY AIDS

CHEMICAL	PURPOSE	TOXICITY
Acrylates	Artificial nails	Neurotoxins[50]
Aluminum	Antiperspirant	Potential connection to Alzheimer's disease[51]
Formaldehyde	Shampoos, nail polish, hair gel, nail and eyelash glue, body wash, color cosmetics	Cancer,[52] allergic reactions[53]

CHEMICAL	PURPOSE	TOXICITY
Fragrance	Shampoos, liquid baby soap, nail polish, glues, hair smoothing, body wash, color cosmetics	Cancer, endocrine disruption, allergic reactions
Oxybenzone	Sunscreen	Hormone disruption, lowers sperm count, skin allergies
Parabens	Preservative, fragrance in cosmetics (eye shadow, foundation, mascara), shampoos, conditioners, lotions, facial/body cleansers	Hormone issues, breast cancer,[54] developmental problems in kids, reproductive problems, allergies
Phthalates (banned in Europe)	Fragrances in cosmetics *Also used in plasticizers (plastic wrap, packaging)*	Hormone disruption;[55] lower IQ;[56] decreases BDNF in males,[57] which helps neurons grow and connect
Polyethylene glycols (PEGs)	Create suds in shampoos, bubble baths, liquid soap	Cancer,[58] birth defects,[59] hair loss, allergies
Triclosan	Antimicrobial cleanser, toothpaste	Hormone disruption,[60] harmful to the microbiome[61]
Lead	Lipstick (kiss of death)	Neurotoxin, damage to hippocampus and prefrontal cortex[62]

Source: Dr. Joseph Pizzorno, ND, *The Toxin Solution*. Used with permission.

9. Household items: when home sweet home becomes "home toxic home"

Many of the common items in your home may harbor potentially harmful chemicals, and tackling DIY home projects can increase your exposure to toxic substances. For example, carpeting, flame-retardant bedding and furniture, flooring, and paints can have high concentrations of chemicals. In 2019, researchers from Duke University presented evidence showing that children who grow up in homes with a flame-retardant sofa had six times more polybrominated diphenyl ethers (PBDEs) in their blood serum.[63] These chemicals have been associated with neurodevelopmental delays, interference with the endocrine system, thyroid disruption, obesity, cancer, and other conditions.

Pamela: The Surprising Source of Her Depression, Migraines, and Memory Problems

Before coming to Amen Clinics, Pamela would spend most of each day in bed:

> My kids would go out; I'd be lying in bed and missing out on everything. I would have migraines. I was down to 116 pounds. I couldn't eat; I couldn't think; I had memory loss. I couldn't finish a sentence. I couldn't come up with a word. There were times I couldn't even remember my children's names. Nobody could give me a reason for that. This just wasn't the person I was before. I was vibrant. I was a successful businesswoman. I had it all together and then all of a sudden, I was falling apart and everything was getting progressively worse. . . .
>
> I tried everything. You name it, I've tried it . . . but more things would keep happening. Something else would add to my list of illnesses. I'd end up getting depressed, because it didn't seem like anybody really understood. I was on 21 prescription medications, because that's all they would give me. "Well, if you feel this, that's not working. Well, here, I'll add this drug to you, and I'll add that drug to you." I felt that somewhere out there, there had to be an answer, and I just had to find the answer. A lot of times, some of these doctors would tell me it was in my head. I'm thinking, *No, this is physical. I can't breathe. I've got migraines. These are not mental issues. These are all physical problems.* . . .
>
> When I started having these memory issues, at that point, I thought, You know what, I need to go to Amen Clinics. When I went to Dr. [Muneer] Ali, I walked in with my 21 prescriptions: my 11 in the morning and my 10 in the evening. He said, "Oh, we're not doing that anymore." He got rid of all of my prescriptions but five of them.

Pamela spent three days at the Amen Clinic in Atlanta, where the staff took a thorough history and SPECT scans, and did extensive laboratory testing. Dr. Ali found a genetic abnormality that made it harder for Pamela to fight off viruses. Pamela also discovered she had Lyme. When Dr. Ali found out that Pamela had a leaky roof, he did a mold test, which came back positive for black mold, one of the worst kinds. The Lyme and mold explained a great deal about her symptoms.

> When I walked in here, I was so sick, and I do not look like
> I do now. I've got a smile, and I'm sitting up. I have energy,
> and I'm completing my sentences. . . . I can remember
> everything. It's like a rebirth. I wanted to be a better mom
> for my kids. That was my goal.

Disturbing Fact: *One of the most effective ways for a woman to decrease her toxic load is through breastfeeding, which decreases breast cancer risk.*[64] *Unfortunately, the baby gets the brunt of it.*

Gone but not Forgotten: PCBs and Their Lingering Effects on Brain/Mental Health

Polychlorinated biphenyls, better known as PCBs, were industrial chemicals used in electrical products and appliances. Though they were banned in 1979, they don't break down well so they are still pervasive in our water, soil, and air. And because of this, they continue to cause problems. A 2014 study found that people with higher levels of work-related exposure to PCBs had an increased risk for developing depression.[65] Other studies show possible links to changes in the brain associated with autism, ADD/ADHD, schizophrenia, and learning problems.[66] PCBs also inhibit the workings of the thyroid, so you feel tired all the time. In addition, PCBs can build up in the fatty tissue of fish that live in contaminated rivers or coastal areas. Eating those fish cause a build-up of PCBs in your fatty tissue as well. Limit your exposure by trimming the skin and fat from raw and cooked fish and avoid fried fish.

B CHECKUP FOR TOXIN ISSUES

Your detoxification organs include your gut, liver, kidneys, and skin. To operate as intended, they must be healthy. Your liver, for instance, filters blood to identify and hold toxins. Its enzyme systems break them down, and the liver produces bile to excrete them. Your liver has finite toxin-processing capacity, which means it is highly vulnerable to toxic overload.

Your kidneys filter all your blood 60 times per day. Because kidney function decreases with age—about 50 percent from age 20 to 85—your support is critical.[67]

Chapter 7 offers ways to check up on your gut. For the other organs, keep reading.

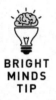

BRIGHT MINDS TIP

Note: If you have limited resources, skip the expensive lab tests and spend your money on high-quality, detoxifying food.

Lab tests
LIVER FUNCTION
- **ALT (SGPT)**—normal range: 7–56 units per liter (U/L)
- **AST (SGOT)**—normal range: 5–40 U/L
- **Bilirubin**—normal range: 0.2–1.2 mg/dL
- **Zinc**—normal range: 60–110 mcg/dL (low zinc will limit detoxification in the liver)

If liver function tests are high, check for excessive sugar and simple carbohydrate intake, alcohol use/abuse, hepatitis or medications that raise liver enzymes, such as acetaminophen (Tylenol).

KIDNEY FUNCTION
- **BUN**—normal range: 7–20 mg/dL
- **Creatinine**—normal range: 0.5–1.2 mg/dL

SKIN
- **Check for rashes, acne, and rosacea**—may be signs of detoxification problems

If mold is suspected

- **TGF Beta-1**—This blood test measures a protein found throughout the body that plays a role in immune system function and is often high in mold exposure (also called mycotoxin exposure). It can also be raised because of certain infections, such as Lyme disease. The normal level is below 2,380; 0 is optimal. Mold exposure can raise this to greater than 15,000.
- **Real Time Labs mycotoxin test** (http://www.realtimelab.com/home)

If heavy metals are suspected

- **Hair sample and urinary "challenge" tests are common**—for these urine tests, a chelating agent is administered prior to collecting the specimen

PRESCRIPTIONS FOR REDUCING YOUR TOXINS RISK FACTORS (AND THE FOUR CIRCLES THEY REPRESENT)

The Strategies

You can reduce your toxic load with three simple strategies:

(SP) 1. **Care about your detoxification organs.**

(B)(P)(S)(SP) 2. **Avoid toxins as much as possible:**

- **Quit smoking** (social circle if you smoke because others are doing it, psychological circle because you have to believe you can quit, and spiritual circle because you have to know why you want to quit). Hypnosis, nicotine patches, or the medication bupropion can help you quit.

- **Address drug and/or alcohol abuse.** What are the underlying causes of why you use? Determine if something such as anxiety or depression is leading you to self-medicate with drugs or alcohol. I recommend going off marijuana completely. (See explanation for social, psychological, and spiritual circles at the end of "Quit smoking" section above.)

- **Gradually replace "silver" dental fillings.** Do not get any new silver amalgams; ask for ceramic fillings. Remove amalgam fillings as soon as possible, but not all at once because of the risk of releasing toxins into the bloodstream. Do just one or two at a time.

- Avoid aluminum and Teflon cookware.

- Buy and store foods in glass jars when possible; plastic containers may contain phthalates and BPAs. Never reheat foods in plastic containers.

B S 3. **Reduce toxin-contaminated foods in your diet** (social circle because your friends and family influence your eating habits).

- **Go organic** (and always wash your produce). When a family switched to organic food for two weeks, a study found that the pesticides levels in their urine went down by 95 percent.[68] Another study revealed that children who ate conventionally grown foods had neurotoxic pesticide levels nine times higher than those who ate organic.[69] The Environmental Working Group publishes an annual list of the foods that have the highest/lowest pesticide levels; check it out at the EWG website (www.ewg.org).

- **Always read food labels.** If you do not know what an ingredient is, don't eat it or put it on your body. Here are chemicals, additives, and preservatives to avoid:

  - Potassium bromate—carcinogenic

  - BHA, BHT—linked to tumors

  - Sodium benzoate—may damage DNA

  - Sodium nitrate—linked to cancer

  - Tartrazine dye (makes cheese yellow)—linked to asthma

  - Monosodium glutamate (MSG)—linked to seizures and heart issues. (MSG is also called glutamic acid, hydrolyzed protein, autolyzed protein, autolyzed yeast extract, and textured protein.)

  - Red Dye #40

  - Artificial sweeteners—Aspartame (blue packets) and saccharin (pink packets) are both linked to obesity,[70] diabetes,[71] and cancer.[72] Sucralose (yellow packets) has the potential of direct toxic effects. It may also induce glucose intolerance by disrupting gut health.[73]

- **Ignore the word *natural* on labels.** It means nothing. (After all, arsenic and cyanide are natural.)

- **Limit or eliminate produce grown with pesticides and herbicides**; dairy raised with hormones and antibiotics; meats raised with hormones, antibiotics, or grain-fed; and farm-raised fish that is grain-fed or includes PCBs.

- **Avoid processed meats**, such as bacon and deli meats (they contain nitrosamines, which cause the liver to produce fats that are toxic to the brain).

- **Drink** no more than two to four normal-size alcoholic drinks a week; choose wine and beer over aged liquors.

- **Do a food detox.** For two weeks, eliminate:[74]

  - Processed foods

  - Glutens (found in flour, triticale, triticum, semolina, durum, Kamut, wheat, rye, and barley, this substance can increase gut permeability—even in people who are not sensitive to them.)

  - Dairy

  - Nonorganic beef and chicken (to avoid hormones, antibiotics, and arsenic)

  - Farm-raised fish

  - "Dirty Dozen" produce items, designated by the EWG (go to https://www.ewg.org/foodnews/summary.php)

  - Soy (high levels of arsenic, cadmium; 96 percent in United States is genetically modified)

  - Artificial sweeteners

  - Alcohol and recreational drugs

  - Water that has not been purified or proven to be clean

B 4. **Purify your air.**

- **Have your home tested for mold,** and eliminate it whether or not you have any symptoms.

- Avoid burning wood fires in fireplaces; they release toxic compounds.

- Regularly swap out the filters on your heating and cooling systems.

B 5. Reduce your use of unsafe health and beauty aids.[75]

- **Do a bathroom cleanse.** Download the Think Dirty app (www.thinkdirtyapp.com), which rates products on a scale of 1–10 (10 = the most toxic), and scan all the products in your bathroom. If you love yourself, throw out toxic products. After downloading this app, I threw away more than 70 percent of the products in my bathroom.

- **Use natural products without fragrance that are low in chemicals and free of phthalates.** This can really make a difference: 100 teenage girls who avoided these chemicals for just three days had significantly lower toxins in their urine.[76] These products may be more expensive in the short run, but they will be cheaper in the long run as you will spend less money on doctors and medicine.

B 6. Really clean the house.

- **Install carbon monoxide alarms and nonradioactive smoke alarms.**

- **Clean with fragrance-free, chemical-free, natural household cleansers.**

- **Clean, dust, and vacuum regularly.**

- **Do not Scotchgard anything in the home.**

- **Periodically check for black mold** in any part of your home that is exposed to water (e.g., under sinks).

- **Limit volatile organic compounds (VOCs) at home** by using VOC-free cleaning products, no- or low-VOC bedding materials made from natural products, low-VOC paints, and throw rugs instead of new carpeting.

B 7. Engage in habits to strengthen your detoxification systems.

- **Support your gut.** (See chapter 7, "I is for Inflammation.")

- Add fiber and fiber-rich foods, which bind to toxins and help your gastrointestinal system get rid of them. In the past, humans ate 100–150 grams of fiber a day. Americans now eat an average of 15 grams.[77] Women should consume at least 25 grams; men, 30 grams.

- **Support your liver.**

  - Limit alcohol and eat brassicas (detoxifying vegetables, such as brussels sprouts, cabbage, broccoli, and cauliflower).

  - Take the nutraceuticals that support your liver.

    - N-acetylcysteine (NAC)—NAC raises blood, liver, cellular, and mitochondrial levels of cysteine and the super-antioxidant glutathione. It also helps decrease the toxicity of chemotherapeutic drugs and antibiotics.[78]
    Dose suggestion: 600 mg twice a day

    - Vitamin C
    Dose suggestion: 1,000 mg twice a day

    - Artichoke extract—significantly increases bile excretion from the liver for two to three hours.[79]
    Dose suggestion: 500 mg twice a day

- **Support your kidneys.**

  - Drink three to four quarts of clean water a day. "The solution to pollution is dilution." Water helps flush toxins from your kidneys. Filter your water with charcoal or reverse osmosis. Check the purity of your local water supply with this EPA link: https://ofmpub.epa.gov/apex/safewater/f?p=136:102.

  - Take the nutraceuticals that support your kidneys.

    - Magnesium glycinate, citrate or malate
    Dose suggestion: 200 mg twice a day

    - Ginkgo biloba extract—increases blood flow to brain and kidneys[80] and helps protect against glyphosates.[81]
    Dose suggestion: 60–120 mg twice a day

B • **Support your skin.**
Your skin is the largest organ in your body.[82] It reflects the
health of your brain.

- Work up a sweat during exercise. Sweating naturally
  cleanses your system. The concentration of most toxins—
  including arsenic, cadmium, lead, and mercury—is 2 to
  10 times higher in sweat than in blood, which indicates
  that the body is effectively using sweating as a significant
  detoxification process.[83] The more you sweat with
  exercise,[84] the more you increase glutathione production,
  one of the most important detoxifiers;[85] protect against
  PCB exposure;[86] and eliminate phthalates[87] and BPA;[88] plus
  it keeps your skin healthy.

- Take a sauna. Research shows that saunas lower toxins
  in firefighters.[89] In a follow-up study over 20 years, the
  findings revealed an inverse relationship between sauna
  bathing and serious memory problems. Men who only had
  one sauna session per week versus those who had two to
  seven saunas were, respectively, 22 percent or 66 percent
  less likely to have dementia.[90] In other research, those who
  had frequent sauna baths also had a lower incidence of
  sudden cardiac death and death from all causes,[91] reduced
  depression;[92] increased endorphins,[93] testosterone, and
  growth hormone; and lowered cortisol[94] and blood sugar.[95]
  When you take a sauna, sweat profusely for 20 to 30
  minutes.[96]

- Take the nutraceuticals that support your skin.

  - Vitamin D
    Dose suggestion: 2,000 IUs a day or more, depending on your level

  - Vitamin E
    Dose suggestion: 60 mg of mixed tocopherols

  - Omega-3 fatty acids
    *Dose suggestion: 1,400 mg or more with a ratio of approximately
    60/40 EPA to DHA*

BRIGHT MINDS: TOXINS

STEPS TO CREATE MENTAL ILLNESS ... AND MAKE MY NIECES, ALIZÉ AND AMELIE, SUFFER	STEPS TO END MENTAL ILLNESS ... AND KEEP MY NIECES, ALIZÉ AND AMELIE, HEALTHY
1. Don't care about your detoxification organs.	1. Care about your detoxification organs.
2. Engage in habits that increase your exposure to toxins.	2. Avoid toxins as much as possible.
	3. Engage in habits to strengthen your detoxification systems.
• Smoke cigarettes, use marijuana, and drink excessive amounts of alcohol.	• Quit smoking, stop using marijuana, and limit alcohol to two to four glasses a week.
• Eat pesticide-laden foods.	• Remove "silver" dental fillings.
• Consume processed foods with chemicals, additives, and preservatives.	• Reduce your consumption of toxin-contaminated foods.
• Eat meat and dairy treated with hormones and antibiotics.	• Choose organic foods when possible.
• Eat fish containing PCBs.	• Always wash your fruits and vegetables.
• Use plastic food containers and reheat food in them.	• Avoid processed foods and those with chemical ingredients.
• Don't bother thinking about how much water you drink.	• Choose meat and dairy that is antibiotic and hormone-free.
• Expose yourself to mold.	• Drink three to four quarts of clean water a day.
• Routinely light a fire in the fireplace at home.	• Check your home for mold and eliminate it.
• Don't change the filters of your heating and cooling systems.	• Do a bathroom cleanse to eliminate unsafe cleaning and personal care products.
• Use cleaning products and personal care products with chemicals and fragrances.	• Support your gut (see chapter 7, "I is for Inflammation").
3. Avoid the strategies that strengthen your detoxification systems.	• Exercise to work up a sweat and detoxify your skin.
	• Consider nutraceuticals to support your liver, kidneys, and skin.

Pick One BRIGHT MINDS Toxins Tiny Habit to Start Today

TINY HABITS

1. When I go grocery shopping, I will buy organic whenever possible.

2. When pumping gas, I will not stand at the pump and breathe in any fumes.

3. When I visit friends and family, I will avoid secondhand smoke.

4. When I drink alcohol, I will limit my intake to no more than two to four glasses a week.

5. When I take my supplements, I will include N-acetyl-cysteine (NAC).

6. When I make meals, I will include brassicas for their detoxifying ability.

7. When I go shopping, I will avoid handling cash register receipts (the BPA in their plastic coating can get through your skin).

8. When I drink, I won't use plastic straws.

9. When I go to the store, I will not buy anything with MSG, artificial dyes, or preservatives.

10. When I am about to buy or use a cleaning or personal care product, I will scan it first on an app like Think Dirty or Healthy Living (ewg.org) and will not use any that contain toxins.

CHAPTER 11

M IS FOR MIND STORMS

SOOTHING THE ABNORMAL ELECTRICAL ACTIVITY THAT DRIVES MOOD SWINGS, ANXIETY, AND AGGRESSION

There was always one instant just before the epileptic fit . . . when suddenly in the midst of sadness, spiritual darkness and oppression, his brain seemed momentarily to catch fire, and in an extraordinary rush, all his vital forces were at their highest tension. The sense of life, the consciousness of self, were multiplied almost ten times at these moments which lasted no longer than a flash of lightning. His mind and his heart were flooded with extraordinary light; all his uneasiness, all his doubts, all his anxieties were relieved at once; they were all resolved in a lofty calm, full of serene, harmonious joy and hope, full of reason and ultimate meaning. But these moments, these flashes, were only a premonition of that final second (it was never more than a second) with which the fit began.

FYODOR DOSTOEVSKY (WHO SUFFERED WITH TEMPORAL LOBE EPILEPSY), *THE IDIOT*

I walked into my California clinic one day, and my office manager quickly pulled me aside and said, "Daniel, you have to see Tommy." I let her know that I already had 14 people on my schedule. But she just dismissed me and said, "Daniel, you need to see Tommy. He's really cute. He's nine years old. He's from Orlando, Florida. And he's read your book *Change Your Brain, Change Your Life*." Okay, a nine-year-old who read my book? Now I was paying attention.

I found Tommy in one of the other doctor's offices, and when the young boy saw me, he yelled, "Hey, you're Dr. Amen!" What he said next absolutely floored me. "Dr. Amen, I have a left temporal lobe problem."

"Really?" I asked. "How do you know?"

He said he had taken the checklist in the book. "I have a really bad temper, and you write that people who have bad tempers often have temporal lobe problems." He was right. Then he added, "And I used to see ghosts." I asked him what he meant, and he said, "I used to see these green things float in front of my eyes. I thought they were ghosts, and they would scare me until I read your book and realized they were just illusions that people with temporal lobe problems get." Then he looked at me with his big, beautiful blue eyes and said, "Last year, to get rid of the bad thoughts in my head, I tried to kill myself."

The thought of this sweet young boy trying to kill himself because he thought he was seeing monsters broke my heart. But he was right. People who have temporal lobe problems do tend to have dark, evil, awful thoughts; I think of them as mind storms. And sadly, they often try to kill themselves. Tommy completely blew me away. I asked him if he had seen his scan yet, and he said no.

"Want to?" I asked.

"Oh, yeah!" he replied.

So I took him and his parents to the imaging center, and when I showed him his scan, it was very clear that he had a left temporal lobe abnormality.

TOMMY'S SURFACE SPECT SCAN

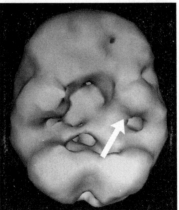

Decreased activity left temporal lobe

"See, I was right," he said. A nine-year-old had accurately predicted what his own brain scan would look like. When he was able to confirm that his mind storms were actually just temporal lobe problems, it gave him hope that we could help him get rid of those bad illusions. That's where the power is in this—you can figure out your brain health/mental health issues even without being scanned. In my mind, that's so exciting and powerful, leading to what's most important—you getting well.

TIM AND WENDY

Since 51 percent of the population will have a mental health issue at some point in life,[1] I often say during lectures that "normal" is a myth. It is more normal to have an issue than to not have an issue. "Normal" is a setting on your dryer or a city in Illinois. I once gave a lecture in Normal, Illinois. It was fun to go to the Normal grocery store, be interviewed on the Normal radio station, and finally meet Normal people. Since I'm from California, that was a treat. Yet I found the Normal people there actually had the same problems I had seen everywhere else. At the lecture, I met a psychologist, Wendy, who told me her husband, Tim, was really struggling. He had been arrested for domestic violence, and Wendy was on the verge of divorcing him, which was breaking her heart. She loved him and knew something was the matter with his brain, even though her own therapist said he had a personality disorder and she should leave as soon as possible. So Wendy and Tim flew to California to see me.

Tim was 54 years old and told me he struggled with memory problems, depression, and irritability. He also frequently saw shadows out of the corner of his eyes and heard an annoying buzzing sound, for which his doctor could not find a cause. His temper flare-ups just seemed to come out of the blue. "The littlest things set me off. Then I feel terribly guilty," he said, crying. "If she leaves me, I don't know what I will do, even though I understand why everyone tells her she should go. Please help me stop these rage attacks."

When Tim was six years old, he fell out of a second-story window. He didn't remember if he lost consciousness, and his parents were no longer alive to ask. As a child, he had learning problems and had gone to the principal's office a lot for fighting. He had tried antidepressant medications, psychotherapy, and couples counseling, but they didn't help. His brain SPECT study showed significantly low activity in his prefrontal cortex (PFC) and left temporal lobe. Low PFC activity often is associated with poor forethought and impulse control. Abnormal activity in the temporal lobes, especially the left side, is associated with mood instability, irritability, learning and memory problems, illusions (such as seeing shadows and hearing buzzing), and rage for little to no reason. It can cause storms of activity in the brain that hijack the mind.

As a young psychiatrist, I was inspired by the story of the late Jack Dreyfus, the financier who founded the successful Dreyfus Fund. In his 1981 book, *A Remarkable Medicine Has Been Overlooked*, he told the story of how, despite his fame and fortune, he awakened in terror and fell into a deep depression that conventional treatments didn't help. He sensed electricity in his body that intensified his feelings of fear, anger, and anxiety, and it reminded him of epileptics he had seen. He asked his doctor if he could try the anti-seizure medication phenytoin (Dilantin), and within a day of taking it, his symptoms of emotional distress began to dissipate. In his book, he wrote, "A few days later my need for psychotherapy was gone."[2] Dreyfus went on to spend $60 million of his own money to study the usefulness of Dilantin for a variety of "mental health" conditions, such as anxiety, violence, and mood swings.

When I first learned about brain SPECT in 1991, one of its primary uses was in evaluating seizure disorders. When patients were having seizures, there was increased activity on SPECT; in between seizures, there was decreased activity. Neurosurgeons often used SPECT to know where to operate on patients with uncontrollable seizures. I thought of Jack's story while working with Wendy and Tim.

On the anti-seizure medication lamotrigine (Lamictal) to stabilize Tim's left temporal lobe, then a stimulant to activate his PFC, along with neurofeedback and our other BRIGHT MINDS strategies, Tim's rage attacks stopped, his memory improved, and his relationship with Wendy became the best it had been in 20 years. Wendy later told me that our work together completely changed how she worked with her own clients.

TIM'S SURFACE SPECT SCAN

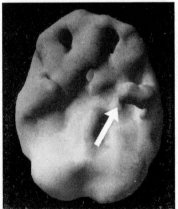

Decreased PFC and left temporal lobe activity (arrow)

THE WORLD'S MOST POWERFUL HYBRID ELECTROCHEMICAL ENGINE

Your brain is the world's most powerful hybrid electrochemical engine. It uses electricity and neurotransmitters to help you think, feel, and act. Electricity (the flow of charged ions) is constantly moving throughout your body, causing your heart to beat and your muscles to contract. Yet nowhere is electricity better documented than in the roughly 100 billion biological wires (neurons) in your brain.

A neuron's main job is to generate an electrical signal called an action potential, which occurs if it is sufficiently "excited" by other nerve cells. The action potential of a single neuron is like a tiny lightning bolt—this is part of the reason why neuroscientists talk about neurons "firing" when they're active—and it may stimulate many other neurons. The stimulated neurons can then generate their own action potentials, which travel to and stimulate still more neurons, creating a coordinated network that performs a specific brain function.

Action potentials race down axons at about 60 miles per hour. The signals can travel this quickly because, as the human brain develops from childhood to adulthood, axons are wrapped and insulated by a special fatty substance called myelin that enhances transmission speeds. Axons that are not insulated by myelin, either by design or disease, transmit signals 10 times slower.

ACTION POTENTIAL

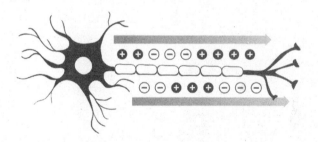

A neuron's main job is to generate an electrical signal called an action potential, which occurs if it is sufficiently "excited" by other nerve cells.

The Actors in Your Brain

An axon branches thousands of times, with each branch forming an electrical or chemical contact, called a synapse, to another neuron. The synaptic space is the tiny area between connecting neurons. At the end of each of the axon's many branches is a mushroom-shaped terminal, which contains molecules called neurotransmitters. Neurotransmitters can excite or quiet (inhibit) other neurons. Each neuron makes a single type of neurotransmitter, such as glutamate, gamma-aminobutyric acid (GABA), dopamine, norepinephrine, serotonin, acetylcholine, or histamine. The primary excitatory neurotransmitter, glutamate, is released by 75 percent of all neurons in the brain, and the primary inhibitory neurotransmitter, GABA, is released by about 20 percent of all neurons in the brain. When the action potential reaches the end of the axon, it stimulates the release of thousands of neurotransmitter molecules into the synaptic space. The neurotransmitters float across this space, and some of them will bind to receptors on the receiving ends of neurons and may stimulate or inhibit action in the receiving neurons.

All of this electrical activity is taking place inside your skull on a millisecond-by-millisecond basis. And it needs to occur precisely for optimal brain functioning and good mental health.

HOW DISEASES IMPAIR BRAIN FUNCTION

Some diseases of the brain start by damaging the brain's wiring or impairing the ability to create the right amount of electricity. In a sort of Goldilocks scenario, too much electricity or too little electricity can be a problem. It needs to be just right. Brain trouble can occur because of

- Fewer synapses in a network, which is common in depression or a lack of mental or physical exercise
- Fewer neurons in a network, which happens in Alzheimer's disease
- Impaired generation of action potentials, which can happen if you have three or more alcoholic drinks at a time
- Damage to neurons that slow the speed of action potentials, common in head trauma or strokes
- Excessive electrical activity, seen in seizure disorders

Abnormal electrical activity not only can change the activity of the brain, but can also change the mind and cause mind storms that can be associated with temper outbursts, depression, suicidal thoughts, panic attacks, distractibility, and confusion. As far back as 1907,[3] Emil Kraepelin discussed interictal dysphoric disorder (IDD)—*ictal* refers to seizure states; *interictal* means between seizures. He observed depressive symptoms mixed with euphoric moods, irritability, fear, and anxiety as well as with intense fatigue, pain, and insomnia in patients with untreated epilepsy.

Abnormal electrical activity can not only change the activity of the brain, but it can also change your mind and cause mind storms that can be associated with temper outbursts, depression, suicidal thoughts, panic attacks, distractibility, and confusion.

Mind Storms Risk Factors
(and the Four Circles They Represent)

- **B** • Seizures or history of seizures

- **P** • Periods of spaciness or confusion

- **B** • Frequent complaints that things look, sound, taste, smell, or feel "funny"

- **P** • Sudden, repeated fear or anger

- **P** • Irritability that tends to build, explode, and then recede, often leaving one feeling tired after a rage

- **P** • Periods of panic and/or fear for no specific reason

- **B** • Visual or auditory changes, such as seeing shadows or hearing muffled sounds

- **P** • Frequent periods of déjà vu (feelings of being somewhere you have been before)

- **P** • Mild paranoia

- **B** • Headaches or abdominal pain of uncertain origin

The tactics of an evil ruler to promote mind storms are simple.

THE EVIL RULER WOULD...	THE BENEVOLENT RULER WOULD...
Discourage the population from getting brain scans or other diagnostic tests to see if their psychiatric symptoms are being caused by abnormal electrical activity.	Encourage people to get brain scans or other diagnostic tests to determine if abnormal electrical activity may be at the root of symptoms of mental illness.

PRESCRIPTIONS FOR REDUCING YOUR MIND STORMS RISK FACTORS
(AND THE FOUR CIRCLES THEY REPRESENT)

The Strategies

SP 1. **Care about how your brain cells fire and talk to each other.**

B P S SP 2. **Avoid anything that increases mind storms.** Are there lifestyle or food choices that make seizures or mind storms more likely? Yes, there are many, including:

- Stress
- Tiredness
- Lack of sleep
- Forgetting medications
- Hyperventilating
- Alcohol and drug abuse
- Low or high blood sugar states
- Missing meals
- Premenstrual syndrome (PMS)
- Illnesses
- Pain
- Video games for vulnerable brains
- Excessive screen time
- Unrecognized Irlen syndrome (see page 167 in chapter 9, "<u>H</u> Is for Head Trauma")

B S 3. **Be aware of the triggering effect of certain foods, food colors, and food preservatives**—especially sugar, MSG, aspartame, and Red Dye #40—on mind storms (social because your family and friends influence what you eat). For example, one of my patients became violent whenever he ate foods prepared with monosodium glutamate (MSG). When we scanned his brain after ingesting MSG, we saw that his brain had changed into a pattern more consistent with our aggressive patients. This is important: MSG doesn't have to be labeled unless it is a single food additive. It can be disguised by being added in with other ingredients and not disclosed. It is commonly hidden in bouillon, soy protein isolate, vegetable protein isolate, and whey protein isolate. Note that anytime the words *yeast extract* appear, it is actually MSG.

When Trey was seven years old, his parents noticed that whenever he ate something bright red or drank a red Slurpee, he had various tics and strange neurological affectations, and his behavior became more aggressive and hostile. He would cry easily and storm off in a huff or throw things. His mother tried to minimize these foods in his diet, but he would often get them at school: Cheetos, Doritos, fruit punch, Red Vines, lollipops, and so on. What she didn't realize was that many of the "healthy" foods she was serving him at home—strawberry yogurt, whole-grain strawberry bars, and even canned pasta sauce and ketchup—contained an ingredient common to those other snack foods: a dye called Red #40.

When Trey reached the age of 14, his folks brought him to the Amen Clinics to confirm their suspicion that he was reacting to this food additive. His brain SPECT scan showed remarkable overall increased activity (mind storms) with exposure to Red Dye #40. After seeing the impact this common food coloring had on their son, Trey's parents became vigilant about reading every nutrition label closely and stayed away from the offending item. By staying away from Red Dye #40, Trey stabilized his moods and behaviors and became a kind, sweet, helpful young man.

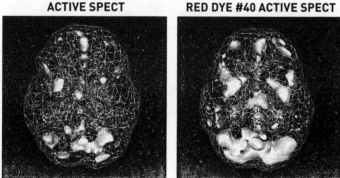

TREY'S BASELINE ACTIVE SPECT

RED DYE #40 ACTIVE SPECT

Mild increased activity

Dramatic increased activity with Red Dye #40

B P S 4. **Be cautious with video games and flashing lights.** If you have a vulnerable brain, avoid flashing lights and excessive video game playing. I've had a number of patients who have had seizures while playing video games even though they did not have prior seizures, and others who became violent or highly emotional from video game play. It is a phenomenon called *photophobic seizures*, which happened to 685 children in Japan on December 16, 1997, while they were watching a Pokémon animated series.[4]

In the show, the animators used a rare rapid strobing technique that flashed red and blue lights to make an explosion look especially cool. Suddenly, children across Japan passed out, had blurred vision, felt dizzy or nauseous, had seizures, or experienced temporary blindness. The incident, which became known in Japan as Pokémon Shock, was a disaster for children's animation in Japan, and Pokémon and Nintendo stocks took a hit.[5]

Other patients of mine have become violent after playing video games. Granted, these cases may be extreme, but I cannot see much good that comes from playing these games for hours a day, and I believe they have the potential for harm. My best advice at this point is be careful and limit screen time and video game exposure to no more than one hour a day.

5. **Engage in behaviors that decrease mind storms.**

(SP) • **Spend time in prayer or meditation every day.** I mentioned this in chapter 5 to help improve blood flow; these practices also help manage stress.

(B) • **Take antiseizure medications:** At Amen Clinics, we use antiseizure medications, when appropriate, to calm the mind storms of our patients. We tend to use

  • Lamotrigine and valproic acid for bipolar disorder

  • Lamotrigine for resistant depression

  • Gabapentin for social anxiety, irritability, insomnia, and pain

  • Pregabalin for pain

  • Oxcarbazepine for irritability and moodiness

  • Topiramate for binge eating disorders and migraines

  It's also important to note that prescribing treatment and medications in the right order is critical for healing. For example, for some people with mind storms, we start with antiseizure medications, then recommend a ketogenic diet (see below), then proceed with other therapies. Doing it the other way around may not have been as effective.

B   • **The ketogenic diet:** This diet has been used in treatment-resistant epilepsy since the 1920s. It cuts seizure frequency in children by more than 50 percent.[6] There are a number of studies showing it may also be helpful for mood stabilization.[7] One of my patients who had a severe case of premenstrual dysphoric disorder (PMDD) noticed her moods were significantly better on the diet. Right before her period, her brain showed severe overactivity, which lessened considerably on the diet.

The ketogenic diet can be challenging to maintain, but when it works it can be powerfully effective. The main idea is for you to get more calories from protein and fat and significantly less from carbohydrates. You cut back on carbohydrates that are easy to digest, like sugar, soda, pastries, and white bread—you should do this anyway. When you eat less than 50 grams of carbohydrates a day, your body runs out of blood sugars and eventually (usually after three to four days) starts to break down protein and fat for energy. This is called ketosis. People use this diet most often to lose weight because it takes more calories to convert fat into energy than it does to convert carbohydrates, and it helps you feel fuller longer, but it has also been shown to help seizures, diabetes,[8] acne,[9] and even some forms of cancer.[10]

B P   • **Neurofeedback:** Neurofeedback can help calm electrical activity in the brain by training you to gain control of your brain waves through self-regulation. See chapter 9 "H Is for Head Trauma" for details.

B P S   6. **Get seven to eight hours of sleep each night** (social because your work, family, or friends may influence how late you stay up or get up). See chapter 15, "S Is for Sleep."

B   7. **Take nutraceuticals that help calm or control the excitability of the brain.** Work with your physician to determine which one is best for you and the right dose.

• **Magnesium** has a calming effect on neuronal function, is involved in more than 300 biochemical reactions in your body, is vital for your body to make energy, and plays a key role in blood sugar regulation. Low magnesium is associated with seizures, inflammation, diabetes, anxiety, and depression.[11] With the standard American diet, 68 percent of Americans do not consume enough magnesium. Some researchers believe that supplementing magnesium can decrease seizure frequency,[12] and others have shown it is helpful for severe stress,[13] migraines, depression, chronic pain, anxiety, and strokes.[14] The mineral is found in green leafy vegetables, such as spinach, kale, and Swiss chard; legumes; nuts; and seeds. In general, foods that contain dietary fiber provide magnesium.

Dose suggestion: The typical adult dose is 50–400 mg a day.

- **GABA** (gamma-aminobutyric acid) is an amino acid that helps to regulate brain excitability and calms overfiring in the brain. GABA and GABA enhancers, such as the anticonvulsant gabapentin and L-theanine (found in green tea), function to inhibit the excessive firing of neurons, which results in a feeling of calmness and more self-control. Low levels of GABA have been found in many mental health disorders, including anxiety and some forms of depression. Rather than overeating or drinking or using drugs to calm your anxiety, natural ways to boost GABA may help. I often recommend GABA supplements. Researchers report that GABA does not cross the blood brain barrier (a network of blood vessels that protect the brain), but the studies are contradictory,[15] with some showing an increase in alpha brain waves (which indicate a relaxed state).[16] Nonetheless, GABA still has a calming influence on the brain imaging studies we have done.

  Dose suggestion: The typical recommended dosage ranges from 100 to 1,500 mg daily for adults and from 50 to 750 mg daily for children. For best effect, GABA should be taken in two or three doses a day.

BRIGHT MINDS: MIND STORMS

STEPS TO CREATE MENTAL ILLNESS . . . AND MAKE MY NIECES, ALIZÉ AND AMELIE, SUFFER	STEPS TO END MENTAL ILLNESS . . . AND KEEP MY NIECES, ALIZÉ AND AMELIE, HEALTHY
1. Don't care about how your brain cells fire with one another.	1. Care about the electrical activity in your brain.
2. Engage in habits that increase your risk for mind storms. • Live a stress-filled life. • Skimp on sleep. • Abuse drugs and alcohol. • Consume a diet high in sugar and skip meals. • Eat foods containing Red Dye #40, MSG, and other food additives • Don't address premenstrual syndrome (PMS) or chronic pain. • Play video games for hours on end. • Use fluorescent lights	2. Avoid anything that increases your risk for mind storms. 3. Engage regularly in healthy habits that decrease the risk for mind storms and treat them when necessary. • Practice stress-management techniques. • Get seven to eight hours of sleep each night. • Eliminate drugs and limit alcohol. • Consider a ketogenic diet. • Seek treatment for PMS or chronic pain conditions. • Limit video games. • Consider neurofeedback and nutraceuticals to calm overfiring in the brain. • Take antiseizure medication, if necessary.
3. Avoid the strategies that decrease your risk for mind storms.	

Pick One BRIGHT MINDS Mind Storms Tiny Habit to Start Today

TINY HABITS

1. When I feel stressed, I will use stress relief techniques like deep breathing and meditation to calm these feelings.

2. When I go shopping, I will avoid foods with a lot of sugar as well as those with dyes and preservatives.

3. When I play video games, I will limit it to one hour per day.

4. When it gets close to bedtime, I will follow a sleep routine to help me fall asleep faster.

5. When I eat, I will consider adopting a ketogenic diet.

CHAPTER 12

I IS FOR IMMUNITY AND INFECTIONS

ATTACKED FROM INSIDE AND OUT

Whenever the immune system deals successfully with an infection, it emerges from the experience stronger and better able to confront similar threats in the future. Our immune competence develops in combat. If, at the first sign of infection, you always jump in with antibiotics, you do not give the system a chance to test itself and grow stronger.

ANDREW WEIL

 JUAN

Juan, 22, was struggling in his studies at the University of Wisconsin, where he was a pre-law student. His family was from Spain, and they had sent many of their family members and friends to our clinic after I first treated the grandfather for depression years before. Juan had been diagnosed with attention deficit hyperactivity disorder (ADHD) as a child and had been taking stimulant medication from the time he was 10 years old. He said his medicine helped him focus, but it also made him more irritable, impatient, and moody. He was in danger of failing, even though he tested with a high IQ. He had recently become depressed and had entertained suicidal thoughts for the first time in his life.

As a young boy, Juan was easily distracted, had difficulty remaining seated, and struggled with following instructions. He remembers sitting in class one day and running out of the room when he saw a bird fly by the window. Once he started taking Ritalin, he was much better able to remain focused, but his mother recalls that once the medication wore out of his system in the evenings, Juan became irritable and agitated. His family described him as having a grumpy personality, especially when taking the medication. When he was an adolescent, he drank heavily, but the alcohol made him aggressive, so he stopped drinking.

During his last semester at school, his anxiety heightened when he realized he might not pass several of his classes. He started worrying more and having difficulty sleeping. He was prescribed Xanax to help him through this stressful time, and it was helpful for sleep, but it also caused memory problems.

His SPECT scan showed overall low activity at rest, in a toxic pattern that was very unusual for someone so young, and it improved with concentration, which is the opposite of what we typically see with people who have ADD/ADHD. We were left asking why his resting SPECT scan looked so bad. The different possibilities were drug and alcohol use, which he denied (we know addicts lie, so we tested him), an environmental toxin, such as mold or carbon monoxide poisoning, a past history of a loss of oxygen (from near drowning or a heart attack, which he did not have), severely low thyroid function or anemia, or an infectious disease process. On an infectious-disease panel, we discovered that Juan had been exposed to multiple past infections, including Lyme, Epstein Barr virus, *Toxoplasma gondii*, *Mycoplasma pneumoniae*, and human herpesvirus 6 (HHV-6). Being exposed to Lyme and HHV-6 decreases immune system function, making Juan more susceptible to other infections. His thyroid function was also low.

Once we treated Juan for the infections and his immune system strengthened, his mood, temper, focus, and grades improved. He no longer needed the stimulant medication and recently graduated with his law degree.

JUAN'S SURFACE SPECT SCAN AT REST

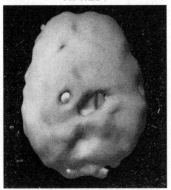

Overall low activity (looks toxic)

SURFACE SPECT SCAN WITH CONCENTRATION

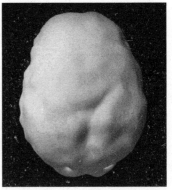

Overall improved (opposite of typical ADD/ADHD)

SPECT scans taught us that when brain health/mental health issues are not improving with standard treatment, it is critical to consider immune system issues and infections. In 30 years, I believe there will be a subspecialty in psychiatry dedicated specifically to these issues.

IMMUNITY: YOUR BODY'S NATURAL PROTECTION SYSTEM

Immunity is your body's natural protection system, and it carries out two primary functions—*defense* and *tolerance*. Your immune system *defends* against external invaders—think bacteria, viruses, and parasites—and it patrols your body for internal troublemakers, such as cancer cells. It also regulates your level of *tolerance* to potential environmental triggers, such as allergens (including pollen, bee stings, grasses, wheat, peanuts, soy, and corn).[1] When your immune system performs these two functions optimally, it helps keep you healthy. However, when your defenses don't do their job, or your body's tolerance level is too low or becomes overwhelmed, it makes you more vulnerable to infections, cancer, and autoimmune disorders, as well as increasing your risk for depression, anxiety, and even psychosis.

Your immune system performs its important mission in four ways:

- Identifies external invaders, internal cells, or tissues that are misbehaving
- Recruits your white blood cells to attack the bad guys
- Tags and decimates external and internal problems
- Remembers invaders and troublemakers in case they return

THE FOUR PRIMARY IMMUNE SYSTEM FUNCTIONS[2]

Defense against external environment	**Defense** against internal environment
If it fails, you get an <u>infection.</u>	If it fails, you get <u>cancer.</u>
Tolerance against external environment	**Tolerance** against internal environment
If it fails, you get <u>allergies.</u>	If it fails, you get an <u>autoimmune disease.</u>

Immune disorders fall into five categories, all of which impact your brain health/mental health:

1. **Immunodeficiency disorders:** These disorders can either be present from birth or result from an illness, such as human immunodeficiency virus (HIV) or acquired autoimmune deficiency syndrome (AIDS), which damages your immune system. People with HIV are twice as likely to experience depression, and they also have an increased risk of anxiety and cognitive disorders, including dementia.[3]

2. **Allergies:** When your immune system views neutral environmental "visitors," such as pollen or pet dander, as enemies, it can lead to allergies, asthma, eczema, or even life-threatening consequences. In a 2018 study including more than 186,000 people, those with asthma, hay fever, and eczema were 66 percent more likely to develop psychiatric disorders compared with those without allergies.[4] And asthma has been shown to increase the risk of dementia by 30 percent.[5]

3. **Cancers of the immune system:** Leukemia and lymphomas are the most common forms of cancer affecting the immune system. Cancer of any kind has long been associated with detrimental changes in emotional health, and research shows that cancer patients are more likely to have a mental health issue than people without the disease.[6] In fact, as many as 25 percent of cancer patients have clinical depression.[7]

4. **Autoimmune disorders:** When your immune system mistakes your own internal tissues for troublemakers and attacks them, it can create an autoimmune disorder. I typically refer to this as "friendly fire."

5. **Persistent infections:** When you experience recurring infections, it may be an indicator of a compromised immune system.

This chapter will go into greater detail about autoimmune disorders and infections, which have been associated with an increased risk for many different brain health/mental health issues. They will make people more likely to be unfocused, depressed, or anxious.

AUTOIMMUNE DISORDERS: THE INCREASED RISK FOR BRAIN ILLNESS/MENTAL ILLNESS

When the body's immune system is impaired, it can turn on you and attack and destroy your own healthy tissues by mistake, resulting in an autoimmune disorder. There are more than 100 different autoimmune disorders—including multiple sclerosis (MS), rheumatoid arthritis, systemic lupus erythematosus, Crohn's disease, psoriasis, Hashimoto's thyroiditis, and type 1 diabetes—affecting 80 million Americans. More than 75 percent of those suffering from an autoimmune disease are women.[8]

Lady Gaga, who suffers from fibromyalgia, is one of them. In 2019, while accepting an award from the Screen Actors Guild-American Federation of Television and Radio Artists Foundation, she said the chronic pain she felt was also accompanied by "panic attacks, acute trauma responses, and debilitating mental spirals that have included suicidal ideation and masochistic behavior."[9] She called mental health issues "a crisis of epic proportions" and advocated that the foundation implement a mental health program for actors. As in Lady Gaga's case, many autoimmune illnesses are linked with psychiatric issues. For example, having an autoimmune disease is associated with an increased risk for:

- Mood disorders (45 percent increased risk)[10]
- Schizophrenia (45 percent increased risk)[11]
- Bipolar disorder[12]
- ADD/ADHD[13]
- Dementia, including Alzheimer's disease[14]

Researchers are still trying to pinpoint the exact causes of autoimmune disorders, but many factors can play a role in their development, which I wrote about in *Memory Rescue*:

- Leaky gut (see chapter 7, "I Is for Inflammation")
- Environmental allergens—pollen, dust mites, mold
- Food allergens—dairy, eggs, fish, shellfish, tree nuts, peanuts, wheat, and soybeans are the top eight, according to the FDA
- Toxins (see chapter 10, "T Is for Toxins")
- Obesity (see chapter 14, "D Is for Diabesity")
- Head trauma (see chapter 9, "H Is for Head Trauma")
- Lack of exercise or excessive exercise
- Poor diet (see chapter 18, "Food Made Insanely Simple")
- Nutrient deficiencies
- Stress
- Sleep disorders (see chapter 15, "S Is for Sleep")
- Hidden infections (see section on infections on the following page)

The traditional treatment protocol for autoimmune disorders centers on suppressing the immune system with strong medications, such as nonsteroidal anti-inflammatory drugs (NSAIDs), corticosteroids, or anticancer drugs like methotrexate. A doctor might give you one medicine to treat arthritis and another one for Crohn's disease, but this isn't the best approach, according to my friend and colleague Mark Hyman, MD, director of the Center for Functional Medicine at the Cleveland Clinic. He says it is a mistake to think of these illnesses as separate conditions. In his view, it makes more sense to address all of them as one single disorder—your immune system attacking itself. If you suffer from any autoimmune disorder, he believes the first question to ask yourself is: *What is making my immune system so angry at me?* In my view, the best approach to get your immune system to stop attacking your body and start cooperating with it is to address all of your BRIGHT MINDS risk factors discussed in this book.[15]

INFECTIOUS DISEASES: INFECTING THE BRAIN, TOO

Infectious illnesses, including Lyme disease, *Streptococcus* (strep throat), *toxoplasmosis*, syphilis, *Helicobacter pylori (H. pylori)*, HIV/AIDS, herpes, and others, are a major cause of psychiatric and cognitive problems that few medical professionals recognize. In a large study from Denmark, researchers correlated infectious diseases in children with a significant increase in psychiatric problems later in life.[16] Another study from Denmark followed more than 3.5 million people, not necessarily children, and found that hospitalization for any infection increased the risk for later mood disorders by 62 percent.[17]

Back in 1991, when I first began using SPECT scans in my practice, I saw many patients who had been diagnosed with conditions like chronic fatigue syndrome (CFS) and fibromyalgia. Sadly, they were often made to feel that their illness was "all in their head" and were regarded by health-care professionals as "psychiatric patients." The medical community was either blaming their condition on stress or basically labeling them as "hysterical" and referring them to me. (It's very frustrating when doctors can't determine what's causing a person's condition, so they simply categorize them as "psychiatric." *Hey*, I think, *that's my job!*). Many of these patients' scans looked terrible (see the next scan), showing overall low blood flow caused by undiagnosed infections. Of course, these patients would seem hysterical, sad, irritable, or stressed! The organ of their behavior—the brain—was being damaged by an infection.[18] Clinical evidence now shows that CFS is an infectious disease,[19] and I hope more physicians will start testing for infections.

CHRONIC FATIGUE SYNDROME BRAIN SPECT SCAN

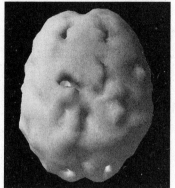

Overall low activity

Scientists have speculated that syphilis changed the course of history,[20] believing that Christopher Columbus and his sailing crew brought it with them to Europe. Thereafter, a number of notable rulers, musicians, and literary greats (King Charles VIII, Queen Mary I, Catherine the Great, Paul I, Vladimir Lenin) contracted it. Syphilis has been linked to psychological effects and a condition called neurosyphilis that can trigger psychiatric symptoms.[21]

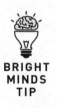

BRIGHT MINDS TIP

Your vulnerability to illness depends on many factors—the strength of your immune system, the level of exposure, stress, and daily habits. Addressing your BRIGHT MINDS risk factors can strengthen your immune system to reduce your risk.

In 2016, 33 scientists from around the world came together to write an editorial in the *Journal of Alzheimer's Disease*,[22] suggesting the medical community was overlooking infectious diseases as a root cause of many memory problems and dementia. Drawing on findings from more than 100 studies, they claimed that significant stress or anything else that suppresses the immune system can activate viruses that were dormant in the brain. Of course, exposure to infectious diseases doesn't mean you will get sick. Your vulnerability to illness depends on many factors—the strength of your immune system, the level of exposure, stress, and daily habits. Addressing your BRIGHT MINDS risk factors can strengthen your immune system to reduce your risk.

In the following section, you will see some of the most common infectious diseases we see at Amen Clinics that create psychiatric symptoms.

> *Infectious illnesses are a major cause of mental health issues that few medical professionals recognize.*

LYME DISEASE: THE TICK THAT CAN CREATE MENTAL ILLNESS

ADRIANNA

Adrianna, age 16, was a healthy, beautiful, honor-roll student when she went with her family on vacation to Yosemite National Park. When they arrived at their cabin, they were surrounded by six deer. It was a beautiful moment.

Ten days later, Adrianna became agitated and started having auditory hallucinations. Her parents sought help for Adrianna who was admitted to a psychiatric hospital and prescribed antipsychotic medications, which didn't help. The next three months were a torturous road of 25 doctors and multiple medications—all at a cost of tens of thousands of dollars. Adrianna had become a shadow of her former self. A doctor at Stanford University told her mother, "Your daughter will be schizophrenic for the rest of her life and will need medication for as long as she lives."

Unwilling to accept that diagnosis and desperate for a different path forward for her daughter, her mother, Deb, found my book *Change Your Brain, Change Your Life* and brought Adrianna to our clinic in Northern California for a scan. It showed evidence of inflammation with areas of unusually high activity. It caused us to look deeper at the potential causes of her symptoms, such as an infection or autoimmune system disorder. It turned out Adrianna had Lyme disease, an infection caused by deer ticks. Treatment with antibiotics helped her get her life back. She subsequently graduated from Pepperdine University and then Queen Mary University of London with a master's degree in international human resource management. Now, she is living a happy life. Nearly every day around noon, I get a text from Deb asking how she can pray for me.

SCHIZOPHRENIA VERSUS LYME[23]

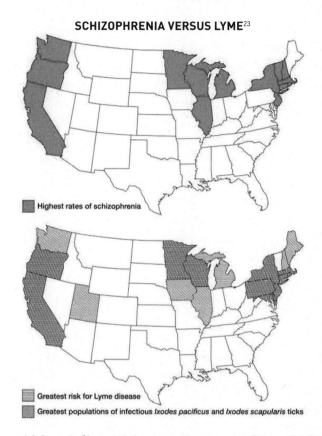

Highest rates of schizophrenia

Greatest risk for Lyme disease

Greatest populations of infectious *Ixodes pacificus* and *Ixodes scapularis* ticks

Source: J. S. Brown Jr., "Geographic Correlation of Schizophrenia to Ticks and Tick-Borne Encephalitis," *Schizophrenia Bulletin* 20, no. 4 (1994), 755–75; used with permission

In an amazing twist of fate, Adrianna's uncle had been committed to Napa State Hospital for 27 years for paranoid schizophrenia. It turned out he also had Lyme disease, which was only discovered after Adrianna's mother had to fight the hospital administration to have him released so he could be tested. Treating Lyme for her brother did not get rid of his hallucinations, but on a small dose of the antipsychotic medication clozapine he has been able to live with his family and is doing well as a free man. Subsequently, Deb has referred countless people to us to be tested for brain infections when their behaviors were off.

Like Adrianna, hundreds of people have come to the Amen Clinics with mental health issues that weren't responding to treatment and tested positive for Lyme disease. Many of them had been infected years or even decades previously, but nobody had ever thought to test them for infectious diseases. With the proper treatment, their symptoms improved significantly. In 2017, scientists from Australia and China reviewed eight clinical trials using the antibiotic minocycline, also used to treat Lyme disease, as an add-on treatment for schizophrenia, concluding it was significantly helpful for both positive symptoms (such as delusions, hallucinations, and agitation) and negative symptoms (decreased motivation, social withdrawal, and lethargy).[24]

For more evidence about the connection between infectious diseases and mental health, look at the two maps on the previous page. In the top image, you will see the highest incidence of schizophrenia in the United States, and in the bottom image, you will see the greatest risk for Lyme disease. It doesn't take an expert cartographer to see that the maps are nearly identical. In a "lifelong" psychotic illness, it is important to rule out infectious diseases and autoimmune disorders as causes of brain health/mental health symptoms.

TOXOPLASMA GONDII:
IS YOUR CAT MAKING YOU CRAZY?[25]

Pop quiz: What do cats have in common with the following?

- Alzheimer's disease
- Anxiety
- Bipolar disorder
- Depression
- Impulsive behavior
- Schizophrenia
- Suicidal thoughts

Answer: *Toxoplasma gondii*

Did you know that more than 40 million Americans may be infected by this tiny single-celled parasite that is often carried in cats and shed in their feces?[26] This infection, called *toxoplasmosis*, has a strong association with schizophrenia and bipolar disorder,[27] anxiety and depression,[28] as well as impulsive behavior and suicidal thoughts. It has also been linked to Alzheimer's and Parkinson's disease, autoimmune disorders, cancer, and heart disease.[29] If a pregnant woman becomes infected, she can pass the infection to her developing fetus, which can lead to brain damage or blindness at birth, or mental disabilities later in life.

Science writer Ed Yong recounts a most unusual love story in an unforgettable TED talk:

Toxo infects a wide variety of mammals, but it can only sexually reproduce in a cat. . . . If Toxo gets into a rat or a mouse, it turns the rodent into a cat-seeking missile. If the infected rat smells the delightful odor of cat piss, it runs toward the source of the smell rather than the more sensible direction of away. The cat eats the rat. Toxo gets to have sex. It's a classic tale of Eat, Prey, Love. . . . Toxo releases an enzyme that makes dopamine, a substance involved in reward and motivation. We know it targets certain parts of a rodent's brain, including those involved in sexual arousal. When you realize that a tiny parasite can control its host's behavior, it makes you wonder just how much control over our behavior we really have.[30]

TOXOPLASMA GONDII

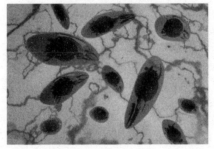

PANS, PANDAS, AND THE MIND

Most people know why it is important to treat strep throat. Left untreated, it can cause rheumatic heart disease and congestive heart failure. In the early 1990s, scientists from the National Institute of Mental Health (NIMH) reported it could also cause new-onset OCD and Tourette's (a tic disorder) in children and teenagers. The new disorder was called *pediatric autoimmune neuropsychiatric disorders associated with streptococcal infections* (PANDAS).

 ## HENRY

When Henry, 10, came to see me, he was on three psychiatric medications for anxiety, depression, ADHD, and Tourette's. His parents, who were going through a divorce, initially blamed his symptoms on the family stress, but his grandfather had been a patient at our clinic in New York, and he encouraged them to bring Henry to us. Henry's scan showed overall increased activity in a pattern that made me think his brain was inflamed. Further testing showed he had both Lyme disease and PANDAS. A year after treatment with anti-biotics and a brain-healthy lifestyle, his father told me Henry picked up four grade levels of learning and was a completely new child off all psychiatric medications.

HENRY'S ACTIVE SPECT SCAN

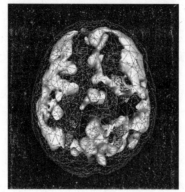

Overall increased activity, looking inflamed

Subsequent to PANDAS, neuroscientists realized other infectious agents, besides strep, could also cause emotional trouble, and they labeled the condition PANS (pediatric acute-onset neuropsychiatric syndrome). Their clinical presentation is almost identical. According to Dr. Susan Swedo at NIMH, "Parents will describe children with PANS as overcome by a 'ferocious' onset of obsessive thoughts, compulsive rituals, and overwhelming fears. Clinicians should consider PANS when children or adolescents present with such acute-onset of OCD or eating restrictions in the absence of a clear link to strep." PANS can be caused by numerous infections, including *Borrelia burgdorferi* (Lyme disease), mycoplasma pneumonia, herpes simplex, common cold, influenza, and other viruses.[31]

In an important study from Denmark,[32] patients who had infections, even those who did not require hospitalization, had a higher incidence of schizophrenia and depression. The researchers did not know if the infections attacking brain tissue were causing the mental health issues or the fact that they had taken antibiotics that changed the gut's microbiome had put people at higher risk of trouble.

FUNGAL INFECTIONS: AN ITCH YOU CAN'T IGNORE

The human body plays host to many types of fungi, including yeasts called *Candida*. One of the most common fungi is *Candida albicans*, which typically resides in small amounts in the gut microbiome and mouth. The good bugs (bacteria) in your gut usually keep *C. albicans* levels in check. However, some people with weakened immune systems can experience an overgrowth of the fungus—especially in warm, moist areas like the genitals or mouth—leading to a fungal infection called candidiasis that causes burning and itching (such as a vaginal yeast infection). These obvious symptoms may not be the only consequences of fungal infections. Emerging research shows a connection between these infections and brain health/mental health disorders.

A 2016 study from researchers at Johns Hopkins revealed that *Candida* yeast infections are more prevalent in men with bipolar disorder or schizophrenia compared with men who don't have these conditions. And among women with bipolar disorder or schizophrenia, those with fungal infections performed worse on memory tests than women who had no history of the infections.[33] One of the study authors, Emily Severance, PhD, says, "Most Candida infections can be treated in their early stages, and clinicians should make it a point to look out for these infections in their patients with mental illness."[34]

Fungal infections can impact brain health in other ways. New research on mice shows *Candida* infections can also contribute to memory loss and brain changes similar to those seen in Alzheimer's disease.[35] In this 2019 study, mice that were infected with the yeast infection showed reduced spatial memory, but after the infection was treated, their spatial memory returned to normal. The researchers also found that *C. albicans* can cross the blood brain barrier and impact the brain's immune cells, producing a sort of brain infection they suggest may play a role in the development of neurodegenerative diseases like Alzheimer's, Parkinson's, and MS.

What makes you more vulnerable to fungal infections?

- Weakened immune system
- Taking immunosuppressant medication
- Taking antibiotics or oral contraceptives
- High alcohol intake
- Consuming a diet high in sugar and refined carbohydrates
- Consuming a lot of fermented foods
- High stress levels
- Uncontrolled diabetes
- Mercury toxicity

If you've got an itch in places where you shouldn't, get it checked out and treated right away.

Immunity and Infections Risk Factors
(and the Four Circles They Represent)

B Autoimmune disorders, such as MS, rheumatoid arthritis, systemic lupus erythematosus, Crohn's disease, psoriasis, Hashimoto's thyroiditis, and type 1 diabetes

B • Unidentified infections, such as Lyme disease, toxoplasmosis, syphilis, *H. pylori*, HIV/AIDS, herpes, PANDAS (or PANS), *Candida* infections, and others

B • Low vitamin D level

B • Asthma and hay fever

B P S • Allergies to gluten, dairy, peanuts, corn, soy, and other foods and substances (psychological circle because you feel as if you "love" these foods, and social circle because you want to eat what everybody else is eating)

THE EVIL RULER WOULD . . .	THE BENEVOLENT RULER WOULD . . .
1. Disallow throat cultures for people with sore throats and never allow health-care professionals to test vitamin D levels.	1. Encourage people with sore throats to get a throat culture and mandate that physicians routinely test patients' vitamin D levels.
2. Encourage the consumption of common allergenic foods—such as gluten, dairy, corn, and soy—that can trigger autoimmune responses.	2. Discourage people from consuming potential allergens—gluten, soy, corn, and dairy—that can trigger autoimmune responses. Encourage food manufacturers to reduce their use of these substances in packaged foods.
3. Tell people to change the cat litter no more than once a week and promote hiking on trails where deer ticks are plentiful.	3. Let cat owners know it's important to change the cat litter on a daily basis, and advise hikers to avoid trails where deer ticks can be found.
4. Promote unprotected sex.	4. Inform the public about the risks of unprotected sex.

PRESCRIPTIONS FOR REDUCING YOUR IMMUNITY AND INFECTIONS RISK FACTORS
(AND THE FOUR CIRCLES THEY REPRESENT)

The Strategies

SP 1. **Love and care about your immune system.** It is critical to your survival.

B 2. **Know your personal history, and check the health of your immune system.** A pattern of allergies, asthma, rashes, or repeated infections could mean your immune system is at risk. The following blood tests can reveal the state of your immune system:

- **Complete blood count (CBC)** with differential looks at your white blood cells, which are necessary to fight infections.

- **Erythrocyte sedimentation rate (ESR)** measures inflammation, which is high in autoimmune disorders.

- **Antinuclear antibodies (ANA)**—antibodies fight infection, but ANAs often attack your body's tissues. ANAs are often high in autoimmune disorders.

- **Vitamin D**—your body converts vitamin D into a hormone that regulates your organs. Only about 25 percent of the US population has healthy levels of vitamin D.[36] The blood test to get: 25-hydroxyvitamin D level. A normal level is 30–100 ng/mL (nanograms per milliliter); optimal is 50–100 ng/mL.

- **Get tested for common infections.** At the Amen Clinics, we do additional testing through Medical Diagnostic Laboratories (mdlab.com) when we see evidence of infections on SPECT scans. Given that most people reading *The End of Mental Illness* won't have the benefit of a SPECT scan, if your mind or a loved one's is not getting better with standard treatment, consider testing for infectious diseases that commonly affect the mind, such as:[37]

  - Lyme-*Borrelia burgdorferi*[38] (the spirochete that causes Lyme)
  - HIV/AIDS[39]
  - Syphilis[40]

- Herpes simplex 1 and 2[41]
- Cytomegalovirus[42]
- Epstein Barr virus[43]
- Herpes 6 (HHV6)
- *Toxoplasma gondii*[44]
- *H. pylori*[45]
- *Chlamydia pneumoniae*[46]
- Candidiasis

- **Consult with an integrative medical provider** to diagnose and treat any immune system issues or infections.

3. **Avoid allergens and infections as much as possible.**

- **Go on an elimination diet for 30 days.** Cut out sugar, gluten, dairy, corn, soy, artificial colors, additives, and preservatives to see if you feel better.

- **Avoid sources of toxoplasmosis:**

  - If you have a cat, change the litter box daily and wear gloves and a mask. The parasite in the feces only becomes infectious after one to five days.

  - Cover children's sandboxes to protect them from stray cats.

  - Help your cat stay healthy by keeping it indoors and feed it dry or canned cat food, not raw meat.

  - Avoid stray cats or kittens as they are more likely to be infected.

  - Wear gloves when you garden or handle soil and wash your hands thoroughly afterwards.

  - Do not eat raw or undercooked meat and avoid raw cured meat, especially lamb, pork, and beef, which can harbor toxoplasmosis.

  - Wash kitchen utensils thoroughly after preparing meat.

  - Do not drink unpasteurized milk as it may contain toxoplasmosis parasites.

4. **Engage in immune-enhancing habits.**

- **Boost your vitamin D level.** See "The Immunity Vitamin" on page 234.

- **Lower your stress** (psychological circle and social circle because the people you spend time with either increase or reduce your stress levels). Stress hurts your immune system and increases the risk of autoimmune diseases.[47] One of my favorite immunity-boosting, stress-management techniques is laughter.[48] "A cheerful heart is good medicine" (Proverbs 17:22). Watching comedies can be healing, literally. Other techniques to soothe stress include diaphragmatic breathing, prayer or meditation, listening to calming music, warming your hands with your mind, hypnosis and guided imagery, and flooding your five senses with positivity. You can read much more about these techniques in my book *Feel Better Fast and Make It Last*.

B 5. **Take nutraceuticals that boost your immunity and stave off infections.** I recommend that everyone start taking a multivitamin and omega-3 fatty acids and optimize their vitamin D levels. Beyond that, work with an integrative practitioner to determine the other supplements from the following list that will improve your immunity.

- **Therapeutic mushrooms:** The unique and diverse compounds in these fungi, not found in other plants, have been found to have immunity-enhancing effects.[49] Studies report they also have antioxidant, antitumor, antivirus, anti-inflammatory, and antidiabetic properties.[50] I recommend eating and cooking with mushrooms (see below) as well as taking them as supplements. Among the most researched are:

  - **Lion's mane**—improves mood[51] and memory in patients with mild cognitive impairment (MCI)[52]

  - **Shiitake**—improves immunity and decreases inflammatory markers[53]

  - *Reishi*—anti-inflammatory, immunity enhancing, and mood promoting[54]

  - **Cordyceps**—a favorite among athletes because it increases ATP production as well as strength, and endurance, and it has anti-aging effects[55]

- Enhance your immune system to fight infections with these nutrients:[56]

  - Aged garlic[57]

  - Anthocyanins—fruit and vegetable extracts, blueberries, cranberries, grapes[58]

  - Echinacea[59]

  - Probiotics[60]

  - Vitamin C[61]

  - Vitamin D[62]—see "The Immunity Vitamin" below

  - Vitamin E[63]

  - Zinc[64]

The Immunity Vitamin

Often referred to as the "sunshine vitamin," vitamin D is actually a hormone that should be called the "immunity vitamin" thanks to its positive effects on the immune system.[65] It also plays an essential role in overall brain health, mood, memory, weight, and other important bodily processes. Low levels of vitamin D have been associated with approximately 200 conditions, including brain health/mental health issues (depression, autism, and psychosis), autoimmune diseases (MS, rheumatoid arthritis, and diabetes), as well as heart disease, cancer, and obesity.[66] The link between vitamin D and mental health is strong, and more than half of psychiatric inpatients are deficient in vitamin D.[67] Low vitamin D has also been associated with memory problems and dementia.[68]

A growing body of research supports the possible role of vitamin D in protecting against autoimmune diseases, depression, cognitive function, and more.[69] A 2008 study followed 441 overweight and obese adults with depression for one year. The individuals who took vitamin D (20,000 IU or 40,000 IU per week) reported a significant decrease in their symptoms, but those who took a placebo did not see such improvement.[70] In a Swiss study, people who took vitamin D over a month had a significant drop in fatigue.[71]

At Amen Clinics, we test the vitamin D levels of all of our patients, and a staggering number of them have low levels. A report that looked at vitamin D levels for American adults in 1988–1994 compared with 2001–2004 showed that our levels are dropping. The percentage of people with levels of 30 ng/mL or more fell from 45 percent to 23 percent.[72] This means that three out of four Americans have low levels of this important vitamin. In part, this is due to the fact that we are spending more time indoors and using more sunscreen when we're outdoors. The following groups are more likely to experience vitamin D deficiency:[73]

- Older adults
- People with darker skin (which reduces ability to make vitamin D from sunlight)
- People with limited sun exposure (think northern latitudes)
- People taking certain medications, such as antihypertensives, antidiabetics, or benzodiazepines[74]
- People with fat malabsorption syndrome, which can occur with liver disease, cystic fibrosis, and Crohn's disease
- People who are obese or who have undergone gastric bypass surgery

BRIGHT MINDS: IMMUNITY AND INFECTIONS

STEPS TO CREATE MENTAL ILLNESS . . . AND MAKE MY NIECES, ALIZÉ AND AMELIE, SUFFER	STEPS TO END MENTAL ILLNESS . . . AND KEEP MY NIECES, ALIZÉ AND AMELIE, HEALTHY
1. Don't care about your immune system. 2. Engage in habits that damage your immune system and increase your risk for infections. • Ignore your allergies, skin rashes, or recurring infections. • Don't pay attention to the allergens in your environment. • Consume a diet high in sugar, gluten, dairy, and other allergens. • Let stress rule your life. • Don't get screened for vitamin D levels or for possible infections. 3. Avoid the strategies that strengthen your immune system.	1. Care about your immune system. 2. Avoid things that impair your immune system. 3. Engage in habits to strengthen your immune system and minimize your risk for infections. • Know your history of asthma, eczema, and past infections. • Eliminate allergens from your home. • Avoid eating foods with allergens like sugar, gluten, dairy, corn, soy, artificial colors, additives, and preservatives. • Add immunity-enhancing mushrooms to your diet. • Practice stress management techniques. • Get screened for possible infections. • Check your vitamin D levels and optimize them if they are low. • Empty the cat litter box every day.

Pick One BRIGHT MINDS Immunity and Infections Tiny Habit to Start Today

1. When I experience treatment-resistant anxiety or depression, I will get tested for exposure to infectious diseases.

2. When I am not responding to traditional treatment, I will do an elimination diet for a month to see if I have food allergies that might be damaging my immune system.

3. When I go hiking, I will avoid areas where deer ticks are common. I will wear long sleeves and pants, and I will check my body for ticks after a hike.

4. When I go to the doctor for my annual physical, I will ask him or her to check my vitamin D level.

5. When I take my daily supplements, I will add extra vitamin C.

6. When I cook, I will occasionally add shiitake mushrooms to my meal.

7. When I go out, I will limit my alcohol consumption because drinking excessive alcohol can upset the gut microbiome,[75] which is critical to immunity.

8. When I want to give my immune system a natural boost, I will watch a comedy or go to a comedy club.

9. If I have a cat, I'll keep it indoors and change the litter box on a daily basis.

CHAPTER 13

<u>N</u> IS FOR NEUROHORMONE ISSUES

MIRACLE GROW FOR YOUR MIND

Many marriages break up over hormonal imbalance, which is truly sad because it comes from a lack of understanding. When hormones are put back in balance . . . a woman or man resumes their normal life of feeling good and having days filled with quality.

SUZANNE SOMERS

 JENNY

Jenny, 42, was struggling in her marriage. She was anxious, tired, irritable, depressed, and couldn't sleep. Two years prior to seeing us, she had started drinking more wine, which upset her husband. She struggled with a low libido, which was not helping her marriage, and she was frequently volatile with the children, which made her husband incredibly frustrated. Her primary care doctor put her on Lexapro (a selective serotonin reuptake inhibitor [SSRI]) for depression, Xanax (a benzodiazepine) for anxiety, and Ambien for sleep, but none of the medication was making her feel better. She and her husband came together to the clinic. To this point, no one had tested her hormones; her thyroid (energy), testosterone (libido, mood, and strength), and progesterone (a sense of calmness) were all low. Most people do not know that progesterone drops ten years before women go into menopause. By replacing her hormones, we were able to take Jenny off all of her medications, and her relationships at home improved within a matter of months.

When the hormones that affect your brain (neurohormones) are off, you are off. Many of the symptoms associated with hormonal imbalances are similar to those seen in brain health/mental health issues. If nobody checks your hormone levels, which is what happened to Jenny, you will never know the root cause of your issues and may be diagnosed with a mental illness. But when your hormones are the problem, no amount of psychiatric medications will get you right. In the following chart, you'll see common complaints from patients with hormonal problems and how they can be mistaken for mental illnesses.

HORMONAL IMBALANCE COMPLAINTS	CAN BE MISTAKEN FOR . . .
"I'm anxious."	Anxiety
"I'm sad all the time."	Depression
"I just don't feel like myself."	Depression
"My brain is foggy."	Dementia
"My memory is worse than ever."	Dementia
"Everything in my body hurts."	Pain disorder
"I can't stay asleep."	Depression, anxiety
"I'm not interested in sex." "I just yelled at my kids for no reason."	Depression Intermittent explosive disorder
"I feel as if I am going to crawl out of my skin."	Panic attacks, anxiety
"I am hungry all the time." "I'm hearing things." "I can't concentrate."	Binge-eating disorder Psychosis Attention deficit hyperactivity disorder

Hormones are chemical messengers produced in the body that control and regulate the activity of certain cells or organs. *Neurohormones* have an important impact on the brain. When they are healthy, you tend to feel young and energetic. When they are out of balance, you feel older, may experience symptoms similar to those associated with mental health issues, and become more vulnerable to brain health/mental health conditions like anxiety, depression, and even psychosis. Dr. Mark Gordon, medical director for Millennium Health Centers and author of *Traumatic Brain Injury: A Clinical Approach to Diagnosis and Treatment*, says, "Hormones influence every one of the mood disorders."[1] In his view, "the absolute or relative loss of neurohormones or sudden and precipitous change in their relative balance can lead to alterations in how we react and how we manage our mental well-being."[2] Basically, when your neurohormones are out of balance, you can experience two types of problems that collectively affect all four circles:

P S SP 1. Distressing symptoms that can alter the way you think, the way you feel, and the way you behave, which can impact how you view your purpose in life

B 2. Heightened risk of brain health/mental health issues, such as depression, panic attacks, or Alzheimer's, as well as physical illnesses, such as heart disease, diabetes, and certain cancers

Communication between the brain and hormones goes both ways. The brain sends out signals that instruct the body's glands to produce and release hormones; and hormones from within the body send messages back to the brain that influence its activity. When thyroid activity is low, for example, brain activity is typically low as well. That's why an underactive thyroid often leads to depression, irritability, and brain fog.

SEVEN NEUROHORMONES THAT INFLUENCE BRAIN HEALTH/MENTAL HEALTH

The human body produces hundreds of hormones, but for the purposes of this book, I am going to limit the discussion to the following seven neurohormones that have the most direct influence on brain health/mental health:

- **Thyroid**—regulates energy and mood
- **Cortisol**—helps to manage stress and anxiety
- **DHEA**—fights stress and depression; decreases brain inflammation
- **Estrogen and progesterone**—when balanced, promote stable moods
- **Testosterone**—affects mood, motivation, sexuality, and strength
- **Insulin**—balances blood sugar (insulin is covered in chapter 14 "D Is for Diabesity")

Thyroid: how imbalances can create depression, anxiety, and cognitive impairment

The thyroid is a small, butterfly-shaped gland located in your lower neck. Despite its diminutive size, it plays a powerful role in keeping your brain and body healthy. This gland produces three main thyroid hormones—thyroid stimulating hormone (TSH), T3, and T4—that are among the most influential in your body, regulating how it uses energy. It also has a strong impact on the brain because it controls the production of many neurotransmitters, such as dopamine, serotonin, and gamma-aminobutyric acid (GABA). All of the thyroid hormones must be produced in the proper balance to maintain optimal brain and body function. Problems occur when thyroid dysfunction causes the gland to produce too little hormone (hypothyroidism) or too much hormone (hyperthyroidism).

The symptoms of thyroid dysfunction can be mistaken for psychiatric illnesses[3] and can increase the risk for brain/mental issues. The link between thyroid dysfunction and mental well-being has been recognized for about 200 years. In 1825, physician Caleb Parry reported a higher prevalence of "nervous affectations" in people with thyroid disorders.[4] And by 1969, researchers were already reporting that depression can be one of the first signs of thyroid disorder.[5] Since then, researchers have also found links between thyroid dysfunction and schizophrenia, bipolar disorder, borderline personality disorder, and other psychiatric illnesses.[6]

In some cases, depression can be one of the first signs of thyroid disorder.

Hypothyroidism: When the thyroid is underactive, it does not produce enough of the hormones you need to keep your body's processes humming at optimum speed. Approximately 5 out of every 100 people ages 12 and older in the United States suffer from hypothyroidism.[7] Insufficient thyroid hormone can make you feel sluggish, as if you just want to stay in bed all day with a bowl of ice cream. All of your body's processes—from your heartbeat to your bowel function to your brain activity—operate at a slower pace. SPECT scans of people with hypothyroidism show overall decreased brain activity, which often leads to depression, cognitive impairment, anxiety, and brain fog.[8] Low thyroid and depression have been linked in more than 430,000 scientific articles. Research shows this thyroid condition can also lead to attention problems and even psychosis.[9] Memory problems are present in more than 80 percent of people with low-grade hypothyroidism, and thyroid dysfunction is directly linked to one-third of all depressions.[10]

Hyperthyroidism: An overactive thyroid produces too much hormone, making everything in your body work too fast. It can feel as if you're in hyper-drive—you feel jittery and edgy, as though you've had way too much caffeine.[11] It is associated with anxiety, depression, restlessness, and psychosis and affects about one in every 100 people in the United States.[12]

BRAIN HEALTH/MENTAL HEALTH SYMPTOMS
OF THYROID DYSFUNCTION

UNDERACTIVE THYROID*[13]	OVERACTIVE THYROID[14]
Fatigue	Sleeplessness; restlessness
Difficulty concentrating	Anxiety
Memory problems	Irritability
Depression	Racing thoughts
Attentional problems	Difficulty concentrating
Psychosis	Memory problems
	Depression
	Mania
	Psychosis

*Note: Even if your thyroid is producing low to normal thyroid levels, you can still have symptoms of what's called *subclinical hypothyroidism*, which can be treated to help you feel better.

What causes thyroid disorders? The most common cause of hypothyroidism is Hashimoto's disease, and the most common cause of hyperthyroidism is Graves' disease. Both are autoimmune disorders, which means that the body is attacking itself. This may be due to leaky gut syndrome, a build-up of environmental toxins within the body, or food allergies (especially to gluten and dairy products), among many other things. Because of this, many healthcare professionals consider the thyroid gland to be a type of "canary in the coal mine," alerting us to the possible presence of ingested toxins.[15]

Cortisol and DHEA: the stress connection to brain health/mental health issues

The adrenal glands, located above your kidneys, play a vital role in how your body reacts to stress. When acute stress hits, the adrenals release a cascade of hormones, including adrenaline, DHEA, and cortisol as part of your "fight-or-flight response." Imagine you're hiking on a mountain trail when you come face-to-face with a bear. Instantly, your adrenals start pumping out adrenaline and the other hormones, your heartbeat and breathing quicken, and your muscles tense up. This is all part of a survival mechanism intended to give you the jolt of energy you need to fight off the bear or sprint to safety. When you've successfully avoided getting mauled by the bear and are at a safe distance, your body's processes return to normal—your muscles relax, your heartbeat and breathing slow to their usual rate, and your adrenals cut back on stress hormone production.

In today's society, however, we're faced with nonstop daily stressors that can keep us in a perpetual state of high alert. Money problems, work stress, packed schedules, fear about the future—they can cause our adrenals to spew out high levels of stress hormones on a near-constant basis. When stress becomes chronic, the cocktail of harmful chemicals that come with it can overwhelm our bodies and contribute to brain health/mental health issues.

When cortisol levels get stuck on high, it also causes a spike in blood sugar and insulin levels. This leads to detrimental changes in the brain, including a drop in the calming neurotransmitter serotonin, leading to a range of mental health issues. Researchers from the University of California, Berkeley, found that chronic stress generates other disruptive changes in the brain that contribute to a higher incidence of brain health/mental health disorders later in life.[16] In particular, chronic stress produces more white matter and fewer neurons (gray matter) than normal, skewing their balance and interfering with communication within the brain.[17]

Ultimately, high levels of cortisol increase the likelihood of developing lasting psychiatric conditions, such as anxiety, depression, or post-traumatic stress disorder (PTSD).[18] Early exposure to stress in childhood increases the risk for anxiety-related disorders later in life. For years, scientists have noticed an association between depression and high levels of cortisol, but they didn't know if it was a case of cause and effect, and if so, which one came first. Research from 2006 concluded that it is long-term exposure to cortisol that actually contributes to depression and its symptoms.[19] And if you are already suffering from a mood disorder, recurring stress tends to worsen symptoms.

In a 2017 review of existing research on the link between stress and anxiety and depression, the authors concluded that stress "could play a very detrimental role in our mental health. It should be curbed in the beginning in order to prevent its serious consequences."[20]

Chronic exposure to stress hormones impacts your brain and body in other ways. It can kill cells in your memory center, the hippocampus, especially when DHEA is also low.[21] DHEA levels typically peak in your 20s and gradually decline with each passing decade. When you reach midlife, about age 40, your body is likely producing only half as much of the hormone as before. Falling levels of DHEA have been linked to depression, fatigue, and a case of the "blahs"—feeling less than your best. Untreated chronic stress is also associated with detrimental effects on many of the BRIGHT MINDS risk factors:

- Digestive issues (see chapter 7, "I Is for Inflammation")
- Increased food cravings and belly fat (see chapter 14, "D Is for Diabesity")
- Greater risk of cardiovascular disease (see chapter 5, "B Is for Blood Flow)
- Increased risk of diabetes (see chapter 14, "D Is for Diabesity")
- Higher levels of inflammation (see chapter 7, "I Is for Inflammation")
- Weakened immune system (see chapter 12, "I Is for Immunity and Infections")
- Disrupted sleep (see chapter 15, "S Is for Sleep")

Unrelenting stress that lasts for months and years overtaxes your system and can lead to a condition known as adrenal fatigue, which means your body no longer has the resources necessary to handle everyday stressors. It leaves you feeling exhausted but also interferes with sleep, throwing you into a vicious cycle that drains your energy and leaves you even more vulnerable to brain health/mental health disorders.

Common Signs of Adrenal Fatigue[22]

- Decreased ability to withstand stress
- Morning and afternoon fatigue, lack of stamina
- High blood pressure and rapid heartbeat
- Abdominal fat that doesn't go away, no matter what you do
- Mental fog with poor memory and difficulty concentrating
- Low sex drive
- Cravings for sweets or salty foods
- Dizziness when getting up from a seated or prone position
- Signs of premature aging
- Lowered resistance to infection
- Poor wound healing

Estrogen and Progesterone: When Brain Health/Mental Health Hangs in the Balance

ESTROGEN: THE MOOD MODULATOR

Estrogen and progesterone are the primary hormones involved in a woman's menstrual cycle. These sex hormones influence many bodily processes, including the skeletal and cardiovascular systems, as well as many brain functions. Although we typically associate estrogen and progesterone with females, these hormones are present in men, too, only in much smaller amounts—unless they have a lot of belly fat, which converts healthy testosterone into unhealthy, cancer-promoting forms of estrogen (in lectures, I often ask why we have so many pregnant men in our society . . . guys, it's time to deliver the baby!).[23]

During a woman's typical 28-day menstrual cycle, estrogen and progesterone rise and fall. When hormones are balanced, estrogen gently rises and falls twice during a cycle, while progesterone rises and falls once. The chart below shows the cycle of estradiol, one of the key forms of estrogen, and progesterone. Note that Day 1 in this chart refers to the first day of a woman's period.

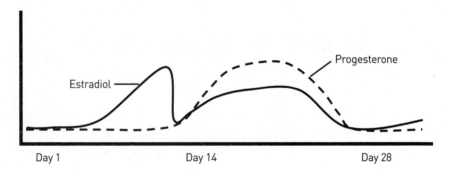

Estrogen affects the brain and your mental well-being in many ways, including:

- Influencing production of neurotransmitters, such as serotonin, dopamine, and GABA, which regulate moods, as well as glutamate, which is involved in memory and learning[24]
- Modulating activity in the hippocampus, the brain region that is critical for healthy moods and memory[25]

When estrogen levels are healthy and balanced, it helps optimize neurotransmitter production and brain function so you feel good all month long. Too much estrogen in relation to progesterone, however, can lead to a condition called estrogen dominance. This causes the gentle monthly hormonal rise and fall to turn into a series of intense spikes and dramatic drop-offs that disrupt important brain processes and make you anxious and irritable. It can also decrease progesterone and GABA, leading to sleep deprivation and all the unpleasant symptoms associated with it. Too little estrogen leads to feeling depressed and confused. The loss of estrogen also hinders critical thinking, short-term memory, and other cognitive functions. These problems can worsen during perimenopause when estrogen levels can fluctuate wildly and during menopause when the hormone drops and stays low (more on this below).

The female body produces three kinds of estrogen: estrone (E1), estradiol (E2) and estriol (E3). (Men produce only E1 and E2.) The health of your liver, gut, and adrenals determines which types of estrogen hormones your body produces. This is yet another reason why addressing all of your BRIGHT MINDS risk factors is critical to your body's systems and your brain health/mental health.

- **Estrone** (E1), the main estrogen produced in women's bodies after menopause, plays a role in breast and uterine cancer. Women make all three estrogens plus progesterone, but the levels of E2, E3, and progesterone drop drastically after menopause, which means women lose the health-protective effects. That's why most breast cancer cases occur postmenopause. Obese women are at higher risk because the fat turns healthy testosterone and estradiol into estrone.[26] Other factors that increase estrone production include taking the antacid cimetidine or birth control pills, hypothyroidism, smoking, pesticide exposure, and the consumption of excess sugar and alcohol, which could explain the link between alcohol intake and breast cancer.[27]

- **Estradiol** (E2), the strongest estrogen, supports healthy moods and cognitive function. The ovaries produce estradiol, which protects bone density, growth hormone production, and cardiovascular function; keeps blood from getting sticky; and improves the lipid profile. Too much estradiol is linked with estrogen-related cancers, but too little can contribute to osteoporosis, heart disease, dementia, and other diseases of aging.

- **Estriol** (E3) protects breast and vaginal tissue, the urinary tract, and bone density. Estriol also helps to reduce hot flashes in women. One compelling study showed women with multiple sclerosis (MS) who took estriol reversed brain lesions.[28]

COMMON SYMPTOMS OF ESTROGEN IMBALANCES[29]

ESTROGEN DOMINANCE	LOW ESTROGEN
Mood swings, depression	Mood changes, depression, weepiness
Fatigue	Fatigue
Sluggish metabolism	Heart palpitations
Low libido	Osteoporosis
Headaches or migraines	Painful intercourse
Brain fog, memory loss	Brain fog, memory loss, focus problems
Weight gain, especially in the belly and hips	Weight gain
Thyroid dysfunction	Bladder incontinence and infections
Sleep disturbances	Sleep disturbances
Fibrocystic breasts	Pain
Bloating	Hot flashes
Vaginal or oral yeast (thrush)	
Heavy bleeding	
Carbohydrate cravings	

PROGESTERONE: NATURE'S ANTI-ANXIETY PILL

Progesterone is the other major hormone in a woman's monthly cycle. This hormone's primary job is to build up the lining of the uterus in anticipation of pregnancy. If a healthy fertilized egg does not implant, progesterone levels fall, the uterine lining is shed during menstruation, and the cycle begins again. Like estrogen, however, progesterone influences more than just a woman's reproductive system. It has a high concentration of receptors in the brain.

Progesterone affects the brain in the following ways:

- Supports GABA, which helps the brain relax
- Protects the nerves
- Supports the myelin that "insulates" and protects neurons

I have always called progesterone the "relaxation hormone." When it is in balance with estrogen, it calms you, brings feelings of peacefulness, and promotes sleep. It has also been shown to reduce inflammation and counteract damage from brain injuries, which makes it important for the head trauma and inflammation BRIGHT MINDS risk factors.

For the first two weeks of the menstrual cycle, progesterone hovers at low levels. It begins climbing during the second half of the cycle, rising and falling along with estrogen. When hormones are balanced, women may notice only a slight shift in mood throughout the month. But when hormones are out of whack or when the relaxation hormone drops too dramatically, calmness can give way to irritability, anxiety, depression, sleepless nights, and brain fog. For some women, when progesterone and estrogen plummet right before menstruation starts, mood stability goes out the window.

Progesterone levels increase during pregnancy, which is why pregnant women often feel so good and have that enviable glow. Some women who have extremes in hormones or moods, in fact, feel so much better thanks to the bump in progesterone that they will deliberately get pregnant multiple times in order to enhance their moods.

Common Symptoms of Low Progesterone[30]

- Anxiety/depression
- Trouble sleeping
- Fibrocystic breasts
- Premenstrual syndrome (PMS)
- Premenstrual headaches
- Postpartum depression
- Bone loss

In a woman's late 30s and 40s, major fluctuations in progesterone can make her feel anxious and out of sorts. A progesterone cream can often be very helpful when used under the care of an experienced health-care provider (see below).

The Pill's Surprising (and Scary) Side Effects

Millions of women take oral contraceptive pills (OCPs), which contain synthetic hormones. If you are taking them, you should be aware of what they do to your hormonal system and the side effects that come with them. OCPs hijack your cyclical hormonal process, replacing it with a steady supply of low levels of synthetic estrogen and progesterone. You may already know that OCPs have been shown to cause problems with blood pressure and blood clots and increase the incidence of strokes, especially if you smoke or have a history of migraine headaches.[31] But did you know that OCPs also affect your brain?

Research shows that taking the pill causes structural changes in the brain, alters neurotransmitter function, and messes with mood regulation.[32] Scientists from Denmark found that women ages 15 to 34 taking OCPs were 23 percent more likely to start taking antidepressants for the first time than non-OCP users.[33] In fact, bouts of depression have been reported by 16 to 56 percent of women on OCPs, which deplete serotonin.[34] Oral contraceptives also put you at greater risk for autoimmune diseases,[35] elevate cortisol levels,[36] and lower levels of testosterone[37] (yes, women produce and need testosterone; more on testosterone to follow), which can decrease your sex drive. And low-testosterone problems can remain even after stopping OCPs, putting you at increased risk for long-term sexual and brain health/mental health problems.[38] Synthetic birth control can also disrupt the gut microbiome[39] and interfere with the absorption of essential vitamins and minerals, which can lead to deficiencies. If you are taking OCPs, supplement your diet with B vitamins (folate, B6, and B12), vitamin E, and magnesium. If you are experiencing mental health symptoms, you may want to ask, is it mental illness or is it the pill?

Stopping OCPs isn't necessarily a quick-fix solution. Some women experience a rash of symptoms—including mood swings, anxiety, and depression—in the months following cessation of hormonal birth control. Some hormonal experts have started calling this effect "post-birth-control syndrome."

PERIMENOPAUSE AND MENOPAUSE: A VULNERABLE TRANSITION PERIOD

As women reach their 30s or 40s, hormones begin to fluctuate as their bodies prepare to exit the baby-making business. It doesn't happen overnight. For up to a decade before entering menopause (when the menstrual cycle ends completely), a woman will go through a transition period called perimenopause.

Most women may not think about this transition until they get hit with hot flashes and night sweats, the most common (and annoying) symptoms. By the time hot flashes arrive, however, women have probably been in perimenopause for up to 10 years.

This transition can be difficult and is often when women start taking psychiatric medications for the first time. With age, a woman's hormonal symphony works less efficiently, leading to estrogen spikes and crashes. The result may be severe PMS symptoms, mood swings, feelings of anxiety, crying spells, or depression. On top of that, short-term memory suffers. With lower estrogen, women can become more sensitive to pain. To stay on top of the changes, a woman should check her hormone levels at about age 35 to establish a baseline, and then recheck them every two to three years. Intervening earlier in the process can help you avoid a lot of problems.

Technically, menopause is the one-year mark after the last menstrual period. Since estrogen and progesterone have fallen to very low levels, women no longer benefit from their protective qualities and are more vulnerable to conditions such as depression, Alzheimer's disease, osteoporosis, heart disease, and stroke. When estrogen levels go low, so does blood flow to the brain, which is associated with depression, anxiety, insomnia, weight gain, and problems with concentration and memory. It is even more critical during this time to take brain health seriously, as the reserve in your brain has declined.[40]

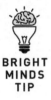

BRIGHT MINDS TIP

It is even more critical during menopause to take brain health seriously, as the reserve in your brain has declined.

Testosterone: Moods, Motivation, and More

Most people associate testosterone with men. It's true that this vital hormone drives the development of the male brain and is responsible for the deep voice, facial hair, and many other features we associate with maleness. But women produce and need testosterone too (just as men have some estrogen), just in smaller amounts. In both men and women, testosterone helps protect the nervous system and wards off depression, cognitive impairment, and Alzheimer's disease. It also seems to protect cells from inflammation, which some researchers believe is why men (who naturally have more of the hormone) are less susceptible than women to inflammatory diseases like rheumatoid arthritis, psoriasis, and asthma, and even why men suffer less from depression.[41]

Testosterone levels peak in a man's late teens and remain strong throughout the 20s, but from age 30 on, they gradually decline. Optimal levels of the hormone promote brain health, energy, strength, motivation, and sex drive. The aging process, however, can leave some men with low testosterone levels that have been shown to increase symptoms of anxiety and depression[42] and a host of other issues.

Common Symptoms of Low Testosterone

- Moodiness
- Depression
- Anxiety
- Difficulty concentrating
- Lack of motivation
- Low libido
- Fatigue
- Trouble sleeping
- Erection problems
- Increased body fat and reduced lean muscle (see chapter 14, "D Is for Diabesity")
- Low bone density
- Hot flashes
- Hair loss

Aging isn't the only thing that leads to low testosterone. In some people, head trauma shuts down production of certain neurohormones and results in the loss of testosterone. See the list on pages 254–255 for additional factors.

Just as low testosterone can be a problem, excessively high levels can cause trouble too. High testosterone levels are associated with lower empathy and a high sex drive, which could be the prescription for having an affair, getting divorced, losing half your net worth, and visiting your children every other weekend.[43]

WHAT INCREASES THE RISK FOR NEUROHORMONAL ISSUES?

A high-sugar diet, head trauma, inflammation, and environmental toxins can damage the production of all of your neurohormones and increase the risk of brain health/mental health issues. One of the big lessons we learned from our work with professional football players was that many of them also had very low hormone levels. It was odd to hear these large, strong men complain of low energy, poor concentration, and a lack of libido. The pituitary gland sits in a bony area of the skull called the sella turcica, making it easily damaged, especially in whiplash injuries.

> *Head trauma is a major cause of hormone disruption,*
> *but few professionals recognize or treat it.*

Would you be surprised to see how an evil ruler would mess with our hormones and keep everyone out of balance?

THE EVIL RULER WOULD . . .	THE BENEVOLENT RULER WOULD . . .
1. Damage neurohormones by subjecting people to chronic stress and having them live in overcrowded cities, feeding them processed foods with a high-sugar content, and encouraging high-risk behaviors that easily damage the pituitary gland.	1. Protect neurohormone production by reducing chronic stress, encouraging schools and work cafeterias to serve brain-healthy foods, and discouraging high-risk behaviors.
2. Flood our environment and our homes with pesticides, plastics, and other products that act as endocrine disruptors.	2. Limit the use of pesticides on crops, outlaw the most toxic pesticides, reduce the use of plastics, and limit products that are endocrine disruptors.
3. Discourage health-care providers from testing thyroid, cortisol, DHEA, estrogen, progesterone, testosterone, human growth hormone, and insulin levels.	3. Encourage the medical community to include testing for thyroid, cortisol, DHEA, estrogen, progesterone, testosterone, human growth hormone, and insulin levels during check-ups.
4. Make policies allowing insurance companies to avoid reimbursing patients for these tests and to deny claims for hormone treatment.	4. Require insurance companies to provide reimbursements for these tests as well as for treatment of hormonal imbalances.

Neurohormone Deficiency Risk Factors
(and the Four Circles They Represent)

(B) • Abnormal levels of thyroid, cortisol, DHEA, estrogen, progesterone, testosterone, human growth hormone, and insulin

(B)(P) • Factors that inhibit thyroid production:[44]
  - Excess stress and cortisol production
  - Deficiencies in vitamins B12 and B9, iron, ferritin, iodine, or selenium
  - Deficient protein; excess sugar
  - Chronic illness
  - Compromised liver or kidney function
  - Cadmium, mercury, lead toxicity
  - Herbicides, pesticides
  - Oral contraceptives; excessive estrogen production

(B)(P)(S) • Factors that contribute to estrogen dominance:
  - Chronic stress and elevated cortisol levels
  - Exposure to environmental toxins
  - Weakened immune system
  - Obesity
  - Diet high in sugar and refined carbohydrates

(B)(P) • Factors that contribute to low estrogen:
  - Perimenopause and menopause
  - Thyroid dysfunction
  - Excessive exercise
  - Eating disorders
  - Low body weight
  - Low-functioning pituitary gland
  - Premature ovarian failure
  - Congenital conditions
  - Chemotherapy

(B)(P)(S) • Factors that contribute to low progesterone:
  - Underactive thyroid
  - Taking antidepressants
  - Chronic stress
  - Deficiencies in vitamins A, B6, C, or zinc
  - A diet high in sugar and refined carbohydrates

(B)(P)(S) • Factors that contribute to low testosterone:
  - Belly fat
  - High stress

- Too much sugar, processed foods, and insulin
- Low zinc
- Alcohol consumption
- Head trauma

PRESCRIPTIONS FOR REDUCING YOUR NEUROHORMONE RISK FACTORS
(AND THE FOUR CIRCLES THEY REPRESENT)

The Strategies

SP 1. **Care about your hormones and test them on a regular basis.** (See chapter 17 on important health numbers.)

B P S 2. **Limit anything that hurts your hormones** (psychological circle because you have to believe that you can change your habits, and social circle because friends and family influence your habits). To keep your hormones healthy, avoid smoking (which lowers the age of menopause),[45] chronic stress, processed food, too much sugar, unhealthy fats, wheat, and obesity.[46] Limit caffeine and alcohol.

B P 3. **Steer clear of "endocrine disrupters"** (psychological circle because you need to change how you think about convenience, pricing, and your own value). In chapter 10, I addressed how toxins can contribute to brain health/mental health issues. The reason is that many toxins, such as pesticides, are known to cause hormonal imbalances and interfere with the body's natural hormone systems, leading to all kinds of health problems.[47] Other endocrine disruptors that can wreak havoc with your hormones include some personal care products, flame retardants, and more. (See chapter 10 for more on how to avoid these chemicals.)

B P S 4. **Boost your healthy hormones.** To optimize your hormones, engage in these healthy behaviors: exercise, lift weights, get adequate sleep, eat a healthy diet, and manage your stress.

B 5. **Use hormone supplements and medication wisely.** For women, go bioidentical when possible because it is the most natural form with generally fewer side effects. Bioidentical hormones are derived from natural sources, such as plant estrogens, and are chemically identical to those produced in the body. The hormones used in traditional replacement therapy are typically derived from horse urine as well as other synthetic substances.

B 6. **Take nutraceuticals that will help support your endocrine system.** Work with a physician to determine which ones are best for you, depending on your hormone levels.

- **L-tyrosine** supports thyroid function.
  Dose suggestion: 500–1,000 mg a day

- **Zinc** helps support healthy testosterone levels.
  Dose suggestion: 25 mg a day

- **DHEA**[48] is available over the counter but is best done under the supervision of your health-care professional. I typically start patients with 10 mg and go up from there. DHEA is usually well tolerated but unwanted side effects, like acne and facial hair, may occur due to DHEA's tendency to increase testosterone levels. These can be avoided by using a specific metabolite of DHEA called 7-keto-DHEA that's more expensive but may be preferable in some cases.
  Dose suggestion: 25–50 mg

- **Diindolylmethane (DIM)**[49] is a phytochemical found in cruciferous vegetables like broccoli and cauliflower. It shifts estrogen metabolism to favor the friendly or harmless estrogen metabolites.[50] DIM can significantly increase the urinary excretion of the "bad" estrogens in as little as four weeks.[51]
  Dose suggestion: 75–300 mg per day

- **Pregnenolone** is a precursor hormone that plays a key role in the healthy production of many of the body's neurohormones, including estrogen, progesterone, testosterone, and cortisol. In supplement form, it has been found to improve depressive symptoms in bipolar disorder,[52] may reduce symptoms of schizophrenia,[53] and may improve memory.[54]
  Dose suggestion: 10–50 mg per day (check with your health-care professional)

- **Calcium D-glucarate**[55] is a natural compound found in fruits and vegetables like apples, brussels sprouts, broccoli, and cabbage. Calcium D-glucarate inhibits the enzyme that contributes to breast, prostate, and colon cancers. It also reduces the reabsorption of estrogen from the digestive tract. *Dose suggestion: 500–1,500 mg per day*

- **Probiotics** help maintain a healthy microbiome and, in turn, healthy hormone levels.

Key Vitamins, Minerals, and Herbs for Hormone Balance[56]

- To support multiple (or all) hormones
  - Multivitamin/mineral complex
  - Omega-3 fatty acids EPA and DHA
  - Probiotics for gut health

- Estrogen (females)
  - DIM—100–200 mg a day
  - Calcium D-glucarate—500 mg a day
  - Plant phytoestrogens, including black cohosh—20–80 mg twice daily
  - Evening primrose oil—500 mg twice a day

- Progesterone (females)
  - Chasteberry—160–400 mg a day

- Testosterone
  - DHEA—need determined by lab testing
  - Zinc—20–30 mg daily

- Thyroid
  - Zinc—20–40 mg daily
  - L-tyrosine—500 mg two to three times a day
  - Iodine—up to 150 mcg a day
  - *Sensoril ashwagandha* extract—250–500 mg once or twice a day

- Cortisol

- L-theanine—200 mg two or three times a day
- Relora—a combination of *Magnolia officialis* and *Phellodendron amurense*, 750 mg one or two times a day
- *Sensoril ashwagandha*—250 mg one or two times a day

- DHEA
  - DHEA—need determined by lab testing
  - 7-Keto-DHEA—need determined by lab testing

BRIGHT MINDS: NEUROHORMONE ISSUES

STEPS TO CREATE MENTAL ILLNESS . . . AND MAKE MY NIECES, ALIZÉ AND AMELIE, SUFFER	STEPS TO END MENTAL ILLNESS . . . AND KEEP MY NIECES, ALIZÉ AND AMELIE, HEALTHY
1. Don't care about your hormones. 2. Engage in habits that promote hormone imbalances and endocrine disruption. • Consume a diet high in sugar, refined carbohydrates, unhealthy fats, and gluten. • Guzzle coffee and other caffeinated drinks throughout the day. • Take up smoking. • Skimp on sleep. • Drink more than a few glasses of alcohol each week. • Overexercise by spending hours doing cardio each day. • Let your weight go until you become obese. • Let chronic stress rule your life. • Expose yourself to environmental toxins and "endocrine disruptors." 3. Avoid the strategies that protect your hormones.	1. Care about your hormones. 2. Avoid anything that hurts your hormone function. 3. Engage regularly in healthy habits that promote healthy hormones. • Starting at age 35, check your hormone levels on an annual basis, or more often if you have imbalances. • Get regular exercise without overdoing it. • Lift weights to build and maintain lean muscle. • Aim for seven to eight hours of sleep each night. • Follow the BRIGHT MINDS diet (see chapter 18). • Practice stress-management techniques. • Limit your exposure to endocrine disruptors. • If you require hormonal supplementation, opt for bio-identical hormones when possible.

Pick One BRIGHT MINDS Neurohormone Issues Tiny Habit to Start Today

TINY HABITS

1. When I turn 35, I will get my hormones tested to establish a baseline.

2. When I shop, I will avoid hormone disruptors, such as BPAs, phthalates, parabens, and pesticides.

3. When I buy eggs, beef, chicken, or other animal proteins, I will avoid products raised with hormones or antibiotics.

4. When I eat my meals, I will add more fiber (to help my body flush out unhealthy forms of estrogen).

5. When I work out, I will lift weights to boost my testosterone levels naturally.

6. When I want something sweet, I will choose fruit instead of sugary snacks.

7. When I take my supplements, I will include zinc to help support healthy testosterone levels.

8. When I take my vitamins, I will include cortisol-reducing supplements, such as ashwagandha, which also supports thyroid function.

9. (For women) When my bloodwork shows my estrogen level is too high, I will avoid eating estrogenic foods like soy and will add cruciferous vegetables like broccoli and brussels sprouts to help filter excess estrogen from my system.

10. (For women) When I am suffering from hormonal imbalances, I will consider bio-identical hormone replacement.

CHAPTER 14

<u>D</u> IS FOR DIABESITY

REVERSE THE EPIDEMIC THAT'S DESTROYING BRAINS, MINDS, AND BODIES

As your weight goes up, the size and function of your brain go down.[1]
CYRUS RAJI, MD, PHD, ASSISTANT PROFESSOR OF RADIOLOGY, WASHINGTON UNIVERSITY

My wife and I saw you on Facebook and decided to give your program a try. We knew we had to make some changes for our family. My wife has Hashimoto's disease [neurohormones]. My daughter has polycystic ovarian syndrome [neurohormones] and struggled with moodiness, and I had not felt great about myself in a long time.

We made a commitment as a family to do what you said and give it two weeks. If it hadn't been for my wife pushing us, I would have quit. I admit we struggled with cravings for the first few days. After one week the cravings were gone! In fact, real food started to taste delicious. I was surprised how much the flavor was magnified in a carrot. I never noticed before. After two weeks on the program, we couldn't have been happier. We all felt fantastic and had each lost between 10 and 12 pounds [diabesity] and no longer thought about quitting. Each week on the program gets better and better, and we feel more energetic [blood flow] than ever! In fact, I can't remember the last time I have ever felt this wonderful. I lost 20 pounds after four weeks. People tell me that my skin looks great. I am more confident, more energetic, and I sleep so much better.

Now we are all mentoring our family and friends to live this way. Both my wife and daughter had struggled with weight loss in the past in spite of exercising twice a day at times. My wife has lost 24 pounds since she started eating this way, and her skin is also more vibrant. My 18-year-old daughter has lost 22 pounds and feels happier and much more confident. As soon as they started eating according to your food rules, they were able to exercise a fraction of the time and get more results. What you eat matters!

One of the amazing things we've noticed is how many other people ask us for help after seeing our family's transformation. My mother, who lives with us after suffering several strokes [blood flow], is now eating this way. Her moods and energy are much better. She is more social and no longer isolates herself to her room as much. My mother-in-law, who suffers from fibromyalgia [immunity/infection], also reports less pain and is able to walk more easily. Even our two younger sons, who don't seem to have much interest in learning about our new lifestyle yet, are eating better without even realizing it because we no longer have junk food in the house. We know this will have a long-term effect on their health. As a family we are healthier and happier.

Several of my coworkers noticed the changes and have started the program. Now they are asking me a ton of questions. When you feel good, you look better. I even walk differently, and I think people notice. It's hard not to share what you learn when the changes are so obvious.
—Bobby L.

Diabesity is having high blood sugar and/or being overweight or obese. In the United States, it has become an epidemic that continues to get worse, with half the population affected by prediabetes (36 percent) or diabetes (14 percent),[2] 70 percent considered overweight, and 40 percent falling into the obese category. The annual medical costs of obesity alone top more than $150 billion.[3] Diabesity is destroying brains, minds, and bodies, and it's robbing our children and grandchildren of their future. They will not be able to afford the tsunami of illness that is headed their way unless we get serious and do something about it. The increase in diabesity is one of the main reasons brain health/mental health issues are increasing. Both high blood sugar and being overweight take a toll on the brain and mind and negatively impact the BRIGHT MINDS risk factors.

Excess fat on your body is not your friend. Obesity is detrimental to brain health/mental health and is associated with a greater risk of depression, bipolar disorder, panic disorder, agoraphobia (fear of going out), and addictions.[4] Untreated attention deficit disorder/attention deficit hyperactivity disorder (ADD/ADHD),[5] lower self-esteem, and poor body image[6] are also associated with being overweight.[7] Among women, increased body mass index (BMI) is also linked to a rise in suicidal thoughts.[8] Being overweight or obese also impacts your BRIGHT MINDS risk factors. For example, it has been associated with a smaller brain and decreased blood flow to the brain.[9] It produces chemicals that increase inflammation, store toxins, and disrupt hormonal function. It also makes you more susceptible to developing sleep problems, such as sleep apnea.[10]

High blood sugar is associated with a smaller hippocampus, the seahorse-shaped structure in your temporal lobes associated with mood, learning, and memory. Anxiety and depression are two to three times higher in patients with Type 2 diabetes than in the general population.[11] High blood sugar causes blood vessels to become brittle and break, delays healing, increases the risk of stroke, and causes overall lower blood flow in the brain. In fact, diabetes has been linked to decreased blood flow on SPECT scans.[12] On top of that, high blood sugar and diabetes are also associated with increased inflammation; Alzheimer's disease; strokes, heart disease, hypertension; and accelerated aging.[13] People with diabetes are also at greater risk for eating disorders, such as binge eating.[14] Having diabetes during pregnancy significantly increases the risk of psychosis in the children (auditory and visual hallucinations).[15]

All of the four circles play a role in the diabesity connection to brain health/mental health:

- **B** • **Biological:** Diabesity impacts many of the BRIGHT MINDS risk factors and vice versa, creating a vicious loop of internal dysfunction that conspires to keep the weight on and create brain health/mental health issues.

- **P** • **Psychological:** Diabesity can make you feel bad about yourself and cause you to think you were destined to have weight and blood sugar problems. This type of thinking makes you more likely to perpetuate the habits that leads to being overweight and to ignore other contributing BRIGHT MINDS factors, such as environmental toxins, inflammation, and neurohormonal issues. This mind-set makes you less likely to take action and change your behavior.

- **S** • **Social:** You could be fueling diabesity by eating unhealthy meals with your family at home, alcohol-filled happy hours with coworkers, and by using sweets as a coping mechanism to deal with stress in your relationships.

- **SP** • **Spiritual:** If you lack purpose in life, you may not see why it's important to achieve a healthy weight and healthy blood sugar levels.

By the way that our culture promotes unhealthy food choices and indulgence, you would think an evil ruler has gotten a hold of us and is behind all our weight issues and the diabetes epidemic.

THE EVIL RULER WOULD . . .	THE BENEVOLENT RULER WOULD . . .
1. Demand that high-sugar desserts be served with all school lunches as a way to boost inattention among children.	1. Limit sugar-laden snacks and desserts in school lunches to promote stable blood sugar levels and healthy weight.
2. Encourage companies to put out candy bowls and doughnuts in the break room to raise the risk of diabesity.	2. Encourage corporations to serve brain-healthy snacks to employees to prevent diabesity.
3. Fool people into viewing sweet desserts (which spike blood sugar and contribute to anxiety and other mental health symptoms) as a "reward" for good behavior or a job well done.	3. Tell the truth that drinking and eating foods that make you fat and diabetic is not a smart way to celebrate.
4. Allow unhealthy, artificially flavor-enhanced foods and drinks to be aggressively marketed as desirable (think Coke's "Open Happiness" slogan). In fact, the evil ruler would encourage professional athletes and coaches to visibly drink Coke, Pepsi, or Gatorade (all filled with sugar, artificial colors, and preservatives) on the sidelines of games as a way of marketing these products to children and teens.	4. Prevent food and beverage manufacturers from easily marketing products that increase the risk for diabesity.
5. Tell people that diabetes isn't that bad and discourage making any lifestyle changes because there are drugs they can take for it.	5. Educate people about the consequences of diabetes and encourage lifestyle changes—exercise and diet—to regulate blood sugar levels.
6. Blame genetics for the obesity epidemic, saying there's nothing people can do about it.	6. Inform people that their DNA is not their destiny. Their daily habits can influence their genes, and it is within their power to control their weight.

As your weight goes up, the size and function of the brain goes down; which should scare the fat off everyone.

INSULIN AND THE BLOOD SUGAR-MOOD CONNECTION

In chapter 14, you learned about six of the neurohormones that influence your brain health/mental health. Here, I'll show you how the seventh neurohormone, insulin, is related to diabesity and your mental well-being. In the body, the hormone insulin is involved in regulating blood sugar levels. Your body's cells need sugar (glucose) for energy, but they can't absorb it directly from your bloodstream. That's where insulin comes in. Released by the pancreas when you eat carbohydrates, insulin is like a key that unlocks cell membranes so they can get the glucose they need from the foods you eat.

Now, not all carbohydrates are created equal. Complex carbohydrates (such as vegetables, quinoa, and fruits) help keep insulin working effectively and stabilize blood sugar levels. However, simple sugars (such as cookies, candies, and sodas) as well as highly processed carbohydrates (such as bread, pasta, and crackers) require the pancreas to pump out large amounts of insulin and can cause blood sugar levels to soar. If there's too much sugar in your bloodstream, insulin signals your body to shuttle it to the liver for storage, which can eventually lead to fatty liver disease in some people. Another consequence of high insulin levels is that the body switches from breaking down and flushing dietary fat from the body to storing that fat, which over time can lead to weight problems. One of the main consequences of chronically eating a high-sugar diet and being obese is a decrease in insulin's ability to regulate blood sugar, leading to prediabetes and diabetes.

How do insulin and blood sugar levels affect your mind? Eating sugar or refined carbs causes blood sugar levels to spike and, subsequently, causes them to crash. This roller-coaster effect can impact your moods and mental well-being. Research shows that high-sugar diets and blood sugar issues are associated with:

- Anxiety[16]
- Depression[17]
- Schizophrenia[18]
- Irritability[19]
- Anger[20]
- Addiction to sugar[21]
- Trouble concentrating[22]

If you want to get your brain right, it is imperative to get your food right. Eliminating sugar and other refined carbohydrates from your diet can help regulate your body's production of insulin, stabilize blood sugar levels, and facilitate the fat breakdown process. It can also prevent the depletion of chromium, a mineral required by insulin receptors. In a fascinating study,[23] researchers from the University of Illinois looked at the nutrient levels of patients and compared them to scans of their brains and measurements of executive function (planning and impulse control) and intelligence. Improved executive function was associated with higher levels of omega-3 fatty acids, lycopene, carotenoids, vitamin D, and vitamins B2 (riboflavin), B9 (folate), and B12 (cobalamin). The brain functioned better with higher levels of omega-3s and carotene; and omega-3 levels were associated with higher intelligence.

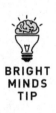

BRIGHT MINDS TIP

Eliminating sugar and other refined carbohydrates from your diet can help regulate your body's production of insulin, stabilize blood sugar levels, and facilitate the fat breakdown process.

Diabesity Risk Factors
(and the Four Circles They Represent)

B • High fasting blood sugar levels, prediabetes, or type 1 or type 2 diabetes[24]

B P S SP • Being overweight or obese[25]

B P S SP • Aging (retirement/aging)

B S • Family history of the disease (genetics)

B P S • Alcohol abuse (toxins)

B • Exposure to environmental toxins (toxins)

B S • Being sedentary (blood flow)

PRESCRIPTIONS FOR REDUCING YOUR DIABESITY RISK FACTORS
(AND THE FOUR CIRCLES THEY REPRESENT)

The Strategies

The good news is that you can significantly lower your risk factor of diabesity.[26] As with all of the BRIGHT MINDS risk factors, you'll need a long-term perspective and lifestyle habits you can feel happy about and maintain for the rest of your life.

(SP)   1. **Care about your weight and blood sugar levels.** As part of caring, you must know your important numbers, including BMI, waist-to-height ratio, fasting blood sugar, hemoglobin A1c (HbA1c), and fasting insulin level. (See chapter 17.)

   2. **Avoid anything that increases the risk of diabesity.**

(B) (P) (S) (SP)   • **Limit or avoid foods that increase the risk of diabesity.** These include:

   • High caloric foods

   • High-glycemic, low-fiber foods (pasta, bread, white potatoes, rice, and sugar), which also promote inflammation

   • Processed foods

   • Artificial dyes, sweeteners, and food additives

   • Potentially allergenic foods (everyone is different), such as gluten, dairy, corn, and soy

   Note: In a disturbing study, children of women with the highest gluten intake (20 g/day or more) versus those with the lowest gluten intake (less than 7 g/day) had double the risk of developing Type 1 diabetes over a follow-up period of 16 years.[27]

(P)   • **Avoid the mind-set of diabesity.** These are beliefs and thoughts you tell yourself that increase the risk you will never truly get healthy, such as:

   • "Everything in moderation," which is generally the

thought just before you are going to eat something that will hurt you.

- "Live a little; you deserve it." Funny, but this is the thought of early death. It should be rephrased as "Live a little shorter."

- "I just want to have fun." But who has more fun? The person with the healthy brain or the one with the troubled brain? No question—the person with the healthy brain.

- "I want what I want when I want it" is a four-year-old's mind-set, but this thought underlies why most people do not get healthy. We need to be good parents to ourselves and be firm about engaging in good behavior if we want to end mental illness.

- "But I always do it this way" is another common thought that tells you that your habits are destroying your mind.

- **(P)** • **Don't fall for every advertising pitch.** Here's what I'd say about some common marketing slogans:

  - Coke's "Open Happiness"—should be rephrased as "Open Illness."

  - Ben and Jerry's "Eat Away Your Feelings"—should be rephrased as "Eat Your Way to Depression."

  - McDonald's "I'm Lovin' It"—should be rephrased as "I'll Start Hating My Mind and Body."

  - McDonald's "You Deserve a Break Today"—should be rephrased as "You Deserve Illness Today."

  - Lay's Potato Chips "Betcha Can't Eat Just One"—should be rephrased as "Bet You Can't Eat Just One Because They Are Addictive."

  - Trix's "Silly Rabbit, Trix Are for Kids!"—should be rephrased as "Silly Rabbit, Trix Are for Kids Who Want to Struggle in School and Be Overweight and Sick!"

3. **Engage in regular brain healthy habits that decrease the risk of diabesity.**

- **Develop a Brain Warrior mind-set.**[28] As my wife, Tana, and I reveal in our book *The Brain Warrior's Way*, you are in a war for the health of your brain. Everywhere you go, someone is trying to shove bad food down your throat that will kill you early. You need to be armed, prepared, and aware to win the fight for your life. In the book, we asked our readers, and I ask you here, "Are you a sheep or a sheepdog?"

  Sheep are best known for their strong flocking behavior. Sheep follow and are easily led. They go with the herd and do what the majority of the other sheep do. When one sheep moves, the rest of the flock tends to follow, even when it's a bad idea. In Turkey in 2005, a sheep jumped off a cliff to its death, then 1,500 others followed.[29] Sheep have two speeds—graze and stampede (group think). Sheep are often annoyed by sheepdogs—they remind them that trouble may be nearby.

  Sheepdogs are serious and purpose-driven to protect their flock. They live to make a difference. Sheepdogs need training to be effective. Sheepdogs love their flock, even when the love is not returned. Sheepdogs will give their lives to protect their sheep. Sheepdogs have a major advantage: They can survive in a hostile environment; sheep cannot. When sheep get attacked, they often give in to death. When sheepdogs are attacked, they fight back and are much more likely to survive.

  Are you a sheep or a sheepdog? If you want to end mental illness, you have to develop a sheepdog's mind-set.

- **Follow the BRIGHT MINDS diet** (see chapter 18). "Eat right to think right" is one of the most important strategies to end mental illness. Over the years, we have developed one overriding food rule that captures all others: "only love and consume foods that love you back." If you can get this one rule right, it will help you feel happy and vibrant for the rest of your life.

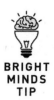

BRIGHT MINDS TIP

The most important food rule is "Only love and consume foods that love you back."

B **P** **S** **SP** • **Lose weight slowly (if you are overweight or obese).** The healthiest way to drop weight and keep it off is to lose one to two pounds a week. Here are more tips:[30]

- Drink more water.

- Have protein for breakfast to balance your blood sugar.

- Add more fiber to your diet to lower the risk of Type 2 diabetes[31] and keep you feeling full longer. Brain-healthy high-fiber foods include vegetables (broccoli and brussels sprouts), berries, chia seeds, and quinoa.

- Green tea has been shown to increase metabolism and decrease the risk of diabetes. It is loaded with antioxidants, but be careful what you put in it and only drink caffeinated green tea in small doses.

- Don't drink your calories. In 1980, Americans drank an average of 225 calories a day; in 2015, it was 450 calories a day. The extra 225 calories a day will put 23 pounds of fat on your body every year! Plus, the calories you drink are more quickly absorbed than those you have to chew.

- Take saunas and eat detoxifying foods. Fat stores toxins, so it's critical to detox when you lose weight.

- Weigh yourself every day because research shows it helps keep you on track.[32]

- Don't overdo your weight loss. Being too thin is definitely not the answer. If your BMI gets too low, you can wind up with cognitive problems.[33]

B **P** **S** • **Start new habits.** You already have daily habits. Start new habits around the foods that promote your mental health rather than the ones that steal it. Most of us have about 20 meals we go to over and over. This week, try to add five brain-healthy meals with foods you love that love you back.

B **S** • **Exercise!** Research shows that working out improves blood sugar levels and weight. Strength training is a must. Compared with women who reported no strength training, women engaging in any strength training reduced the incidence of Type 2 diabetes by 30 percent.[34] Any type of regular movement matters, even walking,[35] but walk as if you are in a hurry.[36] (See chapter 5 "B̲ Is for Blood Flow.")

B • **Check with your physician to see if other treatment is necessary.** Depending on your personal numbers and your genetic risks, you may be able to improve your health without resorting to taking medication.[37]

B 4. **Take nutraceuticals that help balance blood sugar.** Your physician or integrative health-care professional can help determine which of these will work best for you.

• **Omega-3 fatty acids EPA and DHA.**[38] By now, you know that this supplement will help you with many of the BRIGHT MINDS risk factors; that's why I recommend it to all my patients. It helps to maintain proper insulin signaling in the brain, counteract nonalcoholic fatty liver, and decrease the risk of metabolic syndrome.[39] (Metabolic syndrome is defined as having at least three of the following risk factors: high fasting blood sugar levels, abdominal obesity, high triglycerides, low HDL cholesterol, and high blood pressure.) In a large study in older adults, the diabetes risk was 43 percent lower among those with the highest blood concentrations of omega-3 fats compared with those with the lowest concentrations.[40] In a well-designed placebo-controlled trial in overweight type 2 diabetics, supplementing with the omega-3 fatty acid EPA significantly decreased serum insulin, fasting glucose, HbA1c, and insulin resistance.[41] (Check out information on the Omega-3 Index in chapter 7, which will let you know if you're on the right track toward omega-3 protection.)
Dose suggestion: The effective daily dose seems to be 1,400 mg or more with a ratio of approximately 60/40 EPA to DHA.

• **Chromium as chromium picolinate** can help regulate insulin, which boosts the metabolism of glucose and fat. Chromium picolinate also helps decrease carbohydrate cravings and binge eating, thus impacting both blood sugar and weight.[42] Some research shows that chromium picolinate significantly lowers HbA1c in type 2 diabetics.[43]
Dose suggestion: The typical recommended adult dosage is 200–1,000 micrograms (mcg) a day.

- **Cinnamon**[44] offers a bouquet of benefits for those at risk of diabetes. It's been shown to lower fasting glucose levels and HbA1c and improve insulin sensitivity.[45] This sweet and savory spice also lowered cholesterol and improved working memory in older prediabetic[46] adults, while improving blood flow to the prefrontal cortex.[47] Plus, it has been shown to decrease abnormal tau protein aggregation, thought to be one of the major contributors of Alzheimer's disease. Not only can cinnamon help your blood sugar levels, but it can also spice up your love life.

  Dose suggestion: The typical dose for blood sugar control is 1–6 grams a day as a supplement. Use the spice liberally. If you are taking medication to control your blood sugar, talk to your doctor before taking supplemental cinnamon, as it may have an additive effect and lower blood sugar too much.

BRIGHT MINDS: DIABESITY

STEPS TO CREATE MENTAL ILLNESS . . . AND MAKE MY NIECES, ALIZÉ AND AMELIE, SUFFER	STEPS TO END MENTAL ILLNESS . . . AND KEEP MY NIECES, ALIZÉ AND AMELIE, HEALTHY
1. Don't care about your weight or blood sugar levels.	1. Care about your weight and blood sugar levels.
2. Engage in habits that increase the risk of diabesity.	2. Avoid anything that increases the risk of diabesity.
• Don't bother weighing yourself. • Don't get your blood sugar levels or HbA1c levels checked. • Eat a high-sugar, low-fiber diet. • Eat a lot of processed foods. • Skip meals and make up for it by eating twice as much at the next meal. • Overeat on a regular basis. • Adopt a diabesity mind-set that allows you to stay overweight and sick. • When you want to lose weight, go on a crash diet to drop pounds fast. • Be a couch potato.	3. Engage regularly in healthy habits that reduce the risk of diabesity. • Weigh yourself daily. • Get your blood sugar and HbA1c levels checked at least once a year. • Consume a BRIGHT MINDS diet. • Add more fiber to your meals. • Adopt new daily habits to replace the habits that steal your mental health. • Get moving! Engage in strength training and cardio exercise on a regular basis. • Consider supplements that support healthy blood sugar levels.
3. Avoid the strategies that reduce the risk for diabesity.	

Pick One BRIGHT MINDS Diabesity Tiny Habit to Start Today

TINY HABITS

1. I will immediately stop drinking my calories.

2. When I eat lunch and dinner, I will add one serving of a colorful vegetable.

3. At each meal, I'll make sure to include some high-quality protein and fat to stabilize my blood sugar and reduce cravings.

4. When I want to lose weight, I will do it slowly so I can develop lifelong habits.

5. When I take my daily shower, I will weigh myself because it will keep me honest and motivated.

6. I will take omega-3 supplements daily.

CHAPTER 15

S IS FOR SLEEP

WASH YOUR BRAIN EACH NIGHT
TO HAVE BRIGHTER DAYS

The night is the hardest time to be alive and 4 a.m. knows all my secrets.

POPPY Z. BRITE

 CATHY AND KRISTEN

Cathy, 45, was the CEO of a large financial services company and hired us to do a wellness program for her employees. She became passionate about brain health. Over time, I also saw her husband for preventive work. He had a family history of Alzheimer's disease and wanted to do everything he could to avoid it.

Then I saw their teenage daughter, Kristen, who was anxious about starting at a new school and had panic attacks for the first time in her life. She had frequent bouts where she thought she was going to die: Her heart started pounding out of her chest, she hyperventilated and felt as though she couldn't get enough air, her hands were cold and sweaty, and she had a sense that something terrible was about to happen to her. The panic attacks caused her to voice suicidal thoughts to her mother, which is when Cathy called me.

As I got to know Kristen, I learned she had many common brain-damaging teenage habits, including a digital addiction (lots of fights happened around her phone), a junk food addiction (it was hard to get her to eat anything healthy), and very poor sleep habits. Yet when Kristen learned about her brain, she became more interested in taking care of it. I had her take our online course, Brain Thrive by 25 (www.brainthriveby25.com) and had her keep a journal about her food and sleep. After three weeks, it became crystal clear to both of us that when Kristen slept more than seven hours a night, her focus was better at school and the panic attacks vanished. This gave Kristen the motivation to engage in brain-healthy sleep habits. She hated the attacks but now knew she had control over them.

As the chief psychiatrist at the National Training Center (NTC) at Fort Irwin in the Mojave Desert, I often saw the effects of sleep deprivation first-hand. The mission of the NTC was to train soldiers for combat in the desert. The war games went for days, and many soldiers became seriously sleep-deprived. If they went for two or more days without sleep, some were brought to me in psychotic states, seeing visions or being delusional. The prescription was generally not medication but sleep.

While you are sleeping, your brain is hard at work performing some very critical functions necessary to keep it operating at optimal levels. For example, during sleep, your brain cleans or washes itself by eliminating cellular debris and toxins that build up during the day (basically taking out the neural trash), consolidates learning and memory, and prepares for the following day. The brain processes that occur during sleep are also important for the health of your immune system, appetite control, and neurotransmitter production.

BRIGHT MINDS TIP

When you are sleeping, your brain is hard at work performing some very critical functions necessary to keep it operating at optimal levels.

Getting adequate sleep is vital for your brain, but an estimated 50 to 70 million Americans have some form of sleep disorder.[1] Nearly one-third of us suffer from short-term bouts of insomnia, the most common sleep disorder. And chronic insomnia affects approximately one in 10 people.[2] The rates are even higher among people with psychiatric disorders.[3] In fact, more than 50 percent of the time, insomnia is tied to stress, anxiety, or depression.[4]

Sleep and brain health/mental health issues are tightly linked. Research shows that about 75 percent of people with depression also have insomnia.[5] Sixty-nine to 99 percent of people with bipolar disorder experience insomnia or feel a reduced need for sleep during manic episodes.[6] More than half of the people with anxiety have trouble sleeping.[7] And children with attention deficit disorder/attention deficit hyperactivity disorder (ADD/ADHD) are more likely to experience sleep disorders than kids without the condition.[8]

The relationship between sleep and brain health/mental health issues goes both ways. In general, a night of staring at the ceiling can make you wake up feeling angry, irritable, sad, or stressed the next day; lower your ability to concentrate; and impair your judgment. Over time, sleep problems can lead to a higher risk of depression, ADD/ADHD, panic attacks, brain fog, memory problems, and dementia.[9] For example, teenagers who on average get an hour less of sleep at night are 38 percent more likely to feel sad and hopeless, 42 percent more likely to consider suicide, 58 percent more likely to attempt suicide, and 23 percent more likely to engage in substance abuse.[10] Due to a lack of sleep, shift workers have an increased risk of depression, as well as work-related injuries, cardiovascular disease, diabetes, and obesity.[11]

Having too few hours of sleep can have catastrophic consequences, increasing your risk of a traumatic brain injury (TBI). In a report from the Automobile Association of America (AAA), drivers who slept six to seven hours were 30 percent more likely to be in a car crash than those who got more than seven hours; those who slept for five to six hours a night were 90 percent more likely to have an accident; four to five hours, 430 percent more likely; and those who got less than four hours were 1,150 percent more likely to crash.[12] In another study, soldiers who got seven hours of sleep at night were 98 percent accurate on the range; those who got six hours of sleep were only 50 percent accurate; five hours equaled 28 percent accuracy; and four hours equaled only 15 percent accuracy (they were dangerous).[13]

Sleep apnea—when you snore loudly, stop breathing multiple times at night, then feel excessively tired during the day—is bad for your health. It's no good for your partner either, since they can't get a good night's sleep with all that snoring and snorting. Untreated sleep apnea triples your risk of depression and dementia and makes it hard to lose weight. On SPECT scans, sleep apnea often looks like early Alzheimer's disease (see scans on the next page). Getting a diagnosis and treatment for sleep apnea is critical to keeping your brain healthy and preventing or minimizing symptoms of mental disorders. The gold standard for treatment is called a continuous positive airway pressure (CPAP) mask, which delivers a steady stream of air through your passageways. Some people are hesitant to use a CPAP machine because they think the mask will be uncomfortable. This is a mistake. Because the brain is so dependent on oxygen, untreated sleep apnea literally kills brain cells, which doesn't bode well for your mental well-being.

BRAIN SURFACE SPECT SCANS

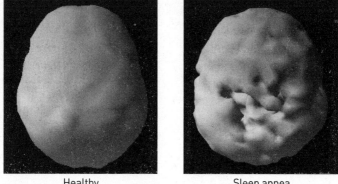

Healthy   Sleep apnea

Sleep Risk Factors
(and the Four Circles They Represent)

All of the four circles contribute to your sleep patterns and can either leave you tossing and turning at night or sleeping peacefully.

 • **Biological:** Conditions like restless leg syndrome or sleep apnea, jet lag, many medications, poor sleep hygiene, or hormonal imbalances (especially hyperthyroidism and low progesterone in women) can get in the way of a good night's sleep.

 • **Psychological:** Worrying about work or finances, relationship problems, or the health of a loved one can keep you up at night. ANTs (automatic negative thoughts) tend to attack before bed and in the middle of the night.

 • **Social:** Doing shift work, having a job that requires a lot of travel across time zones, staying out too late with friends, guzzling coffee day and night, or looking at your email or scrolling through your social media feed at all hours of the night prevents your brain from getting the restorative sleep it needs.

 • **Spiritual:** If you aren't in tune with why you want to make sleep a priority, it will be difficult to adopt the habits that will provide better rest.

Chronic insomnia, less than seven hours of sleep for adults and eight hours for teens (psychological circle if stress is keeping you up at night, and social circle if you are staying out late with friends)

HOW MODERN SOCIETY IS STEALING SLEEP AND SELLING A BROKEN SOLUTION

Companies that are open 24/7 and require employees to work odd hours, bars and nightspots that don't close until 2 a.m., and endless connectivity to the internet can all keep us from getting to bed at a reasonable hour. Similarly, restaurants that serve mega-portions, coffee vendors on nearly every corner selling caffeinated beverages at all hours, and bars pushing alcohol on us can all interfere with a good night's sleep. With increasing insomnia rates, sleep aid medications have skyrocketed. But the sleep solutions our society is pushing come with a cost. Research showed an association between sleep medications—such as zolpidem (Ambien), eszopiclone (Lunesta), and temazepam (Restoril)—and *a more than three-fold increased risk of death.*[14] These sleep aids have also been associated with memory issues, confusion, anxiety, depression, and addiction.[15]

THE EVIL RULER WOULD . . .	THE BENEVOLENT RULER WOULD . . .
1. Mess with people's sleep by making them so addicted to TV and social media that they tune into stressful news before bed, read emails late into the evening, respond to texts in the middle of the night, and tweet outrageous messages and post to Facebook or Instagram at all hours.	1. Limit social media and TV time so people can go to sleep early and get the rest they need.
2. Encourage people to regularly cross several time zones for work, giving them jet lag.	2. Limit excess travel to reduce the incidence of jet lag.
3. Refuse to give up the outdated practice of the twice-a-year time change that messes with people's sleep.	3. Do away with the twice-a-year time change that messes with your sleep.
4. Advocate caffeine consumption morning, noon, and night to disrupt sleep and create an unhealthy cycle that primes people for symptoms of mental illness.	4. Encourage people to adopt a brain-healthy sleep regimen that promotes more restorative sleep.
5. Encourage starting school early to diminish sleep time, which increases many forms of brain health/mental health issues.	5. Start school later to allow children good sleep.
	6. Start days with exercise and hold meetings at work while walking.

PRESCRIPTIONS FOR REDUCING YOUR SLEEP RISK FACTORS
(AND THE FOUR CIRCLES THEY REPRESENT)

The Strategies

SP 1. **Love and care about your sleep.** Make it a priority and keep track of your sleep each night. There are many apps that can help. I often use Sleep Cycle on my phone or my Fitbit watch. Strive to get seven to nine hours, which is a healthy amount for most people.

2. **Avoid anything that hurts your sleep.** Beware of health problems that steal your sleep. These include:

B • Sleep apnea. It leads you to stop breathing for short periods throughout the night, which robs you of restful sleep and leaves you dragging, unfocused, and forgetful throughout the day.

B • Restless leg syndrome.

B • Thyroid conditions. Both hypo- and hyperthyroidism can cause sleep problems. See chapter 13 to find out about testing for thyroid issues.

B • Congestive heart failure.

B • Chronic pain.

B **P** • Untreated or undertreated mental health issues, such as obsessive-compulsive disorder (OCD), depression, or anxiety.

B **P** • Alzheimer's disease. Dementia patients "sundown" or rev up at night and wander.

B • Chronic gastrointestinal problems, such as acid reflux.

(B) • Enlarged prostate gland (benign prostatic hypertrophy). It causes many trips to the bathroom at night, which interrupts slumber.

If you suffer from any of these and you find yourself struggling with getting adequate rest, speak with your health-care provider about possible solutions.

(B) (P) (S) (SP) 3. **Beware of bad sleep habits.** In our hectic, 24/7 society, we could just as easily ask, "What *doesn't* cause sleep deprivation?" A seemingly endless number of reasons cause millions of us to miss out on a good night's sleep. This list includes some of the most common factors.

- A bedroom that is too warm. The ideal temperature is personal, but it should be on the cool side.

- Light in the bedroom. Consider blackout shades if you live in a city, where light pollution is sometimes hard to avoid.

- Noise. Try earplugs if you live in a noisy neighborhood or sleep with someone who snores.

- Gadgets by the bed. Put your phone, tablet, digital watch, and more in another spot, or at least turn off the volume. Turn your digital clock toward the wall so you aren't distracted by glowing numbers.

- Screens. After sundown, use blue light–blocking glasses or screen settings when you are looking at a screen.

- Going to bed worried or angry.

- Medications. Many drugs, including asthma and cough meds, antihistamines, anticonvulsants, and stimulants (such as Adderall or Concerta, prescribed for ADD/ADHD), as well as others, disturb sleep.[16]

- Naps. Even if you are having trouble sleeping, this is a mistake if you suffer from insomnia. Taking a nap because you feel sleepy during the day interferes with your nighttime sleep cycle.

- Caffeine. Too much of the stimulant from coffee, tea, chocolate, or some herbal preparations—especially when consumed later in the day or at night—can disrupt sleep. Refrain from using them after 2 p.m.

- Alcohol, nicotine, and marijuana. Although these compounds initially induce sleepiness for some people, they have the reverse effect as they wear off, which is why you may wake up several hours after you go to sleep—and not be able to return to slumbering.[17]

- Exercise within four hours of the time you hit the sack. Regular workouts are very beneficial for insomnia, but vigorous exercise late in the evening may energize you and keep you awake.[18]

- Changes in hormones. Whether due to pregnancy, premenstrual syndrome (PMS), perimenopause, or menopause, these changes can disrupt women's sleep.

- Snoring. It can keep you or your spouse awake—or anyone else in the house, if it is really loud.

- Shift work. Nurses, firefighters, security personnel, customer service representatives, truck drivers, airline pilots, and many others toil by night and sleep by day—at least, they try to sleep. Shift workers are especially vulnerable to irregular sleep patterns, which leads to excessive sleepiness, reduced productivity, irritability, and mood problems.[19] To improve sleep, turn on bright lights while on the job and use blackout blinds or curtains while you sleep during the daytime.

- Stressful situations. Death, marital conflict, work deadlines, moving, or an upcoming exam can keep you awake at night.

- Eating close to bedtime. This keeps your GI tract active and your blood pressure high. It also increases the risk of heart attack and stroke.

- Jet lag. Travel between time zones messes with your body's natural sleep rhythm. To minimize sleep disruption when traveling, begin altering your bedtime by one hour each night for a few nights before your trip and then get on local time as soon as you land.

B P S SP 4. **Engage in regular brain-healthy sleep habits.** My nieces, Alizé and Amelie, weren't getting good sleep when they first came to stay with us. Alizé had bad dreams and trouble sleeping, while Amelie wanted anxiously to sleep with her mom. With healthier daily habits, they both began sleeping better. Brain-healthy sleep habits will make it easier to drift off to dreamland and get a good night's sleep. We are all unique, so remember that what works for one person may not work for another. Keep trying new techniques until you find something that works for you.

- Set up your bedroom for sleep: cool, dark, and quiet.

- Don't allow pets in your bedroom—or at least keep them off the bed.

- Address emotional problems before going to sleep. Follow the good advice from Ephesians 4:26 to not "let the sun go down while you are still angry." Send a positive text or email, or set an intention to deal with the issue the next day. If you forgive the other person first, you may just end the argument. Worriers, devote a before-bed time period (about 10 to 15 minutes) to journal or pray about your nagging concerns, and then stop.

- Get into a regular sleep schedule. Try to go to bed at the same time each night and wake up at the same time each morning, every day of the week. Getting up at the same time each day, no matter how long you slept, helps to set your internal body clock and prevent insomnia.

- Read a book—not an e-reader or tablet, as the light keeps your brain alert. Preferably choose something thick or tedious, such as 1 and 2 Chronicles in the Old Testament. If you read Judges in the Old Testament or a murder mystery before bed, it is likely to keep you up.

- Try sound therapy. It can induce a very peaceful mood. Consider turning on soothing nature sounds, wind chimes, a fan, or soft music. Slow classical music, or any music that has a slow rhythm of 60 to 80 beats per minute, can help with sleep.[20] Check out sleep-enhancing music by Grammy Award–winning producer Barry Goldstein at mybrainfitlife.com.

- Drink a cup of warm, unsweetened almond milk. Add a teaspoon of vanilla (genuine, not imitation) and a few drops of stevia. The combination may increase serotonin in your brain and help you sleep.[21]

- Wear socks. Research shows that if your hands and feet are warm, you may fall asleep faster.

- Refrain from checking the clock if you wake up in the night. If you know what time it is, it can make you anxious.

- Restrict use of the bed and bedroom for sleep or sexual activity only. Sexual activity releases muscle tension and a flood of natural hormones and boosts well-being. Adults with healthy sex lives also tend to sleep better. If you are unable to fall asleep or return to sleep easily, get up and go to another room.[22]

- Use lavender to enhance your slumbers. The smell of lavender can decrease anxiety and improve mood and sleep.[23]

- If you have to resort to medication, stay away from benzodiazepines and traditional sleep medications. I often prescribe trazodone, gabapentin, and amitriptyline with my patients.

- Create a soothing nighttime routine that encourages sleep. Turn off all electronic devices at least an hour before bedtime, and lower the lights in your house. A warm bath or shower, prayer, or massage can also help you relax. (Download helpful meditations and sleep-promoting hypnosis audios at mybrainfitlife.com.)

Getting Restful Sleep with Hypnosis

Medical hypnosis is a safe and effective tool that can enhance overall health and well-being and promote more restful sleep. The American Medical Association recognized hypnotherapy as a standard medical treatment back in 1958, and the American Psychological Association followed suit by endorsing it as a branch of psychology in 1960. I have been using hypnosis for decades.

When I was an intern at Walter Reed Army Medical Center, many of my patients wanted sleeping pills. As you can imagine, it's hard to sleep in a busy, noisy hospital. Before I would give them pills, I asked if I could try hypnotizing them first. Almost everyone agreed, and hypnosis was so helpful that many of them did not need sleeping pills at all.

B 5. **Take nutraceuticals that help with sleep.** These are often trial and error to determine which ones will help you most. My patients tend to like a combination of melatonin, magnesium, and gamma-aminobutyric acid (GABA). I suggest trying one of the following for several days and taking it 30 minutes before bedtime.

- **Melatonin** is a neurohormone that helps regulate the sleep cycle. Darkness triggers melatonin production, while light—natural or artificial—reduces it. Too much light at night or too little light during the day can interfere with the production of melatonin. Taking melatonin has been found to decrease the time it takes to fall asleep, increase sleeping hours, and increase feelings of alertness the following day. People with depression, seasonal affective disorder, or panic disorder tend to have low levels of melatonin. Taking melatonin improved depression and anxiety in a study on postmenopausal women. Melatonin boosts serotonin production, which may play a role in its ability to help with sleep and depression.
  Dose suggestion: 0.3–6 mg a day (less is often better)

- **5-HTP** boosts production of the neurotransmitter serotonin and helps to calm activity in the anterior cingulate gyrus. This makes it especially helpful for worriers and people who can't seem to turn off their thoughts at bedtime. Research has shown that 5-HTP can be as effective as antidepressant medication.
  Dose suggestion: 50–200 mg a day

- **Magnesium glycinate or citrate** is a mineral that plays a vital role in more than 300 biochemical processes in the human body. In the brain, it helps activate GABA receptors, which can help calm the brain and reduce anxious thoughts at bedtime.

Dose suggestion: 50–400 mg a day

- **GABA** is an amino acid that has a calming effect for people who struggle with anxiety or stressful thoughts. It promotes relaxation, which can help with sleep.

  Dose suggestion: 250–1,000 mg a day

BRIGHT MINDS: SLEEP

STEPS TO CREATE MENTAL ILLNESS ... AND MAKE MY NIECES, ALIZÉ AND AMELIE, SUFFER	STEPS TO END MENTAL ILLNESS ... AND KEEP MY NIECES, ALIZÉ AND AMELIE, HEALTHY

1. Don't care about sleep.
 	
2. Engage in habits that keep you from getting a good night's rest.
 	
  • Drink coffee or energy drinks in the afternoon and at night.
  • Drink alcohol at night.
  • Don't get tested for sleep apnea, and if you have it, don't use the CPAP machine.
  • Use your smartphone, tablet, or e-reader in bed at night, and keep your phone on the nightstand.
  • Eat a big dinner with fatty foods an hour or two before bedtime to increase the likelihood of nighttime heartburn and acid reflux.
  • Do a hard-core cardio class a couple of hours before you go to bed.
  • Keep a night-light on at all times.
  • Take naps in the afternoon.
  • Volunteer for the night shift at work.
  • Travel across time zones on a regular basis.
  • Rely on sleep medication to get the rest you need.
 	
3. Avoid the strategies that encourage restful sleep.
	1. Care about getting restorative sleep.
	
	2. Avoid anything that hurts your sleep patterns.
	
	3. Engage regularly in healthy habits that promote better sleep.
	
	  • Create a sleep routine and stick to it.
	  • Go to bed at the same time each night.
	  • Keep your bedroom on the cool side at night.
	  • Cut out any caffeinated beverages in the afternoon or evening.
	  • Use soothing music to lull you to sleep.
	  • Try a pillow with the calming scent of lavender.
	  • Aim for seven to eight hours of sleep each night.
	  • Give yourself four hours to digest your dinner before going to bed.
	  • Practice stress-management techniques like meditation and prayer.
	  • Wear a sleep mask to keep light from interrupting your sleep.
	  • Consider taking nutraceuticals that promote calmness and help with the production of sleep hormones.

Pick One BRIGHT MINDS Sleep Tiny Habit to Start Today

TINY HABITS

1. When my spouse complains that I snore and stop breathing at night, I will get assessed for sleep apnea.

2. When I want to sleep better, I will eliminate caffeine during the day (gradually—to avoid headaches).

3. When I use tech gadgets after sundown, I will make sure they have blue light blockers.

4. When it gets close to bedtime, I will cool the bedroom so it's a good temperature for sleeping.

5. When I am ready to go to sleep, I will wear a sleep mask or completely darken the bedroom.

6. When I go to bed, I will turn off my tech gadgets so they do not wake me.

7. When I plan my day, I will write down my sleep routine, so I don't forget it.

8. When I take my supplements, I will include melatonin and magnesium if I have trouble sleeping.

9. When it's time for bed, I will listen to music or a hypnosis sleep audio.

10. When I worry too much, I will supplement with 5-HTP.

PART 3

PRACTICAL STRATEGIES TO END MENTAL ILLNESS NOW

CHAPTER 16

MIND MEDS VERSUS NUTRACEUTICALS

WHAT DOES THE SCIENCE SAY?

> *Millions of Americans today are taking dietary supplements, practicing yoga and integrating other natural therapies into their lives. These are all preventive measures that will keep them out of the doctor's office and drive down the costs of treating serious problems like heart disease and diabetes.*
>
> ANDREW WEIL, MD

 ALICIA

Alicia, 53, was struggling with brain fog, memory problems, anxiety, and symptoms of ADD/ADHD (short attention span, distractibility, disorganization, impulsivity) when she first came to the Amen Clinics. Her SPECT scan showed low overall activity, especially in the prefrontal cortex (see images below). As we attacked each of her BRIGHT MINDS risk factors and used nutraceuticals—including omega-3 fatty acids, multiple vitamins, ginkgo, huperzine A, and phosphatidylserine—her brain fog cleared, and her memory and focus were better. And one more thing that was very important to her— her Ping-Pong game dramatically improved.

ALICIA'S SURFACE SPECT SCANS: BEFORE AND AFTER

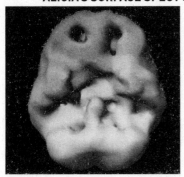 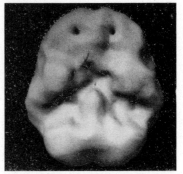

Before: low prefrontal cortex activity   After: overall improved

Alicia had been playing Ping-Pong for months in an effort to boost her brain (I think Ping-Pong is the best sport for your brain), but initially she always lost to her husband because her mind would wander. Her husband even played left-handed in order to give her an advantage. After starting the nutraceuticals, she said, "I was beating my husband in Ping-Pong every game, and it happened overnight . . . my husband was really angry that I was beating him." Alicia then hired a Ping-Pong coach because, "I want to keep beating my husband." About work, she said, "I'm getting a lot more done, and I am happier." Her follow-up scan was also much better. Not to be outdone, her husband started the nutraceuticals, lost 30 pounds, and became serious about his brain health. I'll bet they have a fierce Ping-Pong competition now. In addition, her adult children, who saw the benefit in their mother, started eating better, exercising, and taking nutraceuticals.

> *After starting the nutraceuticals, she said, "I was beating my husband in Ping-Pong every game, and it happened overnight."*

At Amen Clinics we are not opposed to medications for your mind and prescribe them when necessary. However, we are opposed to medications being the first and only thing you do to help your brain and your mind. As you've seen throughout this book, there is so much more that can and needs to be done to end mental illness now.

The pharmaceutical revolution has consumed psychiatry for the past 50 years, but unfortunately, outcomes have not improved along with the enthusiasm. As discussed earlier, one of the reasons outcomes lag behind is that medical professionals are working within the wrong paradigm—making diagnoses based on symptom clusters without any biological information while ignoring overall brain health and the BRIGHT MINDS risk factors.

I first became interested in using nutraceuticals for brain health/mental health issues once I started using SPECT scans. I could see that some of the medications I was taught to prescribe, especially benzodiazepines for anxiety and opiates for pain, were clearly associated with unhealthy looking scans.

TOXICITY ON SURFACE SPECT SCANS OF SOME MEDICATIONS

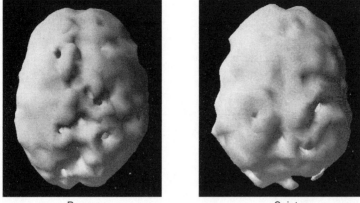

Benzos   Opiates

Thinking of the principle all physicians are taught the first year of medical school—*Primum non nocere*, which is Latin for "First do no harm"—I started looking for less toxic options for my patients and was surprised to find a growing body of scientific literature to support the use of supplements for many brain health/mental health issues. In making treatment recommendations for our patients, we always try to keep a number of principles in mind:

- First, do no harm.

- Use the least toxic, most effective, science-based treatments.

- Consider short-term pain versus long-term gain (don't fix one problem just to cause another one).

- Don't start something a patient will have a hard time stopping (withdrawing from many anti-anxiety or antidepressant medications can be very hard), just to deal with the anxiety of the moment.

- Nutraceuticals or medications should never be the first and only thing people do. Until we understand this concept, we will never truly get well as a society.

I always consider, *What would I prescribe if this were my mother, my wife, or my child?* After nearly 40 years as a psychiatrist, I recommend more and more treatments from nature, including foods and nutraceuticals. We want you to use all the tools available, especially if they are science based, effective, and cheaper, and have minimal side effects.

A number of websites are dedicated to the extensive science of nutraceuticals for health, including brain health, such as MedlinePlus from the National Library of Medicine (medlineplus.gov) and Natural Medicines (naturalmedicines.therapeuticresearch.com). They often grade nutraceuticals from the clinical science evidence similarly to how they rate pharmaceuticals (see chart below).

GRADE	SCIENTIFIC EVIDENCE
A	Robust research conducted with more than two placebo-controlled, double-blind clinical trials
B	Multiple studies where at least two are placebo-controlled, double-blind trials
C	Single double-blind, placebo-controlled trial (only one study so far)
D	Open-label trials (participants and researchers know who is getting the drug or the placebo)
F	Research suggests it does not work

A second chart on the next page shows nutraceuticals with A or B evidence ratings for specific brain health/mental health issues. One major flaw in prescribing nutraceuticals, as with medications, is that they are generally recommended based on symptoms, rather than biology. Our experience is that treatment is much more effective with nutraceuticals and/or medications when we add the biological information from our brain imaging work. Surveys by the CDC find most people are deficient in one or more of these vital nutraceuticals because of their poor-quality diet, or the nutrients are being depleted from their bodies due to stress or the effects of certain medications. It's important to work with a knowledgeable health-care provider to determine the best approach and nutraceuticals for your particular brain health/mental health issues.

SCIENTIFIC EVIDENCE FOR COMMON CONDITIONS AND NUTRACEUTICALS

SYMPTOM-CLUSTERS	A-LEVEL EVIDENCE	B-LEVEL EVIDENCE	NOTES
Anxiety and Stress (anxious, tense, worried, nervous, obsessive thoughts, panic, OCD, PTSD)	Ashwagandha[1] (OCD)[2] Theanine[3] Omega-3 fatty acids EPA and DHA[4]	Inositol[5] (OCD)[6] (panic)[7] GABA[8] Magnesium[9] (better with 30mg of B6)[10] Saffron[11] Passionflower[12] Lavender[13] 5HTP[14] Multiple vitamins[15] NAC (OCD)[16] (PTSD)[17] Probiotics[18] Rhodiola[19] Ginkgo[20] Relora[21]	Zinc levels low in panic disorder[22] Relora = *Magnolia officinalis* + *Phellodendron amurense* bark extracts
Attention, Focus, and Energy	EPA omega-3s[23] Phosphatidylserine (PS)[24]	Zinc[25] Pycnogenol[26] Magnesium[27] Rhodiola[28] Ginseng[29] Ashwagandha[30] Green tea extract[31] Multiple vitamins[32] Bacopa monnieri[33]	Low zinc levels associated with low mood[34]
Mood	EPA omega-3s[35] St. John's wort[36] Saffron[37] SAMe[38]	Curcumin[39] Zinc[40] Magnesium[41] 5-HTP[42] Folate[43] NAC[44] (16 weeks)[45] PS[46] Rhodiola[47] Multiple vitamins[48] Vitamin D[49] Probiotics[50] Ginkgo[51]	SAMe seems to be more effective in males;[52] a few reports suggest it may trigger mania in bipolar patients;[53] folate as an add-on treatment with SSRIs;[54] NAC more effective when CRP is high[55]

SYMPTOM-CLUSTERS	A-LEVEL EVIDENCE	B-LEVEL EVIDENCE	NOTES
Memory	Ginkgo[56] PS[57] Alpha GPC (also called choline alphoscerate)[58]	Omega-3s[59] Multiple vitamins[60] Huperzine A[61] Bacopa monnieri[62] Cocoa flavanols[63] Pycnogenol[64] Saffron[65] Ashwagandha[66] Vitamin D[67]	
Psychotic symptoms	Sarcosine[68]	NAC[69] Omega-3s[70] (prevention of psychotic disorders) Folate[71]	Sarcosine add-on to antipsychotic medication has been shown to be helpful[72]
Sleep	Melatonin[73] (jet lag)[74]	Theanine[75] Magnesium[76] Valerian[77] Probiotics[78]	Combo of melatonin, magnesium, and zinc[79]
Addictions, cravings		Vitamin D[80] Huperzine A[81] NAC (cravings overall)[82] (tobacco)[83] (alcohol and marijuana)[84] (marijuana in teens)[85] (cocaine)[86] (methamphet-amine)[87] (heroin)[88] (gambling)[89] Chromium picolinate[90] Ashwagandha[91]	NAC may be most useful for preventing relapse[92]

My colleague Dr. Parris Kidd, who has more than 35 years of experience working with supplements, recommends that everyone have a core nutraceutical program that includes a broad-spectrum "multiple" (nutraceutical multiple vitamin-mineral supplement), plus a concentrated fish oil or vegan source of omega-3s EPA and DHA. These are all critical for your enzyme systems to work.

For more severe mental health issues, such as schizophrenia or true bipolar disorder, I usually start with medications, such as antipsychotics, like olanzapine (Zyprexa), aripirazole (Abilify), or risperidone (Risperdal), or mood stabilizers, such as lamotrigine (Lamictal). Yet, even when I am prescribing medication, I am also recommending the support of nutraceuticals, such as omega-3 fatty acids, multiple vitamins, and vitamin D. This is in addition to attacking the BRIGHT MINDS risk factors and making nutritional changes. By supporting overall brain health in this way, people typically get better faster and have fewer relapses. For example, here are interventions we typically recommend for these patients.

SCHIZOPHRENIA, TRUE BIPOLAR DISORDER, AND ANY PSYCHOTIC PROCESS

1. Get any psychotic process under control, using the appropriate medications.

2. Support with basic nutraceuticals, including multiple vitamins, folate, and fish oil.

3. Attack the BRIGHT MINDS risk factors.

4. Eliminate artificial dyes, preservatives, and sweeteners from the diet.

5. Try an elimination diet for three weeks, eliminating sugary food, gluten, dairy, corn, soy, and other categories of potentially allergenic foods. Then add these back one at a time (except for sugar) and be alert for reactions to them, which would indicate that you should permanently avoid that food. In general, it's advisable to keep sugar out of your diet.

6. Begin taking the following nutraceuticals:

   • Longvida curcumin, a formulation much more efficiently absorbed than other curcumin supplements
   • Magnesium
   • Zinc
   • Probiotics

For most other disorders, such as ADD/ADHD, anxiety, depression, insomnia, and addictions, I often start with nutraceuticals. If they are ineffective, *then* I consider medications.

For example, here are the steps I recommend for my patients for some common brain health/mental health issues *before* considering prescription medications.

ADD/ADHD

Symptoms of ADD/ADHD include short attention span, distractibility, disorganization, procrastination, impulsivity, and restlessness.

1. Attack the BRIGHT MINDS risk factors.

2. Eliminate artificial dyes, preservatives, and sweeteners from the family's diet.

3. Minimize or eliminate processed foods (anything in a box).

4. Try an elimination diet for three weeks. (See step 5 on page 297.)

5. Try a higher-protein, lower carbohydrate diet. Boost exercise—30 minutes or more five times a week.

6. Increase sleep and good sleep habits.

7. Decrease screen time.

8. Work closely with an integrative physician to check ferritin, vitamin D, magnesium, zinc, and thyroid levels, as well as all the other lab chemistry tests, and balance any that are not optimal.

9. Begin taking the following nutraceuticals:

   - EPA-rich fish oil
     Dose suggestion: 1,000 mg a day of EPA and DHA per 40 pounds of body weight, to maximum 3,000 mg a day EPA and DHA
   - Phosphatidylserine (PS)
     Dose suggestion: 200–300 mg a day
   - Zinc as citrate or glycinate
     Dose suggestion: 30 mg a day (tolerable upper levels are 40 mg a day for adults, 34 mg a day for adolescents; less for younger kids)
   - Magnesium as glycinate, citrate, or malate
     Dose suggestion: 100–400 mg a day

10. Consider neurofeedback.

11. Start kids a bit later in school (the youngest kids in a class are more likely to be diagnosed with ADD/ADHD).

If someone truly has ADD/ADHD, they will still have it a few months after I first see them, so taking some time to get their brain health/mental health optimized is worth the investment before starting a medication that they may be on for years or even decades. At this point, I'll recommend nutraceuticals or medications targeted to someone's specific type of ADD/ADHD (see *Healing ADD: The Breakthrough Program That Allows You to See and Heal the 7 Types of ADD*).

In the case of ADD/ADHD, which has been one of my primary areas of expertise, there is a great deal of negative bias against medication in our society. I've heard countless parents say:

"I'm not going to drug my kid."
"If you take this drug, you won't be creative."
"You won't be yourself."

The problem is that most physicians assume ADD/ADHD is one thing, so they start everyone on the same class of medications—stimulants, such as Ritalin or Adderall. These medications help many people, but they also make many others much worse.

Both "miracle" and "horror" stories about stimulants abound. One of my own children went from being a mediocre student to getting straight As for ten years while using a stimulant medication to optimize the low activity in her prefrontal cortex, and she was accepted to one of the world's best veterinarian schools. The medication stimulated her frontal lobes, giving her greater access to her own abilities, which also enhanced her self-esteem. On the other hand, I have another patient who was referred to me because he became suicidal on Ritalin. His brain was already overactive to start, so stimulating it only made him more anxious and upset. The problem comes when physicians assume everyone with the same symptoms has the same brain patterns, which is just not true and invites failure and frustration.

ADDICTIONS

1. Stop the addictive substance, which is directly or indirectly a toxin to your brain!

2. Twelve step program, such as Alcoholics Anonymous

3. BRIGHT MINDS brain rehabilitation program, attacking all the risk factors

4. BRIGHT MINDS diet to help prevent relapse—most treatment programs serve very unhealthy foods that promote relapse

5. HALT to prevent relapse—do not get too Hungry (balance blood sugar), Angry (kill the ANTs), Lonely (connect with others), or Tired (sleep).

6. Eliminate the ANTs (automatic negative thoughts).

7. Begin taking the following nutraceuticals:
   - Omega-3 fatty acids
     Dose suggestion: 1,400 mg or more with a ratio of approximately 60/40 EPA to DHA
   - NAC
     Dose suggestion: 1,200–2,400 mg a day; clinical research very promising

If the above interventions are ineffective, I'll try other nutraceuticals or medications targeted to someone's specific type of addiction (see my book *Unchain Your Brain: 10 Steps to Breaking the Addictions That Steal Your Life*).

ANXIETY DISORDERS

1. Attack the BRIGHT MINDS risk factors.

2. Check for hypoglycemia, anemia, and hyperthyroidism.

3. Eliminate artificial dyes, preservatives, and sweeteners from the diet.

4. Try an elimination diet for three weeks. (See step 5 on page 297 for more details.)

5. Practice prayer, meditation, and hypnosis. (Research shows they can calm stress and anxiety, and you can use helpful audio programs for guided meditation and self-hypnosis.)

6. Heart rate variability (HRV) training. (Anxiety is linked to low levels of HRV,[93] but you can hack your way to a healthier HRV with biofeedback apps. Read more about this in my book *Feel Better Fast and Make It Last*.)

7. Diaphragmatic breathing and hand-warming biofeedback. (Read more about these in my book *Feel Better Fast and Make It Last*.)

8. Eliminate the ANTs.

9. Calming exercise, such as yoga, qi gong, and tai chi.

10. Begin taking the following nutraceuticals:
    - L-theanine
      Dose suggestion: 200–400 mg a day
    - GABA
      Dose suggestion: 500–1,000 mg a day
    - Magnesium as glycinate, citrate, or malate
      Dose suggestion: 100–500 mg with 30 mg of vitamin B6 a day
    - Probiotics

11. Check your Omega-3 Index (www.omegaquant.com) and get it above 8 percent using 1,400 mg or more omega-3 fish oil with a ratio of approximately 60/40 EPA to DHA.

12. Consider neurofeedback.

Anxiety disorders are very painful, but too often people reach for marijuana, alcohol, or prescribed benzodiazepines, which can be of short-term benefit but can cause long-term problems with addiction and memory issues. If the above interventions are ineffective or only partly effective, I'll try other nutraceuticals or medications targeted to someone's specific type of anxiety (see my book *Healing Anxiety and Depression*).

DEPRESSION

1. Attack the BRIGHT MINDS risk factors.

2. Check for and correct low thyroid function.

3. Work with a nutritionally informed physician to optimize your folate, vitamin B12, vitamin D, homocysteine, and other nutrient levels.

4. Check your Omega-3 Index (www.omegaquant.com) and get it above 8 percent using 1,400 mg or more omega-3 fish oil with a ratio of approximately 60/40 EPA to DHA. (I'm convinced that without doing these nutritional fixes, patients are very unlikely to respond to the medications.)

5. Eliminate processed foods as well as artificial dyes, preservatives, and sweeteners.

6. Try an elimination diet for three weeks. (See step 5 on page 297 for more details.)

7. Increase protein, lower carbs, and add colorful vegetables into your diet.

8. Eliminate the ANTs.

9. Exercise.[94]

10. Begin taking the following nutraceuticals:
    - Curcumin, not as turmeric root but as Longvida, which is much more efficiently absorbed
    - Magnesium as glycinate, citrate, or malate
      Dose suggestion: 100–500 mg with 30 mg of vitamin B6 a day
    - Zinc as citrate or glycinate
      Dose suggestion: 30 mg (tolerable upper levels are 40 mg a day for adults and 34 mg a day for adolescents; less for younger kids)
    - Probiotics

Depression can be devastating, but too often during quick office visits physicians put patients on SSRIs rather than attack the underlying cause. SSRIs are often very hard medications to stop. If the above interventions are ineffective, I'll try other nutraceuticals or medications targeted to their specific type of depression (see my book *Healing Anxiety and Depression*).

INSOMNIA

1. Care about your sleep. Make it a priority.

2. Avoid anything that hurts sleep, such as caffeine; blue light from gadgets; a light, warm room; noise; alcohol; evening exercise; unchallenged negative thoughts; and worries.

3. Treat any issues that steal your sleep—restless leg syndrome, sleep apnea, hyperthyroidism, low progesterone, or chronic pain.

4. Engage in positive sleep habits, such as blue-light blockers, turning off gadgets, prayer, hypnosis, meditation, soothing music, a warm bath, a cool room and pillow, a regular sleep schedule, and lavender aromatherapy.

5. Begin taking the following nutraceuticals:
    - Melatonin
      Dose suggestion: 0.3–5 mg before bedtime, gradually increasing it until it works for you

- Magnesium
  Dose suggestion: 100–500 mg a day
- Zinc
  Dose suggestion: 15–30 mg a day
- 5-HTP
  Dose suggestion: 100–200 mg a day if you are a worrier
- GABA
  Dose suggestion: 250–1,000 mg a day

Too often, people are prescribed addictive sleeping pills that can affect memory without searching for the underlying cause or doing the simple strategies first. If the above interventions are ineffective, I'll try nonaddictive sleep-promoting medications, such as low-dose trazodone, gabapentin, or amitriptyline.

Remember, whether you use medications or supplements or a combination of them, they are only a part of our Amen Clinics Four Circles BRIGHT MINDS Program. Do not expect that a pill, natural or not, by itself will change your life for the better.

PROS AND CONS OF MEDICATIONS

Based on 40 years of studying and practicing psychiatry, I have compiled the following list of pros and cons of medications for your mind:

Pros

1. For more serious mental health conditions, such as schizophrenia, true bipolar disorder (I say true bipolar because people are often misdiagnosed as having bipolar disorder when they have the lasting effects of traumatic brain injury), severe major depression, and OCD, medications are often the most effective and fastest acting treatments.

2. For ADD/ADHD, stimulant medications work quickly and can be very effective, *if they are given for the right type of ADD/ADHD*. As discussed earlier, stimulants work for two of the seven types of ADD/ADHD.

3. Prazosin (Minipress—a blood pressure medication) is often an effective, quick-acting, safe treatment for nightmares in people with PTSD.

4. Physicians are trained in using medications for mental health issues, so they are used to prescribing them, and they are a part of regular medical practice.

5. Medical insurance plans often cover them.

Cons

1. Mind medications have significantly more side effects than nutraceuticals. Most have a "black box" warning, which is the FDA's strictest warning associated with the labeling of prescription drugs. It is used when there is reasonable evidence of an association of a serious hazard with the drug.

2. They are generally much more expensive than nutraceuticals, although they tend to be covered by medical insurance.

3. Once started, many medications are often hard to stop. Withdrawal from antidepressant and antianxiety medications can be long and painful.

4. Once started, many people feel dependent on them and do not do the work to truly get their brains healthy over time.

5. Some medications change your brain so you then need them in order to feel normal.

6. As awful as it sounds, taking prescription medications can affect your insurability. I know many people who have been denied or made to pay higher rates for health insurance because they have taken certain medications.

7. For ADD/ADHD, if stimulants are prescribed without taking into consideration the particular type of ADD/ADHD you have, they can do more harm than good. For example, for five types of ADD/ADHD, stimulants can make you much worse.

An important note: Check with your health-care provider before stopping any medication.

PROS AND CONS OF NUTRACEUTICALS

Based on more than three decades of diving into the research on nutraceuticals to help the brain and using them in my clinical practice, I have compiled the following list of pros and cons of taking nutraceuticals.

Pros

1. They are often effective when prescribed properly.

2. They have dramatically fewer side effects than most prescription medications.

3. They are significantly less expensive than medications.

4. You never have to tell an insurance company that you have taken them, so they will not affect your insurability.

5. When people start to take supplements to optimize their health, they often start to engage in other healthy habits.

Cons

1. Even though they tend to be less expensive than medications, insurance usually does not cover them.

2. Many people are unaware that nutraceuticals can have side effects and need to be thoughtfully used. Just because something is natural does not mean it is innocuous. Both arsenic and cyanide are natural, but that doesn't mean they are good for you. For example, St. John's wort used to be one of my favorite natural antidepressants, but it can cause sun sensitivity and it can also decrease the effectiveness of a number of other medications, such as birth control pills.[95] Oh great! Get depressed, take St. John's wort from the grocery store, and now you are pregnant when you don't want to be. That may not be the outcome you were planning on.

3. One of the major concerns about nutraceuticals is the lack of quality control. There is variability, so you need to find trustworthy brands. I do my very best to recommend only nutraceuticals that have been put through stringent quality control. You can find the high-quality products and brands we recommend to our patients on our site (www.brainmedhealth.com).

4. Another disadvantage is that many people get their advice about supplements from the teenage clerk at the health food store who may not have the best information, or from secondary sources on the Internet. *You need advice from health-care professionals who are trained and competent to give you the best advice.*

Even though they have limitations, the benefits of nutraceuticals compared with their minimal risks make them worth considering, especially if you can get thoughtful, research-based information.

INFORMED CONSENT

In the first year of medical school, all students are taught about informed consent. When it comes to treatment for any medical or brain health/mental health condition, it is not our job to tell you what to do; it is our job to give you the options and inform you about the pros and cons of each option. This is critical. Too many physicians tell you what treatment they'll prescribe rather than giving you all of the options. Your doctor is not your father, mother, or boss; they should be your partner in wellness. Ask for options.

CHAPTER 17

YOU CANNOT CHANGE WHAT YOU DO NOT MEASURE

PREVENTION STARTS BY KNOWING YOUR IMPORTANT HEALTH NUMBERS

If you can't measure it, you can't improve it.

PETER DRUCKER

To end mental illness, it is essential to know if your brain and body are working right and to optimize them if they are not. I have written about this in several of my books because it is critical to know your important health numbers. Check these numbers annually and whenever you feel out of sorts. The important numbers you need to know are organized below according to the BRIGHT MINDS risk factors.

BLOOD FLOW AND VASCULAR FACTORS (CHAPTER 5)

Days a week you exercise: Aim for 5 days a week for 30 minutes or more.

Blood pressure:[1] Good blood pressure is critical for brain health. High blood pressure is associated with lower overall brain function, which means bad decision-making. Recently, the American Heart Association and the American College of Cardiology announced revised guidelines that now mean anyone with blood pressure of 130/80 milligrams of mercury will be diagnosed with Stage 1 hypertension. Previously, a blood pressure of 140/90 was considered hypertension. (The category of "prehypertension" no longer exists.) That means more Americans than ever—half of all men and 38 percent of women, or 103 million people versus 72 million before this change—are now considered to have hypertension.[2] Here are the blood pressure numbers you should know:

Optimal
Systolic 90–120
Diastolic 60–80

Stage 1 Hypertension
Systolic 130–139
Diastolic 80–89

Stage 2 Hypertension
Systolic >/= 140
Diastolic >/= 90

Hypotension—too low can also be a problem
Systolic < 90
Diastolic < 60

Blood lipid panel: Cholesterol and triglycerides (fats) can impact blood delivery to the brain. Cholesterol that is either too high or too low is bad for the brain. Surprisingly, higher cholesterol later in life has been associated with better cognitive performance[3] and a decreased risk of dementia.[4] Normal levels are:

- Total cholesterol (135–200 mg/dL; below 160 has been associated with depression, suicide, homicide, and death from all causes, so 160–200 mg/dL is optimal)
- HDL (>/= 60 mg/dL)
- LDL (<100 mg/dL)
- Triglycerides (<150 mg/dL)

Ask your health-care professional to also test the particle size of your LDL cholesterol because larger particles are less toxic than smaller ones. If you want to find out more about cholesterol, read *The Great Cholesterol Myth* by Stephen Sinatra and Jonny Bowden.

Complete blood count (CBC): This blood test measures your red and white blood cells. People with a low red blood cell count can feel anxious and tired and have trouble with memory. Enlarged red blood cells can indicate too much alcohol consumption. Too many white blood cells can reveal an infection.

Homocysteine (blood test): High homocysteine levels (>10 micromoles/liter) is linked with atherosclerosis (hardening and narrowing of the arteries) and an increased risk of heart attack, stroke, blood clot formation, and possibly Alzheimer's disease. Homocysteine levels also reveal whether you are deficient in folate (see page 310).

RETIREMENT AND AGING (CHAPTER 6)

General metabolic panel (blood test): This reveals the health of your liver, kidneys, sodium levels, and more.

Ferritin (blood test): This is a measure of your iron stores. High levels are associated with inflammation (chapter 7) and insulin resistance (chapter 14). Low levels are associated with anemia, restless leg syndrome, ADD/ADHD, and low motivation and energy. A level of 50–100 nanograms/mL is ideal. Women often have lower iron stores than men because of menstruation. Some theorize that this is one of the reasons that women tend to live longer than men. If your level is low, consider taking iron. If it is high, donating blood may help.

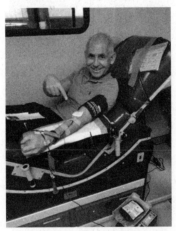
This is me donating blood.

INFLAMMATION AND GUT HEALTH (CHAPTER 7)

C-reactive protein (CRP; blood test): This measures the inflammation level in your body. Inflammation is associated with chronic illnesses such as depression, dementia, and pain syndromes. A healthy CRP range is 0.0–1.0 mg/L.

Omega-3 Index (a drop of blood):[5] This measures the total amount of omega-3 fatty acids EPA and DHA in red blood cells and directly reflects their levels in the brain. The test is a clinically validated biomarker of the health of your brain. Your risk of cognitive decline rises by as much as 77 percent when your Omega-3 Index is low. Aim for a level above 8 percent.

Vitamin B12 (blood test): This is critically important for healthy brain function. A vitamin B12 deficiency can potentially cause severe and irreversible damage, especially to the brain and nervous system. Symptoms such as fatigue, depression, and poor memory can occur at levels only slightly lower than normal. Vitamin B12 also can be depleted by medications, particularly those that impair stomach and intestinal function, such as proton pump inhibitors for acid reflux. Its deficiency can cause symptoms of mania and psychosis and even masquerade as dementia. A normal range is 211 to 946 picograms per milliliter; optimal is greater than 600.

GENETICS (CHAPTER 8)

Know your genetic risks: Diagram your family tree and take notice of any genetic issues that run in your family.

Consider genetic testing: Genomind (www.genomind.com) and GeneSight (www.genesight.com) are two companies our clinicians use at Amen Clinics.

Folate (blood test): This aids in the production of DNA and other genetic material. It is required for the healthy regulation of genes and is especially important when cells and tissues are growing rapidly, such as in infancy, adolescence, and pregnancy. Folate works together with vitamins B6 and B12 and other nutrients to control blood levels of homocysteine. It is common to have low levels of folate as a result of alcoholism, inflammatory bowel disease (IBD), celiac disease, and certain medications. A normal level is 2 to 20 ng/mL; optimal is thought to be greater than 3 nanograms per milliliter.

HEAD TRAUMA (CHAPTER 9)

Number of past concussions with or without loss of consciousness.

TOXINS (CHAPTER 10)

How many alcoholic beverages you consume each day/week, how many cigarettes you smoke, how often you vape, and how often you use drugs (including marijuana).

There are tests for heavy metals and mold, but you do not need to do them routinely unless you are experiencing symptoms or you know you've been exposed to high levels.

MIND STORMS (CHAPTER 11)

QEEG/SPECT tests: There aren't specific numbers associated with mindstorms, but these tests can be extremely helpful if you suspect a problem.

IMMUNITY/INFECTIONS (CHAPTER 12)

CBC to look at your white blood cell count.

Erythrocyte sedimentation rate (ESR) measures inflammation, which is high in autoimmune disorders.

Antinuclear antibodies (ANA)—antibodies fight infection, but ANAs often attack your body's tissues. ANAs are often high in autoimmune disorders.

Vitamin D (blood test):[6] Low levels of vitamin D have been associated with obesity, depression, cognitive impairment, heart disease, reduced immunity, cancer, and all causes of mortality. The blood test to get is 25-hydroxyvitamin D level. A normal vitamin D level is 30–100 ng/mL, with the most optimal range being 50 to 100 ng/mL.

NEUROHORMONES (CHAPTER 13)

Thyroid panel (blood test): If your thyroid hormone levels are abnormal, it could explain the cause of anxiety, depression, forgetfulness, weight problems, and lethargy. Hypothyroidism (low) decreases overall brain activity, which can impair your thinking, judgment, and self-control, and it can make it nearly impossible to manage weight effectively. Hyperthyroidism (high) is associated with anxiety, insomnia, and feeling agitated. If you have symptoms, don't settle for just a TSH test, which measures your thyroid stimulating hormone. TSH levels can be normal even when you have an undiagnosed thyroid problem. Instead, insist that your doctor order all of the following:

- TSH—according to the American Association of Clinical Endocrinologists, anything over 3.0 is abnormal and needs further investigation.
- Free T3—active thyroid; see the normal ranges for the individual laboratory you use.
- Free T4—inactive thyroid; see the normal ranges for the individual laboratory you use.
- Thyroid antibodies
  - Thyroid peroxidase antibodies (TPO)
  - Thyroglobulin antibodies (TG); see the normal ranges for the individual laboratory you use.

- **Liver function tests**—95 percent of T4 is "activated" in the liver, so having a healthy liver is essential.
- **Ferritin level**—Ferritin is like the bus that drives active T3 into the cells; ferritin needs to be above 50 for this to occur.

An important note: While thyroid tests can be helpful, your doctor should treat *you*, not the blood test. I've seen too many hypothyroid patients who haven't been treated because their thyroid numbers were low but "within normal limits." That's a little like saying a vitamin D level of 31 is normal (the normal range is 30 to 100). I have never wanted to be at the bottom of any class I was in. How a patient feels and functions (e.g., low energy, constipation, dry hair, dry skin, poor cognition, low body temperature) is more important in assessing thyroid function than using arbitrary normal ranges on blood tests. All of the above tests could be "normal," and someone could still have a problem.

Cortisol (saliva): This is best done at four intervals throughout the day (to understand your daily cycle): when you first wake up, around lunch time, around dinner time, and just before you go to sleep. Ideally, your cortisol levels are high in the morning (to wake you up) and taper off slowly during the day and evening, allowing you to fall into a restful sleep at night. When cortisol levels are too high, you feel wired. When they are too low, you feel exhausted, spacey, or sluggish.

DHEA-S (blood test): Normal blood levels of DHEA-sulfate can differ by sex and age.
Typical ranges for females:

> Ages 18–19: 145–395 mcg/dL (micrograms per deciliter)
> Ages 20–29: 65–380 mcg/dL
> Ages 30–39: 45–270 mcg/dL
> Ages 40–49: 32–240 mcg/dL
> Ages 50–59: 26–200 mcg/dL
> Ages 60–69: 13–130 mcg/dL
> Ages 70 and older: 17–90 mcg/dL

Typical ranges for males:

> Ages 18–19: 108–441 mcg/dL
> Ages 20–29: 280–640 mcg/dL
> Ages 30–39: 120–520 mcg/dL
> Ages 40–49: 95–530 mcg/dL

Ages 50–59: 70–310 mcg/dL

Ages 60–69: 42–290 mcg/dL

Ages 70 and older: 28–175 mcg/dL

Free and total serum testosterone (blood test): Having an optimal level of testosterone is important for your health and well-being. Too much can cause behavioral problems, such as aggression, but too little is associated with depression, poor memory, and low libido.

Normal levels for adult males:

Total testosterone: 280–800 nanograms ng/dL—optimal is 500–800 ng/dL

Free testosterone: 7.2–24 picograms pg/mL—optimal is 12–24 pg/mL

Normal levels for adult females:

Total testosterone: 6–82 ng/dL—optimal is 40–82 ng/dL

Free testosterone: 0.0–2.2 pg/mL—optimal is 1.0–2.2 pg/mL

Estrogen and progesterone for women:[7] Depending on the circumstances, these are measured in blood or saliva. Menstruating women are usually tested on day 21 of their cycle, while postmenopausal women can be measured any time. Estrogen is responsible for vaginal lubrication, helps with libido and memory—and so much more. Progesterone calms emotions, contributes to a restful sleep, and acts as a diuretic. See the normal ranges for the individual laboratory you use.

DIABESITY (CHAPTER 14)

Body mass index (BMI):[8] This measurement is the result of comparing weight to height. An optimal BMI is between 18.5 and 25; the overweight range falls between 25 and 30; over 30 indicates obesity, and over 40 indicates morbid obesity. Just Google "BMI Calculator" and fill in your height and weight to determine your BMI. Take this number seriously, because being overweight or obese is associated with having a smaller brain, and when it comes to your brain, size matters! Plus, obesity increases the risk for depression and Alzheimer's disease. In a new study, 40 percent of all cancers have been linked to excess weight.[9]

Waist-to-Height Ratio (WHtR):[10] This is another way to measure the health of your weight. Some researchers believe this number is even more accurate than BMI because the most dangerous place to carry weight is in the abdomen. Abdominal fat, which is associated with a larger waist, is metabolically active and produces various hormones that can cause harmful health effects, such as elevated blood pressure, high cholesterol and triglyceride levels, and diabetes.

WHtR is calculated by dividing waist size by height. A woman with a 32-inch waist who is 5'10" (70 inches) would divide 32 by 70 to get a WHtR of 45.7 percent. Generally speaking, it's healthy to stay under 50 percent—in other words, your waist size in inches should be less than half your height. When measuring your waist size, use a tape measure! Don't hazard a guess or rely on your pants' size, which can vary among manufacturers. In my experience, 90 percent of people will underestimate their waist circumference.

Lab tests: Get blood tests for your fasting blood sugar, insulin, and hemoglobin A1c (HbA1c) every year. If they are abnormal, think of it as a health crisis to be taken very seriously.

- **Fasting blood sugar**
  - Normal: 70–105 mg/dL
  - Optimal: 70–89 mg/dL
  - Prediabetes: 105–125 mg/dL
  - Diabetes: 126 mg/dL or higher
- **Hemoglobin A1c:** This test helps diagnose diabetes and prediabetes by revealing average blood sugar levels over the past few months. Normal results for someone without diabetes are in the range of 4 to 5.6 percent; optimal is under 5.3 percent. Levels of 5.7 to 6.4 percent indicate prediabetes. Higher numbers usually indicate diabetes.
- **Fasting insulin:** High insulin levels, usually due to a diet high in simple carbs, are associated with many negative health consequences, including fatty liver, abdominal obesity, excessive cravings, elevated blood sugar, acne, polycystic ovarian syndrome (PCOS), hair loss in women in the male pattern (front and sides), increased risk of gout, high blood pressure, and swollen ankles. Normal is 2.6 to 25; optimal is less than 10. High levels are an early marker for diabetes.

SLEEP (CHAPTER 15)

Number of hours you sleep each night.

Number of sleep disruptions: If you suspect you might have sleep apnea, get a sleep test. Symptoms include daytime fatigue, morning headaches, and irritability; untreated sleep apnea triples your risk of depression and dementia.

KNOW YOUR NUMBERS . . . THEN WHAT?

Knowing your important health numbers is the first step. Optimizing them is critical to helping your brain, emotions, and moods work right. If any of them are abnormal, the function of your brain and mental health can be troubled too. Work with your healthcare provider to help get these numbers into the most optimal range possible.

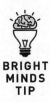

BRIGHT MINDS TIP

Get in the habit of testing your brain and checking out your important health numbers on an annual basis.

CHAPTER 18

FOOD MADE INSANELY SIMPLE

THE BRIGHT MINDS DIET TO END MENTAL ILLNESS

Eating crappy food isn't a reward—it's a punishment.
DREW CAREY (HE GETS IT!)

*No disease that can be treated by diet should
be treated with any other means.*
MAIMONIDES, MEDIEVAL PHILOSOPHER AND PHYSICIAN

When my nieces, Alizé and Amelie, first came under the care of my wife and me, Alizé was obsessed with Flamin' Hot Cheetos. Our first trip to the grocery store together was painful. She wanted junk food (Flamin' Hot Cheetos) for herself and her sister, but I was having none of it. Instead, I tried to teach her how to read the ingredient label on the snack package and understand what each substance does to brain, body, and mental health:

Vegetable oil (corn, canola, and/or sunflower oil)—proinflammatory
Sugar—proinflammatory, promotes aging, increases diabesity
Monosodium glutamate (MSG)—often triggers mind storms
Artificial Color Red Dye #40—often triggers mind storms

She looked at me as if I were an evil ruler. The big breakthrough came a few months later, when we went to Summer House, a fun restaurant frequented by the locals in Corona Del Mar, and she ordered a salmon salad. *And she liked it!* In the two years since, her diet has dramatically improved, and she feels better than ever. When she cheats, she notices how it drains her energy and messes with her mind.

Increasingly, researchers are concluding that the diets of people with brain health/mental health disorders are lacking in key nutrients for brain health. A growing body of evidence suggests that nutritional treatment may help prevent, treat, or improve depression, bipolar disorder, schizophrenia, anxiety, attention deficit disorder/attention deficit hyperactivity disorder (ADD/ADHD), autism, addiction, and eating disorders.[1] And the scientific community is finally beginning to see how food is so strongly linked to brain health/mental health. In 2015, a group of 18 scientists concluded that "the emerging and compelling evidence for nutrition as a crucial factor in the high prevalence and incidence of mental disorders suggests that diet is as important to psychiatry as it is to cardiology, endocrinology, and gastroenterology."[2]

In this chapter, I am going to make food insanely simple and tell you which foods to eat for a better brain and which ones to limit or avoid all together. I've written about many of these foundational food principles before, but here I'll help you connect the dots to your mental health. Yes, there is a lot of conflicting health information about food, but there is also a lot of agreement. If you follow these 11 BRIGHT MINDS rules (details to follow), your brain health/mental health will start to improve within days.

1. Only love foods that love you back.

2. Go for the highest-quality calories you can find—and not too many of them if you need to lose weight.

3. Hydrate, but do not drink your calories.

4. Eat high-quality protein at every meal to balance blood sugar and keep cravings away.

5. Eat and cook with high-quality fat.

6. Go for smart carbohydrates (colorful, low-glycemic, and high-fiber).

7. Use herbs and spices like medicine.

8. Make your food as clean as possible (eliminate artificial sweeteners, colors, preservatives, and foods in plastic containers) and read the labels.

9. If you struggle with any brain health/mental health or physical issue, eliminate any potential allergens or internal attackers, such as sugar, MSG, gluten, corn, soy, and dairy for a month to see if you improve.

10. Use intermittent fasting to supercharge your brain.

11. Get a routine that serves your health rather than hurts it; find 24 foods you love that love you back.

BRIGHT MINDS RULE #1:
Only Love Foods That Love You Back.

If you get this one idea, it will go a long way to ending mental illness in you or your loved ones. But you must first be honest with yourself—you are in a war for the health of your brain. Nearly everywhere you go (schools, work, shopping malls, movie theaters, airports, ball parks, and so on) someone is trying to sell you low-quality, tasty food that will hurt your brain health/mental health and kill you early. The standard American diet (SAD) is filled with pro-inflammatory, allergenic foods laced with artificial chemicals that will damage and prematurely age your brain[3] and increase your risk for depression, ADD/ADHD, anxiety disorders, diabetes, hypertension, heart disease, cancer, and dementia.[4]

The real weapons of mass destruction are foods that are

- highly processed
- pesticide sprayed
- high-glycemic (spikes blood sugar)
- low-fiber
- food-like substances
- artificially colored and sweetened
- laden with hormones
- tainted with antibiotics
- stored in plastic containers

**THE REAL WEAPONS OF MASS DESTRUCTION
DESTROYING THE HEALTH OF AMERICA**

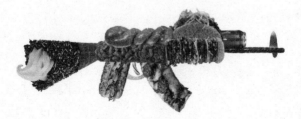

These low-quality "foods" are destroying the brain health/mental health of America, yet corporations pay big money to professional athletes and coaches to visibly drink Coke, Pepsi, or Gatorade (all filled with sugar, artificial colors, and preservatives) on the sidelines of games, effectively marketing these products to children and teens. They also get children hooked on "happy meals" with fun toys that create diabesity and inflammation—definitely not a prescription for happiness. My niece tells me the middle school she attended had days when they would serve Pizza Hut or McDonald's for lunch—foods that can give you brain fog and make it harder to concentrate on learning. Not so smart! Without thinking, we are destroying the mental and physical health of our children.

Many corporations also brag about the addictive nature of their foods: "Bet you can't eat just one." They hire food scientists to combine fat, sugar, and salt with the perfect "texture," "crunchiness," "meltiness," and "aroma" to overwhelm the brain with flavor to trigger the "bliss point" in your brain, which is akin to taking a hit of cocaine, making you literally fall in love with low-quality foods. This is one of the reasons people say they "love" candy, doughnuts, pastries, French fries, and bread—and can't ever conceive of giving them up. They are not eating to live; they are eating for momentary pleasure and to feed addictions that were artificially created for a corporate profit motive. One woman told me that she would rather get Alzheimer's disease than give up sugar. I wondered aloud if she dated the bad boys in high school. Being in love with something that hurts you is an abusive relationship that needs serious intervention. No food of any kind belongs in the same emotional place in your brain as the love you have for your spouse, children, or grandchildren.

We must do better because our children will never be able to afford the tsunami of illness headed their way. Of the health-care dollars in the United States, 75 percent are spent on chronic preventable illnesses,[5] most of which are driven by poor nutrition.

In a fascinating study about diet and depression,[6] researchers went to two remote islands in Australia—one with plentiful fast food and lower fish consumption, the other without fast food and higher fish consumption. Of the people on the island with fast food, 16 percent had moderate-to-severe depression, compared to only 3 percent on the island without, which correlated with the omega-6/omega-3 fatty acid ratio (more on this in rule #5). That is a 500 percent increased risk of depression, based on diet!

Eat This: Foods you love that love you back

Skip or Limit That: Anything you "love" that increases your risk
    of brain health/mental health issues

BRIGHT MINDS RULE #2:

Go for the highest-quality calories you can find—and not too many of them if you need to lose weight.

Calories matter. If you tend to eat when you're feeling depressed, stressed, or anxious and you struggle with your weight, know the amount of calories you consume in a day; but also know that the quality of the calories matters more. If you only eat 800 calories of Twinkies a day, you may lose weight in the short term, but it will definitely make you sicker in the long run. Obesity runs in my family, but I am not overweight because I really care about my health. To counteract the obesity gene, I weigh myself every day (so I always know the truth about my weight), and whenever I gain a few pounds, I start counting calories with a simple note app on my phone. Some professionals will tell you calories don't count, but do not believe them. Supersize your meals, and you'll be supersized too. Calories are like money. I hate wasting money. The same is true for my calories. Maybe you are like me and are a value spender, so spend calories only on high-quality foods.

Eat This: The highest-quality foods you can find that are also calorie smart

Skip or Limit That: Low-quality foods that increase your risk of brain health/mental health issues

BRIGHT MINDS RULE #3:

Hydrate, but do not drink your calories.

Drink 8 to 10 glasses of water a day to stay properly hydrated. Your brain is comprised of 80 percent water, and being even mildly dehydrated can negatively impact your moods—making you feel more anxious, tense, depressed, or angry—in addition to sapping your energy levels and lowering your ability to concentrate.[7] In fact, being dehydrated by just 2 percent impairs performance in tasks that require attention, immediate memory skills, and physical performance.[8] It is also associated with brain atrophy (shrinkage)[9] and performance. Pilots who were dehydrated had poorer performance in the cockpit, especially as it related to working memory, spatial orientation, and cognitive performance.[10]

Replace sugary drinks with water. Just cutting out sugary drinks and fruit juice cuts an average of 400 calories per day from the average American diet! That's either a lot more healthy food you will get to eat instead or a lot of calories you will be losing if you need to lose weight. (Actually, if you do not replace those calories, it equates to losing 40 pounds a year!)

Be deliberate about your water intake, and limit anything that dehydrates you (caffeine, alcohol, and diuretics). When you sweat through exercise, make sure to rehydrate.

> **Drink This:** Water, plain sparkling water, water flavored with slices of fruits (spa water), water with flavored stevia from Sweet Leaf, coconut water, herbal tea, green tea, and black tea (in small amounts if caffeinated)

> **Skip or Limit That:** Calorie-laden drinks, cocktails, energy drinks, sodas, and diet drinks—all of which increase your risk of brain health/mental health issues

BRIGHT MINDS RULE #4:
Eat high-quality protein at every meal to balance blood sugar and keep cravings away.

Protein helps to balance your blood sugar, keeps you full, and provides the building blocks for many neurotransmitters. Protein plays a major role in the healthy growth and functioning of your cells, tissues, and organs. After water, protein is the most abundant substance in your body. At Amen Clinics, we think of protein as medicine that should be taken in small doses with every meal and snack, at least every four to five hours, to help balance your blood sugar levels and decrease cravings. Protein helps you feel fuller longer and burn more calories than you do after eating high-carb, sugar-filled foods.

Your body can produce some of the amino acids it needs, but not all of them—those that can't be manufactured in your body must come from food. These are called essential amino acids, and they are precursors for neurotransmitters, including serotonin and dopamine, which play an important role in brain health/mental health. They must be included in your diet on a regular basis because your body can't store them for future use. Plant foods—such as nuts, seeds, legumes, and some grains, and vegetables—contain only *some* of the 20 amino acids you need. Fish, poultry, and most meats contain *all* of them.[11]

Small amounts of high-quality protein are crucial to good health. But more is not better. Our bodies are simply not designed to effectively process large quantities of protein at a time. Eating too much causes increased stress and inflammation in the body. This contributes to accelerated aging and disease, and it can be hard on some people's kidneys and liver.

Quality is more important than quantity. High-quality animal protein is free of hormones and antibiotics, free range, and grass fed. It is more expensive than industrial farm-raised animal meats, but your brain health/mental health is worth the investment. Compared with grass-fed meat, industrially raised meat is about 30 percent higher in unhealthy fat, which is associated with cardiovascular disease.

Eat This: Healthy proteins include:
- Fish
- Lamb
- Turkey
- Chicken
- Beef
- Pork
- Beans and other legumes
- Raw nuts
- High-protein veggies, such as broccoli and spinach

Skip or Limit That: Low-quality proteins raised with pesticides, hormones, or antibiotics, and excessive protein, which strains your body systems.

BRIGHT MINDS RULE #5:
Eat and cook with high-quality fat.

Of the solid weight of your brain, 60 percent is fat. Low-fat diets are not good for your brain. Focus on healthy fats, such as avocados, nuts, seeds, and sustainable, clean fish. Fat is *not* the enemy. Good fats are essential to your brain health/mental health. For example, omega-3 fatty acids have been found to reduce symptoms of depression. In a study from the Mayo Clinic, people who ate a fat-based diet had a 42 percent lower risk of developing Alzheimer's disease; those who ate a protein-based diet had a 21 percent lower risk of developing Alzheimer's disease; but those who ate a simple-carbohydrate-based diet (think bread, pasta, potatoes, rice, and sugar) had an almost 400 percent *increased* risk of developing Alzheimer's.[12] It's the sugar, and foods that turn to sugar, *not* the fat, that's the problem. However, not all fats are equal. Avoid trans fats (found in foods like processed crackers, baked goods, and frozen pizza), which are associated with an increase in depression. Also skip fats that are higher in omega-6 fatty acids, such as many refined vegetable oils, which are associated with an increase in inflammation.

Eat This: Healthiest fats and oils

Healthiest Fats

- Avocados
- Cocoa butter
- Coconut
- Grass-fed beef, bison, and lamb
- Nuts (walnuts are associated with less depression[13])
- Olives
- Organic free-range poultry
- Seafood—anchovies, arctic char, catfish, herring, king crab, mackerel, wild salmon, sardines, sea bass, snapper, sole, trout, tuna, clams, mussels, oysters, and scallops
- Seeds

Healthiest Oils

- Avocado oil
- Coconut oil
- Flax oil
- Macadamia nut oil
- Olive oil
- Sesame oil
- Walnut oil

Skip or Limit That: Unhealthiest fats and oils
- Canola oil
- Corn oil
- Vegetable oil
- Industrial farm-raised animal fat and dairy
- Processed meats
- Safflower oil
- Soy oil
- Trans fats

BRIGHT MINDS RULE #6:
Go for smart carbohydrates (colorful, low glycemic, and high fiber).

I think of "smart" carbohydrates as those packed with nutrients that balance your blood sugar and reduce cravings. Most vegetables and legumes are low glycemic (unlikely to raise blood sugar). So are many fruits, such as apples, pears, and berries. High-glycemic, low-fiber carbohydrates (sugar, breads, pastas, potatoes, and rice) in significant amounts steal your health because they promote inflammation, diabetes, and depression.[14]

A Swedish study compared the effects on blood sugar of a grain-free diet (Paleo) and a Mediterranean diet, which relies, in part, on whole grains. After 12 weeks, the blood sugar levels were markedly lower in the Paleo group (–26 percent) than in the Mediterranean group (–7 percent). At the end of the study, all patients in the Paleo group had normal blood glucose, which was not true for the Mediterranean group. A diet containing more high-glycemic foods was also associated with a higher incidence of depression and fatigue.[15]

Fiber is a special type of carbohydrate that enhances digestion, reduces the risk of colon cancer, and helps to balance blood pressure and blood sugar. The average American consumes far too little—less than 15 grams of fiber daily. Women should consume 25 to 30 grams of fiber every day; men, 30 to 38 grams. High-fiber foods—such as broccoli, berries, onions, flax seeds, nuts, green beans, cauliflower, celery, and sweet potatoes (the skin of one sweet potato has more fiber than a bowl of oatmeal!)—have the added benefit of making you feel full faster and longer.[16]

Colorful vegetables and fruits are full of brain health/mental health benefits, providing nutrients, vitamins, minerals, and antioxidants. They boost the level of antioxidants in your body, which reduces the risk of developing cognitive impairment and depression. Antioxidants neutralize the production of free radicals in the body, which play a major role in many illnesses, including cardiovascular disease, autoimmune disorders, Alzheimer's disease, Parkinson's,[17] schizophrenia,[18] and depression.[19] Increasing antioxidants has been found to help many conditions, including anxiety and depression.[20]

Here is a list of antioxidant-rich foods and spices, by oxygen radical absorbance capacity (ORAC) value or potency.[21]

Cloves: 290,000+
Oregano (dried): 175,000+
Rosemary: 165,000
Cinnamon: 131,000+
Sage (dried): 119,000+
Acai fruit: 102,000+
Cocoa powder: 80,000+
Parsley (dried): 73,000+
Basil (dried): 61,000+
Ginger root: 14,000+

Walnuts: 13,000+

Artichokes, cooked: 9,400+

Cranberries: 9,000+

Kidney beans: 8,600+

Blackberries: 5,900+

Blueberries: 5,000+

Raspberries: 5,000+

Pomegranates: 4,400+

Red cabbage, cooked: 3,000+

Broccoli, cooked: 2,000+

A recent study found that happiness is correlated to how many fruits and vegetables you eat. The more colorful fruits and vegetables you eat (up to eight servings a day), the happier you become—almost immediately. No antidepressant works this fast![22] I suggest a two-to-one ratio of vegetables to fruits.

Eat This: Smart carbs: colorful, low-glycemic, high-fiber vegetables, fruits, and legumes

Skip or Limit That: High-glycemic, low-fiber foods, such as breads, pasta, potatoes, rice, and sugar that increase your risk of brain health/mental health issues

BRIGHT MINDS RULE #7:
Use herbs and spices like medicine.

Herbs and spices are as powerful as medicines. Hippocrates listed more than 500 medicinal uses for herbs and spices, including ways to prevent illness and increase longevity. Unlike pharmaceutical drugs, which often come with an alarming range of side effects, herbs and spices have minimal consequences. Eighty percent of the developing world still relies on natural and herbal remedies as their primary source of medicines.[23]

Although they are chemically processed, most of today's medications actually come from plants. For example, many pain medications originate from poppy seeds.

Herbs and spices pack a double punch: nutrition *and* flavor. They support your health and tantalize your taste buds. I wonder why we don't store them in the medicine cabinet rather than the spice cabinet. The seasonings we cook with come from some of the same plants for which our ancestors risked their lives or paid a lot of money to obtain pain relief, vitality, and healing.

Here is a short list of herbs and spices to help each of the BRIGHT MINDS risk factors:

- In multiple studies, a saffron extract was found to be as effective as antidepressant medication in treating people with major depression.
- Turmeric, used in curry, contains a chemical that has been shown to decrease the plaques in the brain thought to be responsible for Alzheimer's disease.
- Scientific evidence shows rosemary, thyme, and sage help boost memory.
- Cinnamon has been shown to help improve attention and blood sugar regulation. It is high in antioxidants and is a natural aphrodisiac.
- Garlic and oregano boost blood flow to the brain.
- The hot, spicy taste of ginger, cayenne, and black pepper comes from gingerols, capsaicin, and piperine, compounds that boost metabolism and have an aphrodisiac effect.

Eat This: Lots of herbs and spices tailored to your risk factors and needs

Skip or Limit That: Artificial colors and flavors geared to hijack your brain

BRIGHT MINDS RULE #8:
Make your food as clean as possible (eliminate artificial sweeteners, colors, preservatives, and foods in plastic containers) and read the labels.

Go organic, hormone-free, antibiotic-free, grass-fed, and free-range whenever possible. You are not only what you eat, but you are also what the animals you eat ate. Pesticides used in commercial farming can accumulate in your brain and body, even though the levels in each food may be low. As much as possible, eliminate food additives, preservatives, artificial dyes, and sweeteners. That means you must read food labels. If you do not know what is in a food item or it is not real food, don't eat it. Similarly, it's important to think about how your food is stored. The plastic containers used for many foods and beverages can leech into food and cause issues. Become thoughtful about the food you eat, and your brain will thank you.

I understand that you may not be able to afford to eat solely organic and sustainably raised food. The Environmental Working Group produces an annual list on the foods that are a must to eat organic and those with lower levels of pesticides. Stay updated at www.ewg.org. Here is the current list:

Fifteen foods with the lowest levels of pesticide residues

- Avocados
- Sweet corn
- Pineapples
- Cabbages
- Onions
- Sweet peas (frozen)
- Papayas
- Asparagus
- Mangoes
- Eggplants
- Honeydew melons
- Kiwis
- Cantaloupes
- Cauliflower
- Broccoli

Twelve foods with the highest levels of pesticide residues (buy organic or don't eat them)

- Strawberries
- Spinach
- Nectarines
- Apples
- Grapes
- Peaches
- Cherries
- Pears
- Tomatoes
- Celery
- Potatoes
- Sweet bell peppers

Fish is a great source of healthy protein and fat, but it's important to consider the toxicity in some fish. Here are a couple of general rules to guide you in choosing more healthful fish:

1. The larger the fish, the more mercury it may contain, so go for the smaller varieties.
2. From the safe fish choices, eat a fairly wide variety of fish, preferably those highest in omega-3s, like wild Alaskan salmon, sardines, anchovies, hake, and haddock.[24]

Learn more at www.seafoodwatch.org.

Eat This: Clean, whole foods, sustainably raised, whenever possible

Skip or Limit That: Foods raised with pesticides, hormones, and antibiotics, or containing artificial sweeteners, dyes, and preservatives

BRIGHT MINDS RULE #9:

If you struggle with any brain health/mental health or physical issue, eliminate any potential allergens or internal attackers, such as sugar, MSG, gluten, corn, soy, and dairy for a month to see if you improve.

Subtle but important food allergies may result in brain inflammation that contributes to many of the brain health/mental health issues we see at Amen Clinics. These food allergies can be delayed, in the sense that bodily reactions to the food items may occur up to several days after consuming them. Conventional medicine has tended to ignore these reactions to foods. However, we believe that these food issues create a metabolic disorder that can lead to many "mental" symptoms, including fatigue, brain fog, slowed thinking, irritability, agitation, aggression, anxiety, depression and bipolar conditions, ADD/ADHD, learning disabilities, autism, schizophrenia, and even dementia.

To test the theory that food allergies may be involved in your issues, follow an elimination diet—essentially a dairy-, gluten-, corn-, sugar-, and soy-free diet for one month. See instructions on pages 334–335 detailing how to do an elimination diet.

An example of how effective an elimination diet can be comes from researchers from the Netherlands, who showed a highly restricted diet brought about rapid, lasting improvement in ADD/ADHD and oppositional defiant disorder (ODD) in children.[25] The children ate only rice, turkey, lamb, vegetables, fruits, tea, pear juice, and water. No milk products, wheat, or sugar products. No food additives or artificial colors. In the study, 85 percent of children who followed the diet showed an improvement of 50 percent or more and no longer met criteria for ADD/ADHD, and 67 percent who had ODD no longer met criteria for ODD. The researchers repeated this study and found similar results. In another study using the same diet, physical symptoms (headaches and bellyaches) and sleep also improved.[26]

Food additives and colorings can cause hyperactivity in children with no history of the problem, according to a study in the prestigious journal the *Lancet* (and we believe adults may be affected too).[27] The study, involving nearly 300 children, found that additives caused symptoms of hyperactivity in both young and older children. These effects occurred not just in children diagnosed with ADD/ADHD but also in those with no overt behavior problems.

Over the years, elimination diets have been one of the most important weapons against brain health/mental health issues. If we can get our patients to try an "elimination diet" for just a month, it often makes a dramatic difference. Since we are all unique, not everyone has to lose these substances forever, unless they are sensitive to them. At the moment, I find food allergy lab tests unreliable. The best way to see if you are sensitive to certain foods is to eliminate all the potential culprits and add them back one at a time.

Why you should limit or avoid some foods

1. **Sugar:** When you consume sugar—even if it's natural honey or maple—it causes your blood sugar to spike then drop, impacting your mood and sense of well-being. High-sugar diets increase inflammation, cause fatigue and cravings, lead to erratic brain cell firing that has been implicated in aggression, and alter memory and learning.

Top 15 Names for Sugar

Because two-thirds of packaged goods contain added sugar, it is critical to read food labels when you shop and know all the different aliases for sugar.[28]

1. Sugar
2. Molasses
3. Caramel color
4. Barley malt
5. Corn syrup or corn syrup solids
6. Cane juice
7. High fructose corn syrup
8. Honey
9. Sorbitol
10. Fructose
11. Cane juice crystals
12. Maltose
13. Fruit juice concentrate
14. Maltodextrin
15. Dextrose

Read food labels!

---

2. **Artificial sweeteners:** Artificial sweeteners—including aspartame (NutraSweet, Equal), saccharine (Sweet'N Low), and sucralose (Splenda)—can lead to chronically elevated insulin levels, which raises your risk for depression, Alzheimer's disease, heart disease, diabetes, and other health problems. And they are associated with metabolic syndrome and may actually be contributing to obesity.[29]

3. **Gluten:** Gluten—found in breads, cereals, and pasta, as well as everything from salad dressings and chicken broth to spice mixes and veggie burgers—has been linked to a rising number of health issues, including celiac disease, Type 1 diabetes, and Hashimoto's thyroiditis—all of which are autoimmune conditions. And approximately 18 million Americans have gluten sensitivity, according to the Center for Celiac Research. Gluten sensitivity and celiac disease are related to a number of brain health/mental health symptoms,[30] including:

- Anxiety disorders
- Depression
- Mood disorders
- ADD/ADHD

- Autism spectrum disorders
- Schizophrenia

Indeed, adopting a gluten-free diet has been associated with improvements in people with mental health conditions. Research found a decrease, or even full remission, of symptoms in a subset of patients with schizophrenia.[31] And going gluten-free produced a decrease in symptoms in some people with autism, ADD/ADHD, and depression.[32] In a summary of 13 studies involving 1,139 subjects, a gluten-free diet significantly improved depressive symptoms.[33] The evidence is clear: If you are suffering from a brain health/mental health disorder, it's a good idea to try getting rid of gluten to see if it minimizes your symptoms.

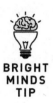

BRIGHT MINDS TIP

When combined with stomach acid, gluten in wheat, casein in dairy, albumin in rice, and zein in corn turn into exorphins, which can have opiate-like effects on the brain, making it very hard to stop eating them.

In a fascinating article titled, "Bread and Other Edible Agents of Mental Disease,"[34] Italian researchers Drs. Peter Kramer and Paolo Bressan argue that because of their lack of training in gastroenterology and nutrition, psychologists and psychiatrists typically fail to appreciate the impact food has on their patients. They argue that bread

1. Makes the gut lining and the blood brain barrier more permeable, allowing food particles and toxins to enter into the blood-stream.

2. Sets off the immune system reaction to attack these substances, which can cause brain fog, depression, inflammation, and allergic reactions.

3. Releases opioid-like compounds, capable of causing brain health/mental health issues, including cravings for the substances that are causing harm.

Of note, not only gluten in wheat, but also casein in dairy, albumin in rice, and zein in corn have opiate-like effects, which is why it can be so hard to stop eating them.[35] Kramer and Bressan also argue that something is changing in the population where blood markers for celiac disease and gluten sensitivity have quadrupled in the United States in the last 50 years and doubled in Finland in the last 20 years. They conclude that "the evidence is overpowering that hypersensitivity to gluten can bring with it mental disturbances like schizophrenia, bipolar disorder, depression, anxiety, and autism in vulnerable individuals. . . . A grain-free diet, although difficult to maintain (especially for those who need it the most), could improve the mental health of many and be a complete cure for others."[36]

On brain SPECT scans, patients with celiac disease (severe gluten sensitivity) also show lower blood flow, especially to the front part of the brain (focus, forethought, and impulse control).[37] When gluten was removed, blood flow to the frontal lobes improved.[38] Gluten has also been implicated in up to 40 percent of cases with cerebellar ataxia (severe coordination issues), which improves when gluten is eliminated.[39] If you want to think right and be able to run in a straight line, hold the gluten!

Is Schizophrenia Rare Where Grains Are Rare?

If grains like wheat are one of the causes of schizophrenia, then it should be rare in societies where grains are rare. In an article by Dr. F. C. Dohan and colleagues, they tested this idea by examining the work of anthropologists on people who ate little or no grain. "Only two overtly insane chronic schizophrenics were found among over 65,000 examined or closely observed adults in remote regions of Papua New Guinea, Malaita, Solomon Islands, and Yap, Micronesia." Yet, when these populations started to eat wheat, barley, beer, and rice, the numbers of schizophrenics rose to Western society levels.[40]

Dr. Dohan also published a study comparing 59 hospitalized schizophrenic men treated with a dairy-free, wheat-free diet to 56 controls who continued to eat dairy and wheat. The dairy-free, wheat-free group was discharged from the hospital about twice as fast as the control group. When wheat was secretly added to the cereal-free diet, it eliminated the positive effect.[41]

4. **Soy:** Soy, a protein derived from soybeans, contains components that may impact some of the BRIGHT MINDS risk factors, including:

- a high concentration of lectins, carbohydrate-binding proteins that can be toxic, allergenic, and inflammatory (Toxins, Inflammation)
- large amounts of omega-6 fatty acids (Inflammation)
- phytoestrogens that may contribute to the development of cancer, early puberty in girls, and impotence in men (Neurohormones)

5. **Corn:** Corn's fatty acid profile is among the most unhealthy of all grains and can have a negative effect on the BRIGHT MINDS risk factors because it is:

- High in omega-6s and very low in omega-3s (Inflammation)
- Damaging to the intestinal lining and triggers intestinal permeability issues (Inflammation)
- Often sprayed with the glyphosate pesticide Roundup, one of the most toxic substances to human cells[42] that is associated with ADD/ADHD,[43] depression, Parkinson's disease, MS, hypothyroidism, cancer, and liver disease[44] (Toxins)

6. **Milk:** Milk can raise the risk for several of the BRIGHT MINDS risk factors. For example, it is converted to galactose and glucose, which raises blood sugar levels and can lead to inflammation and diabesity. And a milk protein called casein is an excitotoxin that can lead to brain inflammation and neurodegenerative diseases. (Inflammation)

HOW TO FOLLOW AN ELIMINATION DIET

1. Cut out the six potential food allergens (sugar, artificial sweeteners, gluten, soy, corn, and milk) for one month.

2. After a month, slowly reintroduce food items one at a time every

three to four days. Eat the reintroduced food at least two to three times a day for three days to see if you notice a reaction.

3. Look for symptoms, which can occur within a few minutes or up to 72 hours later. (If you notice a problem right away, stop consuming that food immediately.) Reactions to foods to which you have allergies can include:

   - brain fog
   - difficulty remembering
   - mood issues (anxiety, depression, and anger)
   - nasal congestion
   - chest congestion
   - headaches
   - sleep problems
   - joint aches
   - muscle aches
   - pain
   - fatigue
   - skin changes
   - changes in digestion and bowel functioning

4. If you have a reaction, note the food and eliminate it for 90 days—and maybe forever. This will give your immune system a chance to cool off and your gut a chance to heal.

   When our patients follow an elimination diet, it often makes a dramatic difference. Remember, you don't have to lose all of these foods forever, unless you are sensitive to them.

Eat This: Clean whole foods

Skip or Limit That: Sugar, artificial sweeteners, preservatives and dyes, gluten, corn, soy, and dairy

BRIGHT MINDS RULE #10:
Use intermittent fasting to supercharge your brain.

Focus on brain-healthy eating throughout the day, but fast for at least 12 hours between dinner and breakfast. Intermittent fasting, or "time-restricted feeding," has been shown to significantly improve memory,[45] mood,[46] fat loss,[47] weight, blood pressure, and inflammatory markers.[48] Nightly 12-to-16-hour fasts turn on a process called autophagy, which helps your brain "take out the trash" it accumulates during the day.[49] This can help you think more clearly and feel more energetic. This type of fasting is simple—if you eat dinner at 6 p.m., don't eat again until 6 to 10 a.m. the next day. Your brain will have the time it needs to cleanse itself.

Not eating within two to three hours of bedtime also reduces your risk of heart attack and stroke.[50] In healthy people, blood pressure drops by at least 10 percent when they go to sleep, but blood pressure in late-night eaters stays high, increasing the risk of vascular problems. New research also suggests that if you have more calories at lunch and then eat a light dinner, you are more likely to lose weight than the other way around.[51]

BRIGHT MINDS RULE #11:
Get a routine that serves your health rather than hurts it; find 24 foods you love that love you back.

We are all creatures of habit. Once you allow your brain to do something, it will want to do it again, whether or not it is good for you. The secret to changing your foods is to find ones you love that love you back. A diet full of nutrition is not boring. On the contrary, it can be loaded with meals that taste amazing. Once you eliminate the adulterated foods loaded with sugar, salt, unhealthy fat, and artificial chemicals, in about 10 days, your taste buds will come back to life, and whole foods will taste amazing.

Here are 24 foods I love that love me back (four breakfasts, four lunches, four snacks, four dinners, five desserts, three drinks). Make a list of your own from the rules given above. For more suggestions check out my wife Tana's cookbooks, especially *The Brain Warrior's Way Cookbook*, and the recipes on her website at www.tanaamen.com, where you can find all of the recipes of the foods listed on the next page.

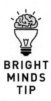

BRIGHT MINDS TIP

For more suggestions, check out my wife Tana's cookbooks, especially *The Brain Warrior's Way Cookbook*, and the recipes on her website at www.tanaamen.com, where you can find many of the recipes of the foods listed below.

Breakfasts

1. Smoothie—Mint Cherry Blast (yum)
2. Super Simple Tanana Pancakes (delicious and filling)
3. Delicious Low Carb Waffles
4. One-Minute Avocado Egg Basket (so quick and easy)

Lunches

5. Spiced Cacao Turkey Chili (a longtime favorite)
6. Kale Citrus Salad (unbelievable; people steal my leftovers)
7. Brain Fit Fajitas (loaded with nutrients)
8. Guiltless Chicken Breast Tenders (kids love them—even big kids)

Snacks (carry them with you in your car, purse, or computer bag)

9. Nuts or seeds (especially pumpkin seeds)
10. Go-Well Trail Mix
11. Cut veggies with hummus or guacamole
12. Whole fruit and nut butter

Dinner

13. Rosemary Thyme Chicken, Sweet Potatoes, and Asparagus
14. Pan-Seared Salmon with Vegetables
15. Cauliflower Pizza
16. Lentil Vegetable Soup

Desserts

17. Nutty Butter Cups
18. Fudgy Brownie Bites
19. Healthy Apple Cinnamon Crisp
20. Fresh Berries with Macadamia-Nut Sauce
21. Amazing Avocado Gelato

Drinks

22. Water flavored with fresh cuts of fruit, such as peaches, oranges, or watermelon
23. Sparkling water with chocolate stevia from Sweet Leaf
24. Pumpkin Spice-Up Cappuccino

BRIGHT MINDS FOOD STARS

Below is a simple chart of foods to choose and foods to lose, based on each of the 11 BRIGHT MINDS risk factors. Focus on your personal risk factors.

FOOD MADE INSANELY SIMPLE[52]

Blood Flow

EAT THIS	SKIP OR LIMIT THAT
Herbs and spices: cayenne, cinnamon, parsley, rosemary, turmeric	**Caffeine and alcohol**
	Sugary sodas
Beets, beet juice, celery, radishes, green, leafy, and colorful vegetables	**Baked goods**
	Foods fried in vegetable or animal fat
Pumpkin seeds, almonds, hazelnuts, and sunflower seeds	**Powdered coffee creamers**

Retirement/Aging

EAT THIS	SKIP OR LIMIT THAT
Antioxidant-rich herbs and spices: cloves, oregano, thyme, cinnamon, rosemary, turmeric	**Sugar**
	High-glycemic foods
Antioxidant-rich foods: cocoa, acai, berries, artichokes, pomegranates, olive oil, green tea	**Charred foods**
	Trans fats
Choline-rich foods to support memory:[53] shrimp, eggs, scallops, chicken, turkey, beef, cod, salmon, shiitake mushrooms, chickpeas, lentils, collard greens	**Red meat** if ferritin levels are high

Inflammation

EAT THIS	SKIP OR LIMIT THAT
Anti-inflammatory spices: turmeric, cayenne, ginger, cloves, cinnamon, oregano, pumpkin pie spice	**Low-quality omega-6 fatty acids,** corn, soy, processed foods
Omega-3 foods: salmon, sardines, avocados, flaxseeds	
Prebiotic-rich foods: asparagus, chia seeds, beans, cabbage, artichokes, raw garlic, onions, leeks	
Probiotic-rich foods: sauerkraut, kimchi, kefir, miso soup, pickles, spirulina, kombucha tea	

Genetics

EAT THIS

Polyphenol rich foods: chocolate, green tea, blueberries, kale, onions, apples, cherries, cabbage

SKIP OR LIMIT THAT

High-glycemic foods with lots of saturated fat—think fast-food pizza, ribeye steak and mashed potatoes, pancakes with syrup and bacon

Processed cheeses and microwave popcorn

Head Trauma

EAT THIS

Spices to support brain healing: turmeric, peppermint

Choline-rich foods: shrimp, eggs, scallops, sardines, chicken, turkey, tuna, cod, beef, collard greens, brussels sprouts

Omega-3-rich foods

SKIP OR LIMIT THAT

Alcohol

Caffeine

Sugar

Fried foods

Processed foods

Toxins

EAT THIS

Liver nourishing foods: green, leafy vegetables, brassicas (any color cabbage, brussels sprouts, cauliflower, broccoli, kale), oranges and tangerines

Kidney-nourishing foods: water, nuts and seeds— such as cashews, almonds, and pumpkin seeds for magnesium; green, leafy vegetables; blueberries

Skin-nourishing foods: green tea, colorful fruits and vegetables, avocados, olive oil, wild salmon

SKIP OR LIMIT THAT

Foods that inhibit detoxification

Processed meats, such as bacon and smoked turkey

Conventionally raised produce (pesticides and herbicides), dairy (hormones and antibiotics), meats (hormones, antibiotics, grain-fed), farmed fish (grain-fed, PCBs)

Excess phosphates (processed cheeses, canned fish, processed meats, flavored water, sodas, nondairy creamers, bottled coffee drinks, iced teas)

Mind Storms

EAT THIS	SKIP OR LIMIT THAT
GABA-rich foods—to stabilize brain electrical activity: broccoli, almonds, walnuts, lentils, bananas, beef liver, brown rice, halibut, gluten-free whole oats, oranges, rice bran, spinach	**High-glycemic foods** **MSG** **Red Dye #40**

Immunity/Infections

EAT THIS	SKIP OR LIMIT THAT
Immunity-boosting spices: cinnamon, garlic, turmeric, thyme, ginger, coriander	**Western diet**—including fast foods and processed foods
Allicin-rich foods: raw, crushed garlic, onions, shallots	**Sodas and diet sodas** **Alcohol**
Vitamin C–rich foods: oranges, tangerines, kiwi, berries, red and yellow bell peppers, dark green leafy vegetables (such as spinach and kale), broccoli, brussels sprouts, cauliflower, cabbage, tomatoes, peas	**Simple sugars**—including table sugar and honey
Vitamin D–rich foods: fatty fish, including salmon, sardines, tuna; eggs; mushrooms (maitake, shiitake); beef liver, cod liver oil	**High Omega-6s**—found in most vegetable oils (corn, soybean, sunflower, safflower)
Zinc-rich foods: oysters, beef, lamb, spinach, shiitake and cremini mushrooms, asparagus, sesame and pumpkin seeds	**Fried foods** **Pesticide-laden foods**—choose organically grown/raised food whenever possible
Mushrooms: shiitake,[54] white button, portabella[55]	**Dairy**
Selenium-rich foods: nuts (especially Brazil nuts), seeds, fish, grass-fed meats, mushrooms	**Gluten**

Neurohormone Issues

EAT THIS	SKIP OR LIMIT THAT
Fiber-rich foods containing lignin: green beans, peas, carrots, seeds, and Brazil nuts Lignin binds harmful estrogens in the digestive tract, so they can be excreted in the feces instead of being reabsorbed. Dietary fiber also improves the composition of intestinal bacteria, so that harmful estrogen metabolites can be excreted from the body. It also decreases the conversion of testosterone into estrogens, maintaining a healthy testosterone level.	**Sugar and simple carbohydrates** **Protein** from animals raised with hormones or antibiotics **Processed foods** **Gluten**

Hormone-supporting spices: turmeric, ginger, garlic, sage, parsley, anise seed, red clover, hops

Eggs: Many hormones are made from cholesterol, so make sure you have enough cholesterol in your diet

Testosterone-boosting foods: pomegranate, olive oil, oysters, coconut, brassicas (including cabbage, broccoli, Brussels sprouts, cauliflower), garlic

Estrogen-boosting foods: whole soybeans, flaxseeds, sunflower seeds, beans, garlic, yams, foods rich in vitamins C and B, beets, parsley, aniseed, red clover, licorice, hops, sage

Thyroid-boosting foods (selenium-rich): seaweed and sea vegetables, brassicas, maca

Soy protein isolate

Excitoxins—substances that can kill neurons, including MSG, aspartame, hydrolyzed vegetable protein, sucralose, "natural flavors" (these often contain MSG)

Foods/drinks that lower testosterone levels: spearmint tea, soy products and licorice

Diabesity

EAT THIS

Spices: cinnamon, sage, nutmeg

Fiber-rich foods to balance blood sugar: raspberries, broccoli, spinach, lentils, green peas, pears, winter squash, cabbage, green beans, avocados, coconut, figs, artichokes, chickpeas, hemp and chia seeds

Best vegetables: low-glycemic, such as celery, spinach, broccoli, brassicas (broccoli, brussels sprouts, cauliflower)

Best fruits: low-glycemic, such as apples, oranges, blueberries, raspberries, blackberries, strawberries

SKIP OR LIMIT THAT

High-glycemic, low-fiber foods, such as white and wheat bread, pasta, white potatoes, rice

Sugar—no nutritional benefit, depletes chromium and other valuable vitamins and minerals

Corn

Processed foods

Dried fruits: prunes, apricots, figs, cranberries; raisins, dates

High-glycemic fruits—such as pineapple, watermelon, ripe bananas

Sleep

EAT THIS

Sleep-enhancing spices: ginger root

SKIP OR LIMIT THAT

Alcohol, including wine—hard liquor is worse for your brain;

Foods rich in melatonin—the hormone of sleep: tart cherry juice concentrate, sour cherries, walnuts, ginger root, asparagus, tomatoes

Serotonin-rich foods: combine tryptophan-containing foods, such as eggs, turkey, seafood, chickpeas, nuts and seeds (building blocks for serotonin), with healthy carbohydrates, such as sweet potatoes and quinoa, to elicit a short-term insulin response that drives tryptophan into the brain. Dark chocolate also increases serotonin

Chamomile or passion fruit tea

snoring is worse with alcohol

Caffeine—including dark chocolate (which also contains theobromine)

Energy drinks (duh!)

Spicy foods—especially at night

Grapefruit—due to acidity may cause heartburn at night

Foods that contain diuretics—celery, cucumbers, radishes, watermelon (they will keep you up going to the bathroom)

Foods that contain tyramine—it increases norepinephrine, a stimulating neurotransmitter: tomatoes, eggplant, soy, red wine, aged cheeses

Unhealthy fatty foods, such as burgers, fries, and cheese pizza, which all have harder-to-digest saturated fats

Black bean chili—it will keep your GI tract rumbling

High-protein foods—they are harder to digest

CHAPTER 19

HOW TO MAKE A MASSIVE DIFFERENCE

BRAIN HEALTH IN FAMILIES, SCHOOLS, BUSINESSES, CHURCHES, AND ANYWHERE PEOPLE CONGREGATE

You never change things by fighting the existing reality. To change something, build a new model that makes the existing model obsolete.

R. BUCKMINSTER FULLER

Brain health issues do not just affect the person who suffers. They affect everyone around them, and nearly a million families every year break apart under the stress. When I first started scanning people, I realized that I needed to be concerned about all of the brains in the family. Family dynamics are never based on just one brain, so I needed to understand all of them. For example, my nieces, Alizé and Amelie, were seriously impacted by the brain dysfunction of their parents. Their mother, Tamara, had been impacted by the brain health of her mom and dad. If you spend a lot of time with parents who are depressed, anxious, or abusing drugs, the stress can reshape your brain to make you more vulnerable to depression and substance abuse. If you have a spouse or an adult child with brain health/mental health issues, you know the impact it can have on everyone in the family.

Few people talk about the incredible toll these brain health/mental health issues take on families: from being blamed as the cause of the problem to the chronic stress they feel, the financial pressure, and the grief and sadness they experience. Helping families help each other is such an important part of the healing process.

If we want to truly end mental illness, we must work to support everyone in the family by:

- Encouraging communication. People cannot read your mind. They haven't had your experiences, so they likely don't know what you're going through unless you tell them. Here are some magic words to open communication:
  - "I'm concerned about you."
  - "I'm here for you."
  - "Can we talk about how you're feeling?"
  - "Is there someone else you might feel more comfortable talking to?"

- Teaching everyone about brain health. Just focusing on the person who suffers invites frustration and failure.

- Showing people that asking for help is a sign of strength, *not* weakness. Imagine if a business was having problems and the owners just ignored them or denied them. The business would go bankrupt. The same thing happens when brain health/mental health issues are ignored. This is one of the reasons so many families break apart.

- Being cautious with tough love—it works for people whose brains work right, but for people who have brains that are struggling, tough love is like smashing your computer when it has a problem. It can cause lasting damage.

- Teaching family members to be curious, *not* furious and judgmental, when one family member has a setback. As you have seen in this book, behavior is much more complicated than most people think.

BRAIN HEALTH EDUCATION IN SOCIETY

In 2017, I was invited to the White House to discuss prison reform, the opiate epidemic, and mental illness in America. In the same way our society can work against us to create mental illness, it can also enable us to enhance brain health and end mental illness. My central recommendation was to create a national campaign that teaches brain health in schools, prisons, churches, recovery programs, and workplaces. This recommendation was based on three large-scale programs I helped to create. Here are details of these programs.

1. Brain Thrive by 25

In 2005, Dr. Jesse Payne and I created a high school and college course to teach students how to love and care for their brains. Called Brain Thrive by 25 (www.brainthriveby25.com), it has been taught in all 50 states and in seven countries. Independent research has shown that it reduces drug, alcohol, and tobacco use; decreases depression; and improves self-esteem. In the course, we teach kids to love and care for their brains, including lessons on basic brain facts, the developing brain, gender differences, the impact of drugs and alcohol on the brain, nutrition, stress management, killing ANTs (automatic negative thoughts), and how to throw a brain-healthy party. It has been a popular course that has changed lives.

I am confident that teaching brain health in schools on a nationwide basis would have a huge positive effect on our young people and could help them avoid developing brain disorders/mental illnesses. And by ending mental illness in young people like my nieces, Alizé and Amelie, it would help end it in their children, grandchildren, and so on.

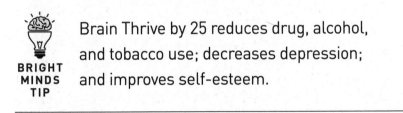

BRIGHT MINDS TIP

Brain Thrive by 25 reduces drug, alcohol, and tobacco use; decreases depression; and improves self-esteem.

Here are just a few of the testimonials from students who have taken Brain Thrive by 25:

I was told my whole childhood that I was stupid by my dad. Now, I am on a quest to learn how to hack life, and this course has made a huge difference for me. I am making my brain stronger and becoming healthier overall.

I noticed that I had a pretty big social media addiction that was harming my ability to process emotions and control my impulses. I have now minimized my addiction, which has helped me feel better overall.

My dream is to be a musician, and I am nervous about the drug and alcohol culture within the music industry. It will be easier staying clean from drugs now that I realize how bad they are for me and, most importantly, for my brain.

2. The Daniel Plan

In 2010, I went to my own church and saw them serving doughnuts, bacon, hot dogs, and ice cream, and I was horrified that I was going there to get my soul fed, yet these people were trying to kill my body. At that service, I prayed that God would use me to change the culture of food at church. Two weeks later, Pastor Rick Warren, the senior pastor at Saddleback Church, one of the largest churches in America with 20 campuses around the world, called me and said, "I'm fat; my church is fat. Will you help me?" Together with Pastor Warren, Dr. Mehmet Oz, and my friend Dr. Mark Hyman, we created The Daniel Plan, based on the principles of the four circles.

The first week, 15,000 people signed up, and over the first year they lost *more than 250,000 pounds* and reported better energy, focus, creativity, sleep, and mood, plus reductions in stress, blood pressure, blood sugar, sexual dysfunction, and many medications. Together, we went on to write a #1 *New York Times* and international bestselling book, *The Daniel Plan: 40 Days to a Healthier Life*. The Daniel Plan has been implemented in thousands of churches worldwide. Whenever I am on one of the Saddleback campuses, I hear story after story of how people's lives have been changed.

As you've seen in this book, diabesity is a BRIGHT MINDS risk factor that contributes to brain health/mental health. If all churches implemented simple strategies that minimize these risk factors—such as serving brain-healthy foods and encouraging physical activity—it could help millions of people reduce symptoms of anxiety and depression, improve focus and attention, and more. And if each of those people shared what they learned with their family and friends, it would improve brain health/mental health on a national level.

I no longer take antidepressant medication. My mood is so much more stable and positive.

I just finished chemo. Everyone is amazed at how much energy I have and how fast my hair is returning. I am running circles around a friend who is 10 years younger and doesn't have cancer. (He is not on the plan.)

I'm off my high blood pressure meds . . . and am working on getting off of my type 2 diabetes and cholesterol meds.

Odd to say this in church, but my sex life has dramatically improved!

The Daniel Plan helps people get better together.

3. Creating BRIGHT MINDS at Work

If you are like many Americans, work creates stress and sours their mood. You grind your teeth in traffic to get to the office where you have an inbox full of urgent emails waiting for you. But before you get to your cubicle, you pass by the break room where you find doughnuts, leftover cake from yesterday's birthday celebration, coffee with artificial creamer and sugar, and a bowl of jelly beans. Helping yourself to them just sets your brain up for more stress, a lack of focus, and mood swings, as well as increasing your BRIGHT MINDS risk factors. It's not a recipe for success. It doesn't have to be this way.

The BRIGHT MINDS at Work program gives companies and other organizations the tools needed to help teams boost brain health and create a more positive, productive environment where everyone is happier, less stressed, and primed for success. When incorporated as part of a comprehensive wellness program, this brain-healthy approach has also been shown to contribute to improved immune systems and a decrease in absenteeism. Imagine if every workplace promoted a brain-healthy lifestyle. It could greatly cut down on the risk factors that make people vulnerable to brain health/mental health issues.

Just a few of our many testimonials show how this information can change lives.

Discovering Dr. Amen's brain health initiative could not have come at a more opportune time for me. My mother was recently diagnosed with predementia, meaning I have a higher risk for dementia or Alzheimer's disease. Dr. Amen's BRIGHT MINDS approach helped me to understand key risk factors for memory decline and behavioral changes that I can make to help mitigate my risk. Starting with simple things like eliminating caffeine, becoming more disciplined about diet and exercise, and introducing supplements, I have already seen a reduction in my cholesterol and triglycerides (the source of restricted blood flow to the brain in my mother's case). Learning that there are things I can do to delay the inevitable decline in memory function is empowering, and

I am thankful to have been introduced to Dr. Amen while there is still time for me to implement these changes.

I can't say thank you enough to express how grateful I am for the opportunity that our company provided us to meet Dr. Amen. He inspired me to be the best version of myself. He taught me how to love my mind and my body. Since I have started his classes, I no longer blame myself for not being the best. I no longer let my body have nonhealthy and chemical foods. And also, I no longer judge people and overthink, which was killing me in the past few years. I just lost 17 pounds and reached my weight goal! 140 pounds! I'm so happy!

When I started the BRIGHT MINDS program six months ago, I had no idea how profoundly it would affect my life. Because of Dr. Amen's recommendation to 'Know Your Numbers,' I got lab work done that showed a serious problem with my cardiovascular system, putting both my brain and my heart at risk. As a 50-year-old woman with no health symptoms, I would have never known that I was at risk without the encouragement of Dr. Amen to take charge of my own health and live my best possible life. Thank you, Dr. Amen and our company, for this wonderful program!

To end mental illness, we must create brain health in ourselves, in our families, in our communities, and in our organizations.

How to Find a BRIGHT MINDS Brain Health Practitioner

My mission has always been to teach other medical and mental health professionals the techniques we have learned at Amen Clinics. We have trained more than 3,000 brain health certified coaches (www.brainhealthcoaching.com). To find professionals who will have a similar integrative mind-set to the one expressed in this book, visit https://AmenUniversity.com/Referral Directory. You can also go to the Institute for Functional Medicine (www.ifm.org) or American Academy of Anti-Aging Medicine (www.a4m.com) websites to see if there is a functional medicine doctor near you.

10 Common Genes That May Influence Brain Health/Mental Health

GENES	IMPORTANCE/INTERVENTIONS FOR VARIANTS
1. MTHFR—methylenetetrahydrofolate reductase Enzyme critical for making methylfolate, essential for making neurotransmitters such as norepinephrine, dopamine, and serotonin.	Nonideal variants associated with depression,[1] bipolar disorder, schizophrenia,[2] and autism.[3] Leads to high homocysteine and vascular disease. Associated with brain shrinkage.[4] *Supplementing with methylfolate (0.4–15 mg a day) can improve depression.[5]*
2. COMT—catechol-O-methyltransferase (warrior or worrier gene) Enzyme that breaks down dopamine in prefrontal cortex (PFC). Estrogen decreases COMT, increasing dopamine in PFC. Females have higher anxiety, fewer ADD/ADHD diagnoses.	One variant breaks down dopamine faster in PFC, which leads to lower dopamine levels and higher impulsivity, risk-taking behavior, extroversion, poorer working memory, being less of a rule follower, and less neuroticism. It has been associated with ADD/ADHD.[6] *Performs better under stress* (more likely to run toward fires). *Responds better to stimulant medications, modafinil, green tea, tyrosine, exercise, and transcranial magnetic stimulation (TMS).* *Some studies show that teens with a variant of COMT have an increased risk of psychosis with marijuana use.[7]*

GENES	IMPORTANCE/INTERVENTIONS FOR VARIANTS
	Another variant breaks down dopamine slower in PFC, leading to higher levels of dopamine and lower risk-taking behavior, less impulsivity, being more of a rule follower, more introversion, more neuroticism, better working memory. OCD and bipolar disorder are higher in this group.[8] Performs worse under stress (less likely to run toward fires). *More likely to benefit from early interventions to prevent the onset of panic after childhood adversities.*[9]
3. BDNF—brain derived neurotrophic factor Protein involved in neurogenesis and neuroplasticity, helping to encourage the growth of new neurons.	One variant is associated with impaired working memory, depression, increased stress response, and PTSD. *Physical exercise helps to ameliorate the trouble it can cause.*[10] Another variant had a three times better response to SSRI medications.[11] *Lithium (300 mcg) has been shown to increase BDNF levels.* *High saturated fat and sugar decrease BDNF.*
4. MAOA—monoamine oxidase A Involved in dopamine, norepinephrine, and serotonin levels that affect mood, focus, energy, addictions, sleep, and carb cravings.	One variant tends toward carb cravings, addictions, ADD/ADHD, depression, weight gain, being depressed on diet, and wakefulness at night Another variant can lead to being easily startled, aggression, headaches from cheese or wine, difficulty falling asleep, mood swings, irritability, and addictions.
5. DAO—diamine oxidase Decreases histamine, mainly in gut. Affects allergic response to various foods; may be associated with food sensitivity.	Variants associated with food sensitivities, leaky gut, allergic reactions, autoimmune risk, headaches, irritability, racing heart, itchy skin, and bloody nose. *Consider low-histamine diet and fresh foods, avoid leftovers, improve gut health, treat leaky gut, manage stress, exercise, have a healthy sleep routine, avoid environmental toxins/allergens, and avoid aspirin/NSAIDs.*

GENES	IMPORTANCE/INTERVENTIONS FOR VARIANTS
6. SLC6A4—serotonin transporter protein Codes for serotonin transporter protein responsible for serotonin uptake. Antidepressant activity of SSRI medications is achieved through inhibition of this protein.	Studies have shown those with one or two copies of the short form allele(s) are more likely to have a poorer or slower response to SSRI medications and more side effects.[12] Not all studies agree. One study found elderly people with the short allele had a better response.[13] Those with the short allele(s) also have more anxiety personality traits[14] and increased activity in the amygdala (an area of the brain more active when anxious).[15] Higher rate of PTSD, mood disorders, and stress reactivity.
7. CACNA1C—gated calcium channel Involved in nerve cell firing.	May lead to excessive glutamate, the most prevalent stimulating neurotransmitter, which can be toxic in high amounts. Found to be higher in those with treatment-resistant depression, bipolar disorder, and schizophrenia.[16] *Mood-stabilizing medications and Omega-3 fatty acids may be helpful.*
8. ANK3—ankyrin-G Belongs to a family of proteins that have a role in nerve-cell firing.	May lead to excessive glutamate, the most prevalent stimulating neurotransmitter, which can be toxic in high amounts. Studies have shown a correlation between this variation and bipolar disorder, mood instability, and schizophrenia.[17] *Mood stabilizing medications and omega-3 fatty acids may be helpful.*
9. APO E—apolipoprotein E gene type Helps in development, repair, and maintenance of nerve cell membranes. Also involved in waste management and clearing cellular debris.	Three versions: *APOE* e2, e3, and e4. *APOE* e4 has been associated with an increased risk of Alzheimer's disease, hypertension, and atherosclerosis.[18] Not everyone with the e4 gene will develop Alzheimer's disease; in fact, 75 percent will not. *APOE* e4 gene is associated with overall lower blood flow to the brain;[19] take care of blood vessels if you have it. *Exercise, vitamin D, Mediterranean diet, and omega-3 fatty acids may help.*

GENES	IMPORTANCE/INTERVENTIONS FOR VARIANTS
10. Cytochrome P450 Metabolism of medications and hormones	Different genotypes code for blood levels that may be significantly higher or lower than predicted based on dose: Poor metabolizers (PM) have two nonfunctional genes so have little to no enzyme activity, increased drug levels, and more side effects. Intermediate metabolizers (IM) have one non-functional gene and one normally functioning gene, therefore, have decreased enzyme activity. Extensive metabolizers (EM)—have two normally functioning genes and normal enzyme activity. Ultrarapid metabolizers (UM) have more than two copies of functional genes that results in increased enzyme activity compared to EM; may have decreased drug levels and a poor response. May need higher than normal dosages. *Practical note: Citalopram (Celexa) should be avoided in CYP2C19 poor metabolizers (2–7 percent of population).*

Gratitude and Appreciation

So many people have been involved in the process of creating *The End of Mental Illness*. I am grateful to them all, especially the tens of thousands of patients and families who have come to Amen Clinics and allowed us to help them on their healing journey.

I am grateful to the amazing staff at Amen Clinics, who work hard every day serving our patients. Special appreciation to Frances Sharpe, who helped me craft the book to make it easily accessible to our readers. Also, to my friends and colleagues Dr. Parris Kidd, Dr. Rob Johnson, and Natalie Buchoz for their input, love, and support. I am also grateful to Jan Long Harris and the team at Tyndale for their belief in the book and help in getting it to the world, and my editor, Andrea Vinley Converse, who helped make this book the best it can be.

I am grateful to my amazing wife, Tana, who is my partner in all I do, and to my family, who has tolerated my obsession with making brains better. I love you all.

About Daniel G. Amen, MD

The *Washington Post* has called Dr. Daniel G. Amen the most popular psychiatrist in America, and Sharecare, a digital health company designed to help people manage their health in one place, named him the web's most influential expert and advocate on mental health.

Dr. Amen is a physician, double board–certified psychiatrist, 10-time *New York Times* bestselling author, and international speaker. He is the founder of Amen Clinics in Costa Mesa, Los Angeles, and San Francisco, California; Bellevue, Washington; Reston, Virginia; Atlanta; New York; and Chicago. Amen Clinics have one of the highest published success rates treating complex psychiatric issues, and they have built the world's largest database of functional brain scans, totaling more than 170,000 scans on patients from 121 countries.

Dr. Amen is the lead researcher on the world's largest brain imaging and rehabilitation study of professional football players. His research has not only demonstrated high levels of brain damage in players, it has also shown the possibility of significant recovery for many with the principles that underlie his work.

Together with Pastor Rick Warren and Mark Hyman, MD, Dr. Amen is also one of the chief architects of Saddleback Church's Daniel Plan, a program to get the world healthy through religious organizations.

Dr. Amen is the author or coauthor of more than 70 professional articles, seven book chapters, and more than 30 books, including the #1 *New York Times* bestsellers *The Daniel Plan* and *Change Your Brain, Change Your Life*; as well as *Magnificent Mind at Any Age*; *Change Your Brain, Change Your Body*; *Use Your Brain to Change Your Age*; *Healing ADD*; *The Brain Warrior's Way*; *The Brain Warrior's Way Cookbook*; *Captain Snout and the Super Power Questions*; *Memory Rescue;* and *Feel Better Fast and Make It Last.*

Dr. Amen's published scientific articles have appeared in the prestigious journals *Brain Imaging and Behavior*, Nature's *Molecular Psychiatry*, *PLOS ONE*, Nature's *Translational Psychiatry*, Nature's *Obesity*, the *Journal of Neuropsychiatry and Clinical Neurosciences*, *Minerva Psichiatrica*, *Journal of Neurotrauma*, the *American Journal of Psychiatry*, *Nuclear Medicine*

Communications, Neurological Research, Journal of the American Academy of Child & Adolescent Psychiatry, Primary Psychiatry, Military Medicine, and *General Hospital Psychiatry.* His research on post-traumatic stress disorder and traumatic brain injury was recognized by *Discover* magazine in its Year in Science issue as one of the "100 Top Stories of 2015."

Dr. Amen has written, produced, and hosted 14 popular shows about the brain on public television. He has appeared in movies, including *After the Last Round* and *The Crash Reel,* and in Emmy Award–winning television shows, such as *The Truth about Drinking* and *The Dr. Oz Show.* He was a consultant on the movie *Concussion,* starring Will Smith. He has also spoken for the National Security Agency (NSA), the National Science Foundation (NSF), Harvard's Learning & the Brain Conference, the Department of the Interior, the National Council of Juvenile and Family Court Judges, and the Supreme Courts of Delaware, Ohio, and Wyoming. Dr. Amen's work has been featured in *Newsweek, Time* magazine, the *Huffington Post,* the BBC, the *Guardian, Parade* magazine, the *New York Times,* the *New York Times Magazine,* the *Washington Post, Los Angeles Times, Men's Health,* and *Cosmopolitan.*

Dr. Amen is married to Tana. He is the father of four children and grandfather to Elias, Emmy, Liam, Louie, and Haven. He is also an avid table tennis player.

Resources

AMEN CLINICS

www.amenclinics.com

Amen Clinics, Inc. (ACI), was established in 1989 by Daniel G. Amen, MD. We specialize in innovative diagnosis and treatment planning for a wide variety of behavioral, learning, emotional, cognitive, and weight issues for children, teenagers, and adults. ACI has an international reputation for evaluating brain-behavior problems, such as ADD/ADHD, depression, anxiety, school failure, traumatic brain injury and concussions, obsessive-compulsive disorder, aggressiveness, marital conflict, cognitive decline, brain toxicity from drugs or alcohol, and obesity. In addition, ACI works with people to optimize brain function and decrease the risk for Alzheimer's disease and other age-related issues.

One of the primary diagnostic tools used at ACI is brain SPECT imaging. ACI has the world's largest database of brain scans for emotional, cognitive, and behavioral problems. ACI welcomes referrals from physicians, psychologists, social workers, marriage and family therapists, drug and alcohol counselors, and individual patients and families.

Our toll-free number is (888) 412-1607.

Amen Clinics Orange County, California
3150 Bristol St., Suite 400
Costa Mesa, CA 92626

Amen Clinics Northern California
350 N. Wiget Ln., Suite 105
Walnut Creek, CA 94598

Amen Clinics Northwest
616 120th Ave. NE, Suite C100
Bellevue, WA 98005

Amen Clinics Los Angeles
5363 Balboa Blvd., Suite 100
Encino, CA 91316

Amen Clinics Washington, D.C.
1875 Campus Commons Dr.
Reston, VA 20191

Amen Clinics New York
16 East 40th St., 9th Floor
New York, NY 10016

Amen Clinics Atlanta
5901-C Peachtree Dunwoody
Road, N.E., Suite 65
Atlanta, GA 30328

Amen Clinics Chicago
2333 Waukegan Rd., Suite 100
Bannockburn, IL 60015

Our website, www.amenclinics.com, is educational and interactive, geared toward mental health and medical professionals, educators, students, and the public. It contains a wealth of information and resources to help you learn about optimizing your brain. The site contains more than 300 color brain SPECT images, thousands of scientific abstracts on brain SPECT imaging for psychiatry, a free brain health assessment, and much, much more.

BRAIN FIT LIFE

www.mybrainfitlife.com

Based on Dr. Amen's 35 years as a clinical psychiatrist, he and his wife, Tana, have developed a sophisticated online community that includes:

- Detailed questionnaires to help you know your brain type and a personalized program targeted to your own needs
- WebNeuro, a neuropsychological test that assesses your brain
- Fun brain games and tools to boost your motivation
- Exclusive, award-winning, 24-7 brain gym membership
- Physical exercises and tutorials led by Tana
- Hundreds of Tana's delicious, brain-healthy recipes
- Exercises to kill the ANTs (automatic negative thoughts)
- Meditation and hypnosis audios for sleep, anxiety, pain, and more
- Brain-enhancing music by Grammy Award winner Barry Goldstein
- Online forum and a community of support
- Access to monthly live coaching calls with Daniel and Tana

BRAINMD

www.brainmdhealth.com

For the highest quality brain health supplements, courses, books, and more.

Notes

BEFORE YOU BEGIN

1. See https://www.facebook.com/Illumeably/videos/283984572006650.

2. Howard Schneider et al., "Conventional SPECT Versus 3D Thresholded SPECT Imaging in the Diagnosis of ADHD: A Retrospective Study," *Journal of Neuropsychiatry and Clinical Neurosciences* 26, no 4 (Fall 2014): 335–43.

   J. F. Thornton et al., "Improved Outcomes Using Brain SPECT-Guided Treatment Versus Treatment-as-Usual in Community Psychiatric Outpatients: A Retrospective Case-Control Study," *Journal of Neuropsychiatry and Clinical Neuroscience* 26, no. 1 (Winter 2014): 51–56.

INTRODUCTION: WHY I HATE THE TERM *MENTAL ILLNESS* AND YOU SHOULD TOO

1. NPR Staff, "The Thomas Eagleton Affair Haunts Candidates Today," NPR, August 4, 2012, www.npr.org/2012/08/04/157670201/the-thomas-eagleton-affair-haunts-candidates -today.

2. Joshua Wolf Shenk, "Lincoln's Great Depression," *Atlantic*, October 2005, www.theatlantic .com/magazine/archive/2005/10/lincolns-great-depression/304247/.

3. Edward J. Kempf, "Abraham Lincoln's Organic and Emotional Neurosis," *A.M.A. Archives of Neurology and Psychiatry* 67, no. 4 (April 1952): 419–33; accessed at www.lincolnportrait .com/emotional_neurosis.html.

   Timothy P. Townsend, "Life of Lincoln, 1809–1865," National Park Service, US Department of the Interior, https://www.nps.gov/liho/learn/historyculture/life.htm.

4. National Institute of Mental Health, "Suicide," updated April 2019, www.nimh.nih.gov /health/statistics/suicide.shtml.

5. Holly Hedegaard, Sally C. Curtin, and Margaret Warner, "Suicide Mortality in the United States, 1999–2017," National Center for Health Statistics Data Brief No. 330, November 2018, www.cdc.gov/nchs/products/databriefs/db330.htm.

6. Jürgen Unützer, "What If We Treated Mental Health Like Cancer?" NEJM Catalyst event, "Expanding the Bounds of Care Delivery: Integrating Mental, Social, and Physical Health," January 25, 2018, Vanderbilt University Medical Center, catalyst.nejm.org/videos/treat -mental-health-like-cancer/.

7. Lawrence Scholl et al., "Drug and Opioid-Involved Overdose Deaths—United States, 2013–2017," *Morbidity and Mortality Weekly Report*, Centers for Disease Control and Prevention, January 4, 2019, www.cdc.gov/mmwr/volumes/67/wr/mm675152e1 .htm?s_cid=mm675152e1_w.

8. J. M. Twenge et al., "Age, Period, and Cohort Trends in Mood Disorder Indicators and Suicide-Related Outcomes in a Nationally Representative Dataset, 2005–2017," *Journal of Abnormal Psychology* 128, no. 3 (April 2019): 185–99.

9. J. Breslau J et al., "Sex Differences in Recent First-Onset Depression in an Epidemiological Sample of Adolescents," *Translational Psychiatry* 7 (2017): 1139.

10. Janice Wood, "Antidepressant Use Up 400 Percent in US," Psych Central, January 8, 2018, psychcentral.com/news/2011/10/25/antidepressant-use-up-400-percent-in-us/30677.html.

11. R. C. Kessler, M. Angermeyer, J. C. Anthony et al. "Lifetime Prevalence and Age-of-Onset Distributions of Mental Disorders in the World Health Organization's World Mental Health Survey Initiative," *World Psychiatry* 6 no. 3 (October 2007):168–76, https://www.ncbi.nlm.nih.gov/pmc/articles/PMC2174588/.

    "Learn about Mental Health," Centers for Disease Control and Prevention, January 26, 2018, https://www.cdc.gov/mentalhealth/learn/.

12. Jürgen Unützer, "What If We Treated Mental Health Like Cancer?" NEJM Catalyst, January 25, 2018, https://catalyst.nejm.org/videos/treat-mental-health-like-cancer/.

    K. Kroenke and J. Unützer, "Closing the False Divide: Sustainable Approaches to Integrating Mental Health Services into Primary Care," *Journal of General Internal Medicine* 32, no. 4 (2017): 404–10.

13. Julia Velten et al., "Lifestyle Choices and Mental Health: A Representative Population Survey," *BMC Psychology* 2, no. 58 (2014): 58.

14. Mitsutaka Takada, Mai Fujimoto, Kouichi Hosomi, "Association between Benzodiazepine Use and Dementia: Data Mining of Different Medical Databases," *International Journal of Medical Sciences* 13, no. 11 (October 18, 2016): 825–34.

15. Thomas R. Insel, "Disruptive Insights in Psychiatry: Transforming a Clinical Discipline," *Journal of Clinical Investigation* 119, no. 4 (April 1, 2009): 700–705.

    I. Kirsch, "Antidepressants and the Placebo Response," *Epidemiologia e Psichiatria Sociale* 18, no. 4 (October–December 2009): 318–22.

16. Steven E. Hyman, "The Daunting Polygenicity of Mental Illness: Making a New Map," *Philosophical Transactions of the Royal Society of London. Series B, Biological Sciences* 373, no. 1742 (March 19, 2018): 20170031.

17. Kate Allsopp et al., "Heterogeneity in Psychiatric Diagnostic Classification," *Psychiatry Research* 279 (September 2019): 15–22.

18. Ibid.

19. Daniel G. Amen et al., "Multi-Site, Six Month Outcome Study of Complex Psychiatric Patients Evaluated with Addition of Brain SPECT Imaging," *Advances in Mind-Body Medicine* 27, no. 2 (January 1996): 6–16.

CHAPTER 1: FROM DEMON POSSESSION TO THE 15-MINUTE MED CHECK

1. John Green, "What Is the Origin of the Word 'Shrink' for Psychologists?" Classroom, last modified July 31, 2019, https://classroom.synonym.com/origin-word-shrink-psychologists-11814.html.

2. Daniel G. Amen et al., "Predicting Positive and Negative Treatment Responses to Stimulants with Brain SPECT Imaging," *Journal of Psychoactive Drugs* 40, no. 2 (June 2008): 131–38.

3. "Psychiatry," Dictionary.com, https://www.dictionary.com/browse/psychiatry.

4. Richard Restak, *Mysteries of the Mind* (National Geographic Society, 2000).

5. Christos F. Kleisiaris et al., "Health Care Practices in Ancient Greece: The Hippocratic Ideal," *Journal of Medical Ethics and History of Medicine* 7, no. 6 (March 15, 2014).

6. Hippocrates, *The Genuine Works of Hippocrates* (New York: W. Wood and Company, 1886).

7. Kleisiaris et al., "Health Care Practices in Ancient Greece: The Hippocratic Ideal."

8. R. J. Hankinson, "Galen's Anatomy of the Soul," *Phronesis* 36, no. 2 (1991): 197–233.

9. D. Brett King, William Douglas Woody, and Wayne Viney, *A History of Psychology: Ideas and Context* (New York: Routledge, 2013), 72.

10. Ingrid G. Farreras, "History of Mental Illness," in R. Biswas-Diener and E. Diener, eds. *Noba Textbook Series: Psychology* (Champaign, IL: DEF Publishers), see http://noba.to/65w3s7ex.

11. Theodore Porter, *Genetics in the Madhouse* (Princeton, NJ: Princeton University Press, 2018).

12. Alexandra Minna Stern, "That Time the United States Sterilized 60,000 of Its Citizens," *Huffington Post*, January 7, 2016, www.huffingtonpost.com/entry/sterilization-united -states_us_568f35f2e4b0c8beacf68713.

13. Farreras, "History of Mental Illness."

14. Joshua Wolf Shenk, *Lincoln's Melancholy* (New York: Houghton Mifflin, 2005), 58.

15. Melissa Fares, "Michael Phelps' Purple Blotches Spotlight 'Cupping' Trend," Reuters, August 8, 2016, www.reuters.com/article/us-olympics-rio-swimming-phelps-cupping -idUSKCN10J214.

16. Joshua Wolf Shenk, *Lincoln's Melancholy*, 58–59.

17. Joshua Wolf Shenk, "Lincoln's Great Depression," *Atlantic*, October 2005.

18. Mayo Clinic Staff, "Electroconvulsive Therapy (ECT)," Mayo Clinic, October 12, 2018, www.mayoclinic.org/tests-procedures/electroconvulsive-therapy/about/pac-20393894.

19. Brendan L. Smith, "Inappropriate Prescribing," *Monitor on Psychology* 43, no. 6 (June 2012): 36, www.apa.org/monitor/2012/06/prescribing.aspx.

20. Daniel G. Amen et al., "Predicting Positive and Negative Treatment Responses to Stimulants with Brain SPECT Imaging."

21. Daniel G. Amen et al., "Deficits in Regional Cerebral Blood Flow on Brain SPECT Predict Treatment Resistant Depression," *Journal of Alzheimer's Disease* 63, no. 2 (2018): 529–38.

22. Lisa M. Schwartz and Steven Woloshin, "Medical Marketing in the United States, 1997–2016," *Journal of American Medical Association* 321, no. 1 (January 1/8, 2019): 80–96.

23. "Review Article Takes Rare Look at Impact of Advertising Psychiatric Drugs," Brown University press release, September 13, 2016, https://www.brown.edu/news/2016-09 -13/advertising.

24. Benedict Carey and Robert Gebeloff, "Many People Taking Antidepressants Discover They Cannot Quit," *New York Times*, April 7, 2018, www.nytimes.com/2018/04/07/health /antidepressants-withdrawal-prozac-cymbalta.html.

25. G. M. Goodwin et al., "Emotional Blunting with Antidepressant Treatments: A Survey among Depressed Patients," *Journal of Affective Disorders* 221 (October 15, 2017): 31–35.

26. Thomas Insel, "Transforming Diagnosis," National Institute of Mental Health, April 29, 2013, https://www.nimh.nih.gov/about/directors/thomas-insel/blog/2013/transforming -diagnosis.shtml.

27. "Mental Illness," National Institute of Mental Health, February 2019, https://www.nimh .nih.gov/health/statistics/mental-illness.shtml.

28. Ramin Mojtabai and M. Olfson, "Proportion of Antidepressants Prescribed without a Psychiatric Diagnosis Is Growing," *Health Affairs* 30, no. 8 (August 2011): 1434–42.

29. Racheli Magnezi et al., "Comparison between Neurostimulation Techniques Repetitive Transcranial Magnetic Stimulation vs Electroconvulsive Therapy for the Treatment of Resistant Depression: Patient Preference and Cost-Effectiveness," *Patient Preference and Adherence* 10 (August 4, 2016): 1481–87.

30. Tarique Perera et al., "The Clinical TMS Society Consensus Review and Treatment Recommendations for TMS Therapy for Major Depressive Disorder," *Brain Stimulation* 9, no. 3 (May–June 2016): 336–46.

31. D. White and S. Tavakoli, "Repetitive Transcranial Magnetic Stimulation for Treatment of Major Depressive Disorder with Comorbid Generalized Anxiety Disorder," *Annals of Clinical Psychiatry* 27, no. 3 (August 2015): 192–96.

32. Marco Ceccanti et al., "Deep TMS on Alcoholics: Effects on Cortisolemia and Dopamine Pathway Modulation. A Pilot Study," *Canadian Journal of Physiology and Pharmacology* 93, no. 4 (April 2015): 283–90.

33. Limor Dinur-Klein et al., "Smoking Cessation Induced by Deep Repetitive Transcranial

Magnetic Stimulation of the Prefrontal and Insular Cortices: A Prospective, Randomized Controlled Trial," *Biological Psychiatry* 76, no. 9 (November 2014): 742–49.

34. Paulo Sergio Boggio et al., "Noninvasive Brain Stimulation with High-Frequency and Low-Intensity Repetitive Transcranial Magnetic Stimulation Treatment for Posttraumatic Stress Disorder," *Journal of Clinical Psychiatry* 71, no. 8 (August 2010): 992–99.

35. Alisson Trevizol et al., "Transcranial Magnetic Stimulation for Obsessive-Compulsive Disorder: An Updated Systematic Review and Meta-Analysis," *Journal of ECT* 32, no. 4 (December 2016): 262–66.

36. Hellen Livia Drumond Marra et al., "Transcranial Magnetic Stimulation to Address Mild Cognitive Impairment in the Elderly: A Randomized Controlled Study," *Behavioural Neurology* (2015).

    William M. McDonald, "Neuromodulation Treatments for Geriatric Mood and Cognitive Disorders," *American Journal of Geriatric Psychiatry* 24, no. 12 (December 2016): 1130–41.

    Jose M. Rabey et al., "Repetitive Transcranial Magnetic Stimulation (rTMS) Combined with Cognitive Training Is a Safe and Effective Modality for the Treatment of Alzheimer's Disease: A Randomized, Double-Blind Study," *Journal of Neural Transmission* 123, no. 12 (December 2016):1449–55.

37. Mehmet Yilmaz et al., "Effectiveness of Transcranial Magnetic Stimulation Application in Treatment of Tinnitus," *Journal of Craniofacial Surgery* 25, no. 4 (July 2014): 1315–18.

38. Daniel G. Amen et al., "Discriminative Properties of Hippocampal Hypoperfusion in Marijuana Users Compared to Healthy Controls: Implications for Marijuana Administration in Alzheimer's Dementia," *Journal of Alzheimer's Disease* 56, no. 1 (2017): 261–73.

39. Daniel G. Amen et al., "Patterns of Regional Cerebral Blood Flow as a Function of Age throughout the Lifespan," *Journal of Alzheimer's Disease* 65, no. 4 (2018): 1087–92.

40. Chittaranjan Andrade, "Ketamine for Depression, 1: Clinical Summary of Issues Related to Efficacy, Adverse Effects, and Mechanism of Action," *Journal of Clinical Psychiatry* 78, no. 4 (April 2017): e415–e419.

    Michael F. Grunebaum et al., "Ketamine for Rapid Reduction of Suicidal Thoughts in Major Depression: A Midazolam-Controlled Randomized Clinical Trial," *American Journal of Psychiatry* 175, no. 4 (April 1, 2018): 327–35.

41. Nolan R. Williams et al., "Attenuation of Antidepressant Effects of Ketamine by Opioid Receptor Antagonism," *American Journal of Psychiatry* 175, no. 12 (December 1, 2018): 1205–15.

42. Nedra Pickler, "Obama Calls for End to Mental Illness Stigma," *San Diego Union-Tribune*, June 3, 2013, www.sandiegouniontribune.com/sdut-obama-calls-for-end-to-mental -illness-stigma-2013jun03-story.html.

CHAPTER 2: MAKING INVISIBLE ILLNESSES VISIBLE

1. Michael B. First et al., "Clinical Applications of Neuroimaging in Psychiatric Disorders," *American Journal of Psychiatry* 175, no. 9 (September 1, 2018): 915–16.

2. Max Planck, *Scientific Autobiography and Other Papers* (New York: Philosophical Library, 1949), 33–34.

3. Fred A. Mettler Jr. et al., "Radiologic and Nuclear Medicine Studies in the United States and Worldwide: Frequency, Radiation Dose, and Comparison with Other Radiation Sources—1950–2007," *Radiology* 253, no. 2 (November 2009): 520–31.

4. Michael D. Devous et al., "Single-Photon Emission Computed Tomography in Neurotherapeutics," *NeuroRx* 2, no. 2 (April 2005): 237–49.

5. Ronald Jack Jaszczak, "The Early Years of Single Photon Emission Computed Tomography (SPECT): An Anthology of Selected Reminiscences," *Physics in Medicine & Biology* 51, no. 13 (July 7, 2006): R99–115.

6. "Brain SPECT," Cedars-Sinai (2019), www.cedars-sinai.edu/Patients/Programs-and -Services/Imaging-Center/For-Patients/Exams-by-Procedure/Nuclear-Medicine/Brain

-SPECT.aspx; Mayo Clinic staff, "SPECT Scan," Mayo Clinic (December 23, 2016), www
.mayoclinic.org/tests-procedures/spect-scan/about/pac-20384925.

7. See PubMed.gov for a list of studies. Type in "Brain SPECT and [the condition]" for
best matches. For example, "Brain SPECT and Strokes" provides the following list:
https://www.ncbi.nlm.nih.gov/pubmed/?term=brain+SPECT+strokes.

8. S. Yassin et al., "Differences in SPECT Perfusion in Children and Adolescents with
ADHD," *Archives of Clinical Neuropsychology* 29, no. 6 (September 2014): 541–42

Daniel G. Amen and B. D. Carmichael, "High-Resolution Brain SPECT Imaging in
Attention Deficit Hyperactivity Disorder," *Annals of Clinical Psychiatry* 9, no. 2 (June 1997):
81–86.

9. Daniel G. Amen et al., "Predicting Positive and Negative Treatment Responses to
Stimulants with Brain SPECT Imaging," *Journal of Psychoactive Drugs* 40, no. 2 (June
2008): 131–38.

10. Daniel G. Amen et al., "Patterns of Regional Cerebral Blood Flow as a Function of Age
throughout the Lifespan," *Journal of Alzheimer's Disease* 65, no. 4 (September 25, 2018):
1087–92.

11. J. Link et al., "SPECT Differences between Those with Higher and Lower Levels of
Aggression: An Exploratory Analysis," *Archives of Clinical Neuropsychology* 29, no. 6
(September 2014): 576.

12. Daniel G. Amen et al., "An Analysis of Regional Cerebral Blood Flow in Impulsive
Murderers Using Single Photon Emission Computed Tomography," *Journal of
Neuropsychiatry and Clinical Neuroscience* 19, no. 3 (Summer 2007): 304–9.

13. Jada J. Stewart et al., "Diagnostic Accuracy of SPECT Scans: Examining Specific Brain
Areas of Regional Hypoperfusion at Baseline in Alzheimer's Disease," *Archives of Clinical
Neuropsychology* (2014).

14. J. Messerly et al., "Preliminary Investigation of SPECT Differences between Individuals
with Varying Levels of Anxiety," *Archives of Clinical Neuropsychology* 29, no. 6 (September
2014): 579.

15. Daniel G. Amen et al., "Functional Neuroimaging Distinguishes Autistic Spectrum
Disorder from Healthy and Comorbid Conditions in Focused and Large Community
Datasets," *Journal of Systems and Integrative Neuroscience* 3 (April 2017).

16. Daniel G. Amen et al., "Deficits in Regional Cerebral Blood Flow on Brain SPECT Predict
Treatment Resistant Depression," *Journal of Alzheimer's Disease* 63, no. 2 (2018): 529–38.

17. Lucas Driskell et al., "A SPECT Exploratory Analysis of Differentiating Mania
Symptomology Severity," *Archives of Clinical Neuropsychology* 29, no. 6 (September 2014):
578.

18. Daniel G. Amen et al., "Classification of Depression, Cognitive Disorders, and Co-Morbid
Depression and Cognitive Disorders with Perfusion SPECT Neuroimaging," *Journal of
Alzheimer's Disease* 57, no. 1 (2017): 253–66.

19. Daniel G. Amen et al., "Gender-Based Cerebral Perfusion Differences in 46,034
Functional Neuroimaging Scans," *Journal of Alzheimer's Disease* 60, no. 2 (2017): 605–14.

20. Daniel G. Amen et al., "Functional Neuroimaging Distinguishes Posttraumatic Stress
Disorder from Traumatic Brain Injury in Focused and Large Community Datasets,"
PLOS One (July 1, 2015), http://journals.plos.org/plosone/article?id=10.1371/journal.
pone.0129659.

Cyrus A. Raji et al., "Functional Neuroimaging with Default Mode Network Regions
Distinguishes PTSD from TBI in a Military Veteran Population," *Brain Imaging and
Behavior* 9, no. 3 (September 2015): 527–34.

21. Daniel G. Amen et al., "Discriminative Properties of Hippocampal Hypoperfusion
in Marijuana Users Compared to Healthy Controls: Implications for Marijuana
Administration in Alzheimer's Dementia," *Journal of Alzheimer's Disease* 56, no. 1 (2017):
261–73.

22. Andrew B. Newberg et al., "Cerebral Blood Flow Differences between Long-Term

Meditators and Non-Meditators," *Consciousness and Cognition* 19, no. 4 (December 2010): 899–905.

Dharma Khalsa et al., "Cerebral Blood Flow Changes during Chanting Meditation," *Nuclear Medicine Communications* 30, no. 12 (December 2009): 956–61.

23. Daniel G. Amen et al., "Quantitative Erythrocyte Omega-3 EPA Plus DHA Levels Are Related to Higher Regional Cerebral Blood Flow on Brain SPECT," *Journal of Alzheimer's Disease* 58, no. 4 (2017): 1189–99.

24. K. Willeumier et al., "Elevated Body Mass in National Football League Players Linked to Cognitive Impairment and Decreased Prefrontal Cortex and Temporal Pole Activity," *Translational Psychiatry* 2, no. 1 (January 2012): e68.

K. Willeumier et al., "Elevated BMI Is Associated with Decreased Blood Flow in the Prefrontal Cortex Using SPECT Imaging in Healthy Adults," *Obesity* 19, no. 5 (May 2011): 1095–97.

25. K. Willeumier et al., "Decreased Cerebral Blood Flow in the Limbic and Prefrontal Cortex Using SPECT Imaging in a Cohort of Completed Suicides," *Translational Psychiatry* 1, no. 8 (August 9, 2011): e28.

Daniel G. Amen et al., "A Comparative Analysis of Completed Suicide Using High Resolution Brain SPECT Imaging," *Journal of Neuropsychiatry and Clinical Neurosciences* 21, no. 4 (Fall 2009): 430–39.

26. Cyrus A. Raji et al., "Clinical Utility of SPECT Neuroimaging in the Diagnosis and Treatment of Traumatic Brain Injury: A Systematic Review," *PLOS One* 9, no. 3 (March 19, 2014): e91088.

27. Daniel G. Amen et al., "Perfusion Neuroimaging Abnormalities Alone Distinguish National Football League Players from a Healthy Population," *Journal of Alzheimer's Disease* 53, no. 1 (April 25, 2016): 237–41.

Daniel G. Amen et al., "Impact of Playing American Professional Football on Long-Term Brain Function," *Journal of Neuropsychiatry and Clinical Neurosciences* 23, no. 1 (Winter 2011): 98–106.

28. Daniel G. Amen et al., "Reversing Brain Damage in Former NFL Players: Implications for Traumatic Brain Injury and Substance Abuse Rehabilitation," *Journal of Psychoactive Drugs* 43, no. 1 (January–March 2011): 1–5.

29. Paul G. Harch et al., "A Phase I Study of Low-Pressure Hyperbaric Oxygen Therapy for Blast-Induced Post-Concussion Syndrome and Post-Traumatic Stress Disorder," *Journal of Neurotrauma* 29, no. 1 (January 1, 2012): 168–85.

30. Daniel G. Amen et al., "Predicting Positive and Negative Treatment Responses to Stimulants with Brain SPECT Imaging."

31. Daniel G. Amen and Blake Carmichael, "Oppositional Children Similar to OCD on SPECT: Implications for Treatment," *Journal of Neurotherapy* 2, no. 2 (August 1997): 1–6.

CHAPTER 3: 12 GUIDING PRINCIPLES TO CHANGE YOUR LIFE

1. Read about these principles in depth in *Change Your Brain, Change Your Life* (New York: Harmony Books, 2015).

2. Jonathan Day et al., "Influence of Paternal Preconception Exposures on Their Offspring: Through Epigenetics to Phenotype," *American Journal of Stem Cells* 5, no. 1 (2016): 11–18.

CHAPTER 4: GET YOUR BRAIN RIGHT AND YOUR MIND WILL FOLLOW

1. Erika L. Sabbath et al., "Time May Not Fully Attenuate Solvent-Associated Cognitive Deficits in Highly Exposed Workers," *Neurology* 82, no. 19 (May 13, 2014): 1716–23.

Samuel Keer et al., "Neuropsychological Performance in Solvent-Exposed Vehicle Collision Repair Workers in New Zealand," *PLOSOne* 12, no. 12 (December 13, 2017): e0189108.

2. Daniel G. Amen et al., *Change Your Brain, Change Your Life* (New York: Harmony Books, 2015), 49.

3. J. Araújo et al., "Prevalence of Optimal Metabolic Health in American Adults: National Health and Nutrition Examination Survey 2009–2016," *Metabolic Syndrome and Related Disorders* 17, no. 1 (February 2019): 46–52.

4. Ibid.

5. Michele Corriston, "Demi Lovato Fights for Mental Health Reform on Capitol Hill: 'I Went through Several Years of Pain and Suffering,'" *People*, October 5, 2015, people .com/celebrity/demi-lovato-fights-for-mental-health-awareness-in-washington-dc/.

6. Amen, *Change Your Brain, Change Your Life*, 51.

7. Kristine Engemann et al., "Residential Green Space in Childhood Is Associated with Lower Risk of Psychiatric Disorders from Adolescence into Adulthood," *Proceedings of the National Academy of Sciences of the United States of America* 116, no. 11 (March 12, 2019): 5188–93.

8. Eckhart Tolle, "Living in Presence with Your Emotional Pain Body," *HuffPost The Blog*, October 6, 2010, www.huffingtonpost.com/eckhart-tolle/living-in-presence-with-y_b _753114.html.

9. Ibid.

10. Ibid.

11. Jean Twenge, "What Might Explain the Current Unhappiness Epidemic?" Ladders.com, (December 7, 2018), www.theladders.com/career-advice/what-might-explain-the -current-unhappiness-epidemic.

12. M. E. Seligman et al., "Positive Psychology Progress: Empirical Validation of Interventions," *American Psychologist* 60, no. 5 (July–August 2005): 410–21.

13. Thomas H. Holmes and Richard H. Rahe, "The Social Readjustment Rating Scale," *Journal of Psychosomatic Research* 11, no. 2 (August 1967): 213–18.

14. Emily J. Jones et al., "Chronic Family Stress and Adolescent Health: The Moderating Role of Emotion Regulation," *Psychosomatic Medicine* 80, no. 8 (2018): 764–73.

15. Scott Stump, "Girl Scout Sells 300 Boxes of Cookies outside Marijuana Dispensary in 6 Hours," Today.com, February 7, 2018, www.today.com/parents/girl-scout-sells-300 -boxes-cookies-outside-marijuana-dispensary-6-t122455.

16. Wendy M. Johnston and Graham C. L. Davey, "The Psychological Impact of Negative TV News Bulletins: The Catastrophizing of Personal Worries," *British Journal of Psychology* 88, pt. 1 (February 1997): 85–91.

17. Janet Adamy and Paul Overberg, "The Loneliest Generation: Americans, More Than Ever, Are Aging Alone," *Wall Street Journal*, December 11, 2018, www.wsj.com/articles /the-loneliest-generation-americans-more-than-ever-are-aging-alone-11544541134.

18. "Loneliness and Alzheimer's," Rush University Medical Center, www.rush.edu/health -wellness/discover-health/loneliness-and-alzheimers.

19. Melissa G. Hunt et al., "No More FOMO: Limiting Social Media Decreases Loneliness and Depression," *Journal of Social and Clinical Psychology* 37, no. 10 (2018): 751–68.

   Denis Campbell, "Depression in Girls Linked to Higher Use of Social Media," *Guardian*, January 3, 2019, www.theguardian.com/society/2019/jan/04/depression-in-girls-linked -to-higher-use-of-social-media?CMP=Share_iOSApp_Other.

20. Jacqueline V. Hogue and Jennifer S. Mills, "The Effects of Active Social Media Engagement with Peers on Body Image in Young Women," *Body Image* 28 (March 2019): 1–5.

21. Lisa Lee, "NIH Study Probes Impact of Heavy Screen Time on Young Brains," *Bloomberg Quint*, December 9, 2018, www.bloombergquint.com/technology/screen-time-changes -structure-of-kids-brains-60-minutes-says#gs.ddq1FHk.

22. Larry Magid, "Dire Warnings about Children Dying because of Apps and Games Are a Form of 'Juvenoia,'" ConnectSafely.org, August 27, 2018, www.connectsafely.org/dire -warnings-about-children-dying-because-of-apps-and-games-are-a-form-of-juvenoia/.

23. Gisele Bündchen, *Lessons: My Path to a Meaningful Life* (New York: Avery, 2018).

24. "Frederick's Experiment," Digma.com, https://www.digma.com/digma-images/video-scripts/fredericks_experiment.pdf.

25. Harry T. Chugani et al., "Local Brain Functional Activity Following Early Deprivation: A Study of Postinstitutionalized Romanian Orphans," *NeuroImage* 14, no. 6 (December 2001): 1290–301.

26. Patricia A. Boyle et al., "Effect of Purpose in Life on Risk of Incident Alzheimer's Disease and Mild Cognitive Impairment in Community-Dwelling Older Persons," *Archives of General Psychiatry* 67, no. 3 (March 2010): 304–10.

27. Ibid.

28. Anthony L. Burrow and Nicolette Rainone, "How Many *Likes* Did I Get?: Purpose Moderates Links between Positive Social Media Feedback and Self-Esteem," *Journal of Experimental Social Psychology* 69 (March 2017): 232–36.

29. Daniel G. Amen, *Change Your Brain, Change Your Life*, 53–54.

CHAPTER 5: B IS FOR BLOOD FLOW

1. "CVD and Mental Health Disorders: Link Established, More Research Needed," *Cardiology Today*, November 2015, www.healio.com/cardiology/vascular-medicine/news/print/cardiology-today/%7Bdfb3be16-c566-43d8-9ee0-fbe553b1c35c%7D/cvd-and-mental-health-disorders-link-established-more-research-needed.

2. Kamen A. Tsvetanov et al., "The Effect of Ageing on fMRI: Correction for the Confounding Effects of Vascular Reactivity Evaluated by Joint fMRI and MEG in 335 Adults," *Human Brain Mapping* 36, no. 6 (June 2015): 2248–69.

3. Y. Iturria-Medina et al., "Early Role of Vascular Dysregulation on Late-Onset Alzheimer's Disease Based on Multifactorial Data-Driven Analysis," *Nature Communications* 7 (June 21, 2016): 11934.

4. Sebastian Köhler et al., "Depression, Vascular Factors, and Risk of Dementia in Primary Care: A Retrospective Cohort Study," *Journal of the American Geriatrics Society* 63, no. 4 (April 2015): 692–98.

5. Justin B. Ng et al., "Heart Disease as a Risk Factor for Dementia," *Clinical Epidemiology* 5 (2013): 135–45.

6. James M. Greenblatt, "The Implications of Low Cholesterol in Depression and Suicide," Great Plains Laboratory, Inc. (November 16, 2015), www.greatplainslaboratory.com/articles-1/2015/11/13/the-implications-of-low-cholesterol-in-depression-and-suicide.

7. Sebastian Köhler et al., "Depression, Vascular Factors, and Risk of Dementia in Primary Care: A Retrospective Cohort Study."

E. Duron and O. Hanon, "Vascular Risk Factors, Cognitive Decline, and Dementia," *Vascular Health and Risk Management* 4, no. 2 (2008): 363–81.

8. Sean P. Kennelly et al., "Blood Pressure and the Risk for Dementia: A Double Edged Sword," *Ageing Research Reviews* 8, no. 2 (April 2009): 61–70.

9. Chun-Ming Yang et al., "Increased Risk of Dementia in Patients with Erectile Dysfunction: A Population-Based, Propensity Score-Matched, Longitudinal Follow-Up Study," *Medicine* 94, no. 24 (June 2015): e990.

10. J. Kulmala et al., "Association between Mid- to Late Life Physical Fitness and Dementia: Evidence from the CAIDE Study," *Journal of Internal Medicine* 276, no. 3 (September 2014): 296–307,

Kay Deckers et al., "Target Risk Factors for Dementia Prevention: A Systematic Review and Delphi Consensus Study on the Evidence from Observational Studies," *International Journal of Geriatric Psychiatry* 30, no. 3 (March 2015): 234–46.

Robert P. Friedland et al., "Patients with Alzheimer's Disease Have Reduced Activities in Midlife Compared with Healthy Control-Group Members," *Proceedings of the National Academy of Sciences of the United States of America* 98, no. 6 (March 13, 2001): 3440–45.

11. Kaigang Li et al., "Changes in Moderate-to-Vigorous Physical Activity among Older Adolescents," *Pediatrics* 138, no. 4 (October 2016): e20161372.

12. "How Does Depression Affect the Heart?" American Heart Association (June 2014), www.heart.org/en/healthy-living/healthy-lifestyle/mental-health-and-wellbeing/how-does-depression-affect-the-heart.

13. Daniel G. Amen et al., "Patterns of Regional Cerebral Blood Flow as a Function of Age throughout the Lifespan," *Journal of Alzheimer's Disease* 65, no. 4 (2018): 1087–92.

14. Kristen C. Willeumier et al., "Elevated BMI Is Associated with Decreased Blood Flow in the Prefrontal Cortex Using SPECT Imaging in Healthy Adults," *Obesity* 19, no. 5 (May 2011): 1095–97.

15. Merideth A. Addicott et al., "The Effect of Daily Caffeine Use on Cerebral Blood Flow: How Much Caffeine Can We Tolerate?" *Human Brain Mapping* 30, no. 10 (October 2009): 3102–14.

16. Edward F. Domino et al., "Regional Cerebral Blood Flow and Plasma Nicotine after Smoking Tobacco Cigarettes," *Progress in Neuropsychopharmacology and Biological Psychiatry* 28, no. 2 (March 2004): 319–27.

17. Daniel G. Amen et al., "Discriminative Properties of Hippocampal Hypoperfusion in Marijuana Users Compared to Healthy Controls: Implications for Marijuana Administration in Alzheimer's Dementia," *Journal of Alzheimer's Disease* 56, no. 1 (2017): 261–73.

18. Giuseppe Faraco et al., "Water Deprivation Induces Neurovascular and Cognitive Dysfunction through Vasopressin-Induced Oxidative Stress," *Journal of Cerebral Blood Flow and Metabolism* 34, no. 5 (May 2014): 852–60.

19. "Stopping Smoking Is Good for Your Mental Health," NHS UK, January 25, 2018, www.nhs.uk/live-well/quit-smoking/stopping-smoking-mental-health-benefits/.

20. Yuan-Hwa Chou et al., "Effects of Video Game Playing on Cerebral Blood Flow in Young Adults: A SPECT Study," *Psychiatry Research* 212, no. 1 (April 30, 2013): 65–72.

21. Goh Matsuda and Kazuo Hiraki, "Sustained Decrease in Oxygenated Hemoglobin during Video Games in the Dorsal Prefrontal Cortex: A NIRS Study of Children," *Neuroimage* 29, no. 3 (February 1, 2006): 706–11.

22. Jack James, "Critical Review of Dietary Caffeine and Blood Pressure: A Relationship That Should Be Taken More Seriously," *Psychosomatic Medicine* 66, no. 1 (January–February 2004): 63–71.

23. Andrew Newberg et al., "Cerebral Blood Flow during Meditative Prayer: Preliminary Findings and Methodological Issues," *Perceptual and Motor Skills* 97, no. 2 (October 2003): 625–30.

24. Huseyin Naci et al., "How Does Exercise Treatment Compare with Antihypertensive Medications? A Network Meta-Analysis of 391 Randomised Controlled Trials Assessing Exercise and Medication Effects on Systolic Blood Pressure," *British Journal of Sports Medicine* 53, no. 14 (July 2019): 859–69.

25. Victoria Allen, "Moderate Exercise Just Three Times a Week and Eating Healthy Can Take 10 Years Off Your Brain Age, Study Says," *Daily Mail* (December 19, 2018), www.dailymail.co.uk/news/article-6514359/Moderate-exercise-just-three-times-week-eating-healthy-10-years-brain-age.html.

26. Karmel W. Choi et al., "Assessment of Bidirectional Relationships between Physical Activity and Depression among Adults: A 2-Sample Mendelian Randomization Study," *JAMA Psychiatry* 76, no. 4 (April 1, 2019): 399–408.

27. Viola Oertel-Knöchel et al., "Effects of Aerobic Exercise on Cognitive Performance and Individual Psychopathology in Depressive and Schizophrenia Patients," *European Archives of Psychiatry and Clinical Neuroscience* 264, no. 7 (October 2014): 589–604.

28. Claudia Battaglia et al., "Participation in a 9-month Selected Physical Exercise Programme Enhances Psychological Well-Being in a Prison Population," *Criminal Behaviour and Mental Health* 25, no. 5 (December 2015): 343–54.

29. Richard A. Rawson et al., "The Impact of Exercise on Depression and Anxiety Symptoms among Abstinent Methamphetamine-Dependent Individuals in a Residential Treatment Setting," *Journal of Substance Abuse Treatment* 57 (October 2015): 36–40.

30. P. Abedi et al., "Effect of Pedometer-Based Walking on Depression, Anxiety and Insomnia among Postmenopausal Women," *Climacteric* 18, no. 6 (2015): 841–45.

31. Laura Q. Rogers et al., "Effects of a Multicomponent Physical Activity Behavior Change Intervention on Fatigue, Anxiety, and Depressive Symptomatology in Breast Cancer Survivors: Randomized Trial," *Psychooncology* 26, no. 11 (November 2017): 1901–6.

32. Lisanne F. ten Brinke et al., "Aerobic Exercise Increases Hippocampal Volume in Older Women with Probable Mild Cognitive Impairment: A 6-Month Randomised Controlled Trial," *British Journal of Sports Medicine* 49, no. 4 (February 2015): 248–54.

    Caterina Rosano et al., "Hippocampal Response to a 24-Month Physical Activity Intervention in Sedentary Older Adults," *American Journal of Geriatric Psychiatry* 25, no. 3 (November 15, 2016): 209–17.

    Maike M. Kleemeyer et al., "Changes in Fitness Are Associated with Changes in Hippocampal Microstructure and Hippocampal Volume among Older Adults," *Neuroimage* 131 (May 1, 2016): 155–61.

    F. G. Pajonk et al., "Hippocampal Plasticity in Response to Exercise in Schizophrenia," *Archives of General Psychiatry* 67, no. 2 (February 2010): 133–43.

33. Kim M. Gerecke et al., "Exercise Protects against Chronic Restraint Stress-Induced Oxidative Stress in the Cortex and Hippocampus," *Brain Research* 1509 (May 6, 2013): 66–78.

34. Vijay R. Varma et al., "Low-Intensity Daily Walking Activity Is Associated with Hippocampal Volume in Older Adults," *Hippocampus* 25, no. 5 (May 2015): 605–15.

35. Francesca Calabrese et al., "Brain-Derived Neurotrophic Factor: A Bridge between Inflammation and Neuroplasticity," *Front Cell Neuroscience* 8 (December 22, 2014): 430.

36. Carl W. Cotman and N. C. Berchtold, "Exercise: A Behavioral Intervention to Enhance Brain Health and Plasticity," *Trends in Neurosciences* 25, no. 6 (June 2002): 295–301.

    William D. S. Killgore et al., "Physical Exercise Habits Correlate with Gray Matter Volume of the Hippocampus in Healthy Adult Humans," *Scientific Reports* 3 (December 12, 2013): 3457.

37. Cell Press, "Physical Activity May Leave the Brain More Open to Change," *ScienceDaily* (December 7, 2015), www.sciencedaily.com/releases/2015/12/151207131508.htm.

38. Ana M. Abrantes et al., "A Pilot Randomized Controlled Trial of Aerobic Exercise as an Adjunct to OCD Treatment," *General Hospital Psychiatry* 49 (November 2017): 51–55.

39. Mathew G. Fetzner and G. J. Asmundson, "Aerobic Exercise Reduces Symptoms of Posttraumatic Stress Disorder: A Randomized Controlled Trial," *Cognitive Behaviour Therapy* 44, no. 4 (2015): 301–13.

40. R. Ryan Patel, "Weight-Lifting, Exercise, and Mental Health," Ohio State University, October 20, 2017, https://u.osu.edu/emotionalfitness/2017/10/20/weight-lifting-exercise-and-mental-health/.

41. Chien-Yu Pan et al., "A Racket-Sport Intervention Improves Behavioral and Cognitive Performance in Children with Attention-Deficit/Hyperactivity Disorder," *Research in Developmental Disabilities* 57 (October 2016): 1–10.

42. Rahav Boussi-Gross et al., "Hyperbaric Oxygen Therapy Can Improve Post Concussion Syndrome Years after Mild Traumatic Brain Injury—Randomized Prospective Trial," *PLoS One* 8, no. 11 (November 15, 2013): e79995.

43. Sigal Tal et al., "Hyperbaric Oxygen May Induce Angiogenesis in Patients Suffering from Prolonged Post-Concussion Syndrome Due to Traumatic Brain Injury," *Restorative Neurology and Neuroscience* 33, no. 6 (2015): 943–51.

44. Paul G. Harch et al., "A Phase I Study of Low-Pressure Hyperbaric Oxygen Therapy for Blast-Induced Post-Concussion Syndrome and Post-Traumatic Stress Disorder," *Journal of Neurotrauma* 29, no. 1 (January 1, 2012): 168–85.

45. Shao-Yuan Chen et al., "Reversible Changes of Brain Perfusion SPECT for Carbon Monoxide Poisoning-Induced Severe Akinetic Mutism," *Clinical Nuclear Medicine* 41, no. 5 (May 2016): e221–27.

46. Shai Efrati et al., "Hyperbaric Oxygen Induces Late Neuroplasticity in Post Stroke Patients—Randomized, Prospective Trial," *PLoS One* 8, no. 1 (2013): e53716.

47. Shai Efrati et al., "Hyperbaric Oxygen Therapy Can Diminish Fibromyalgia Syndrome—Prospective Clinical Trial," *PLoS One* 10, no. 5 (May 26, 2015): e0127012.

48. Chien-Yu Huang et al., "Hyperbaric Oxygen Therapy as an Effective Adjunctive Treatment for Chronic Lyme Disease," *Journal of the Chinese Medical Association* 77, no. 5 (May 2014): 269–71.

49. I-Han Chiang et al., "Adjunctive Hyperbaric Oxygen Therapy in Severe Burns: Experience in Taiwan Formosa Water Park Dust Explosion Disaster," *Burns* 43, no. 4 (June 2017): 852–57.

50. M. Löndahl et al., "Relationship between Ulcer Healing after Hyperbaric Oxygen Therapy and Transcutaneous Oximetry, Toe Blood Pressure and Ankle-Brachial Index in Patients with Diabetes and Chronic Foot Ulcers," *Diabetologia* 54, no. 1 (January 2011): 65–68.

51. Anne M. Eskes et al., "Hyperbaric Oxygen Therapy: Solution for Difficult to Heal Acute Wounds? Systematic Review," *World Journal of Surgery* 35, no. 3 (March 2011): 535–42.

    Joshua J. Shaw et al., "Not Just Full of Hot Air: Hyperbaric Oxygen Therapy Increases Survival in Cases of Necrotizing Soft Tissue Infections," *Surgical Infections* 15, no. 3 (June 2014): 328–35.

52. Mina Taghizadeh Asl et al., "Brain Perfusion Imaging with Voxel-Based Analysis in Secondary Progressive Multiple Sclerosis Patients with a Moderate to Severe Stage of Disease: A Boon for the Workforce," *BMC Neurology* 16 (May 26, 2016): 79.

53. P. S. Dulai et al., "Systematic Review: The Safety and Efficacy of Hyperbaric Oxygen Therapy for Inflammatory Bowel Disease," *Alimentary Pharmacology & Therapeutics* 39, no. 11 (June 2014): 1266–75.

54. David N. Teguh et al., "Early Hyperbaric Oxygen Therapy for Reducing Radiotherapy Side Effects: Early Results of a Randomized Trial in Oropharyngeal and Nasopharyngeal Cancer," *International Journal of Radiation Oncology, Biology, Physics* 75, no. 3 (November 1, 2009): 711–16.

    Nico Schellart et al., "Hyperbaric Oxygen Treatment Improved Neurophysiologic Performance in Brain Tumor Patients after Neurosurgery and Radiotherapy: A Preliminary Report," *Cancer* 117, no. 15 (August 1, 2011): 3434–44.

55. Daniel A. Rossignol et al., "The Effects of Hyperbaric Oxygen Therapy on Oxidative Stress, Inflammation, and Symptoms in Children with Autism: An Open-Label Pilot Study," *BMC Pediatrics* 7, no. 36 (November 16, 2007).

    Daniel A. Rossignol et al., "Hyperbaric Treatment for Children with Autism: A Multicenter, Randomized, DoubleBlind, Controlled Trial," *BMC Pediatrics* 9, no. 21 (March 13, 2009).

56. Arun Mukherjee et al., "Intensive Rehabilitation Combined with HBO2 Therapy in Children with Cerebral Palsy: A Controlled Longitudinal Study," *Undersea & Hyperbaric Medicine* 41, no. 2 (March–April 2014): 77–85.

57. Claudio Borghi and Arrigo F. G. Cicero, "Nutraceuticals with a Clinically Detectable Blood Pressure-Lowering Effect: A Review of Available Randomized Clinical Trials and Their Meta-Analyses," *British Journal of Clinical Pharmacology* 83, no. 1 (January 2017): 163–71.

58. Ameneh Mashayekh et al., "Effects of *Ginkgo biloba* on Cerebral Blood Flow Assessed by Quantitative MR Perfusion Imaging: A Pilot Study," *Neuroradiology* 53, no. 3 (March 2011): 185–91.

    J. Kleijnen and P. Knipschild, "Ginkgo biloba for Cerebral Insufficiency," *British Journal of Clinical Pharmacology* 34, no. 4 (October 1992): 352–58.

    F. Eckmann, "Cerebral Insufficiency—Treatment with Ginkgo-biloba Extract. Time of Onset of Effect in a Double-Blind Study with 60 Inpatients," *Fortschritte der Medizin* 108, no. 29 (October 10, 1990): 557–60.

59. R. F. Santos et al., "Cognitive Performance, SPECT, and Blood Viscosity in Elderly Non-Demented People Using *Ginkgo biloba*," *Pharmacopsychiatry* 36, no. 4 (July 2003): 127–33.

Joseph A. Mix and W. David Crews Jr., "A Double-Blind, Placebo-Controlled, Randomized Trial of *Ginkgo biloba* Extract EGb 761® in a Sample of Cognitively Intact Older Adults: Neuropsychological Findings," *Human Psychopharmacology* 17, no. 6 (August 2002): 267–77.

60. Horst Herrschaft et al., "*Ginkgo Biloba* Extract EGb 761® in Dementia with Neuropsychiatric Features: A Randomised, Placebo-Controlled Trial to Confirm the Efficacy and Safety of a Daily Dose of 240 mg," *Journal of Psychiatric Research* 46, no. 6 (June 2012): 716–23.

61. Chun-Xiao Dai et al., "Role of Ginkgo Biloba Extract as an Adjunctive Treatment of Elderly Patients with Depression and on the Expression of Serum S100B," *Medicine* 97, no. 39 (September 2018): e12421.

62. Helmut Woelk et al., "Ginkgo Biloba Special Extract EGb 761® in Generalized Anxiety Disorder and Adjustment Disorder with Anxious Mood: A Randomized, Double-Blind, Placebo-Controlled Trial," *Journal of Psychiatric Research* 41, no. 6 (September 2007): 472–80.

63. Daniel J. Lamport et al., "The Effect of Flavanol-Rich Cocoa on Cerebral Perfusion in Healthy Older Adults during Conscious Resting State: A Placebo Controlled, Crossover, Acute Trial," *Psychopharmacology* 232, no. 17 (September 2015): 3227–34.

David T. Field et al., "Consumption of Cocoa Flavanols Results in an Acute Improvement in Visual and Cognitive Functions," *Physiology & Behavior* 103, nos. 3–4 (June 2011): 255–60.

S. T. Francis et al., "The Effect of Flavanol-Rich Cocoa on the fMRI Response to a Cognitive Task in Healthy Young People," *Journal of Cardiovascular Pharmacology* 47, suppl 2:S215–20 (June 2006).

Farzaneh A. Sorond et al., "Neurovascular Coupling, Cerebral White Matter Integrity, and Response to Cocoa in Older People," *Neurology* 81, no. 10 (September 3, 2013): 904–9.

64. Karin Ried et al., "Effect of Cocoa on Blood Pressure," *Cochrane Database of Systematic Reviews* 8 (August 15, 2012): CD008893.

Karin Ried et al., "Does Chocolate Reduce Blood Pressure? A Meta-Analysis," *BMC Medicine* 8, no. 39 (June 28, 2010).

65. Giovambattista Desideri et al., "Benefits in Cognitive Function, Blood Pressure, and Insulin Resistance through Cocoa Flavanol Consumption in Elderly Subjects with Mild Cognitive Impairment: The Cocoa, Cognition, and Aging (CoCoA) Study," *Hypertension* 60, no. 3 (September 2012): 794–801.

Daniela Mastroiacovo et al., "Cocoa Flavanol Consumption Improves Cognitive Function, Blood Pressure Control, and Metabolic Profile in Elderly Subjects: The Cocoa, Cognition, and Aging (CoCoA) Study—A Randomized Controlled Trial," *American Journal of Clinical Nutrition* 101, no. 3 (March 2015): 538–48.

66. Davide Grassi et al., "Flavanol-Rich Chocolate Acutely Improves Arterial Function and Working Memory Performance Counteracting the Effects of Sleep Deprivation in Healthy Individuals," *Journal of Hypertension* 34, no. 7 (July 2016): 1298–1308.

67. Mandy Oaklander, "5 Surprising Ways to Help Your Memory," *Time* (June 10, 2015), http://time.com/3915030/boost-memory-exercise/.

Philippa A. Jackson et al., "DHA-Rich Oil Modulates the Cerebral Haemodynamic Response to Cognitive Tasks in Healthy Young Adults: A Near IR Spectroscopy Pilot Study," *British Journal of Nutrition* 107, no. 8 (April 28, 2012): 1093–98.

Tae-Jin Song et al., "Low Levels of Plasma Omega 3-Polyunsaturated Fatty Acids Are Associated with Cerebral Small Vessel Diseases in Acute Ischemic Stroke Patients," *Nutrition Research* 35, no. 5 (May 2015): 368–74.

68. A. Veronica Witte et al., "Long-Chain Omega-3 Fatty Acids Improve Brain Function and Structure in Older Adults," *Cerebral Cortex* 24, no. 11 (November 2014): 3059–68.

69. E. L. Boespflug et al., "Fish Oil Supplementation Increases Event-Related Posterior Cingulate Activation in Older Adults with Subjective Memory Impairment," *Journal of Nutrition, Health & Aging* 20, no. 2 (February 2016): 161–69.

70. Nina Hamazaki-Fujita et al., "Polyunsaturated Fatty Acids and Blood Circulation in the Forebrain during a Mental Arithmetic Task," *Brain Research* 1397 (June 23, 2011): 38–45.

71. Jennifer Mildenberger et al., "N-3 PUFAs Induce Inflammatory Tolerance by Formation of KEAP1-Containing SQSTM1/p62-Bodies and Activation of NFE2L2," *Autophagy* 13, no. 10 (October 3, 2017): 1664–78.

72. Fredrik Jernerén et al., "Brain Atrophy in Cognitively Impaired Elderly: The Importance of Long-Chain ω-3 Fatty Acids and B Vitamin Status in a Randomized Controlled Trial," *American Journal of Clinical Nutrition* 102, no. 1 (July 2015): 215–21.

73. Emma L. Wightman et al., "Epigallocatechin Gallate, Cerebral Blood Flow Parameters, Cognitive Performance and Mood in Healthy Humans: A Double-Blind, Placebo-Controlled, Crossover Investigation," *Human Psychopharmacology* 27, no. 2 (March 2012): 177–86.

74. Xiaoli Peng et al., "Effect of Green Tea Consumption on Blood Pressure: A Meta-Analysis of 13 Randomized Controlled Trials," *Scientific Reports* 4 (September 1, 2014): 6251.

75. Xin-Xin Zheng et al., "Green Tea Intake Lowers Fasting Serum Total and LDL Cholesterol in Adults: A Meta-Analysis of 14 Randomized Controlled Trials," *American Journal of Clinical Nutrition* 94, no. 2 (August 2011): 601–10.

76. Xin-Xin Zheng et al., "Effects of Green Tea Catechins with or without Caffeine on Glycemic Control in Adults: A Meta-Analysis of Randomized Controlled Trials," *American Journal of Clinical Nutrition* 97, no. 4 (April 2013): 750–62.

77. Qiangye Zhang et al., "Effect of Green Tea on Reward Learning in Healthy Individuals: A Randomized, Double-Blind, Placebo-Controlled Pilot Study," *Nutrition Journal* 12, no. 84 (June 18, 2013).

78. Qing-Ping Ma et al., "Meta-Analysis of the Association between Tea Intake and the Risk of Cognitive Disorders," *PLoS One* 11, no. 11 (November 8, 2016): e0165861.

   L. Feng et al., "Tea Consumption Reduces the Incidence of Neurocognitive Disorders: Findings from the Singapore Longitudinal Aging Study," *Journal of Nutrition, Health & Aging* 20, no. 10 (2016): 1002–9.

79. David O. Kennedy et al., "Effects of Resveratrol on Cerebral Blood Flow Variables and Cognitive Performance in Humans: A Double-Blind, Placebo-Controlled, Crossover Investigation," *American Journal of Clinical Nutrition* 91, no. 6 (June 2010): 1590–97.

   Rachel H. X. Wong et al., "Acute Resveratrol Consumption Improves Neurovascular Coupling Capacity in Adults with Type 2 Diabetes Mellitus," *Nutrients* 8, no. 7 (July 12, 2016): 425.

CHAPTER 6: R IS FOR RETIREMENT AND AGING

1. Daniel G. Amen et al., "Patterns of Regional Cerebral Blood Flow as a Function of Age throughout the Lifespan," *Journal of Alzheimer's Disease* 65, no. 4 (2018): 1087–92.

2. D. J. Hare et al., "Is Early-Life Iron Exposure Critical in Neurodegeneration?" *Nature Reviews Neurology* 11, no. 9 (September 2015): 536–44.

3. R. McClelland et al., "Accelerated Ageing and Renal Dysfunction Links Lower Socioeconomic Status and Dietary Phosphate Intake," *Aging* 8, no. 5 (May 2016): 1135–49.

4. L. E. Hebert et al., "Change in Risk of Alzheimer Disease Over Time," *Neurology* 75, no. 9 (August 31, 2010): 786–91.

5. "Mental Health of Older Adults," World Health Organization, December 12, 2017, www.who.int/news-room/fact-sheets/detail/mental-health-of-older-adults.

6. W. Cai et al., "Oral Glycotoxins Are a Modifiable Cause of Dementia and the Metabolic Syndrome in Mice and Humans," *Proceedings of the National Academy of Sciences of the United States of America* 111, no. 13 (April 1, 2014): 4940–45.

7. "National Poll on Healthy Aging," University of Michigan (March 2019), ihpi.umich.edu /sites/default/files/2019-03/NPHA_Loneliness-Report_FINAL-022619.pdf.

8. Gabriel H. Sahlgren, "Work Longer, Live Healthier," IEA discussion paper no. 46 (May 2013), http://iea.org.uk/sites/default/files/publications/files/Work%20Longer,%20Live _Healthier.pdf.

9. Kapil Sayal et al., "Relative Age within the School Year and Diagnosis of Attention-Deficit Hyperactivity Disorder: A Nationwide Population-Based Study," *Lancet Psychiatry* 4, no. 11 (November 1, 2017): 868–75.

10. Corey L. M. Keyes, "Authentic Purpose: The Spiritual Infrastructure of Life," *Journal of Management, Spirituality & Religion* 8, no. 4 (November 2011): 281–97.

11. P. A. Boyle, et al., "Effect of Purpose in Life on Risk of Incident Alzheimer Disease and Mild Cognitive Impairment in Community-Dwelling Older Persons," *Archives of General Psychiatry* 67, no. 3 (March 2010): 304–10.

12. T. J. Holwerda et al., "Feelings of Loneliness, but Not Social Isolation, Predict Dementia Onset: Results from the Amsterdam Study of the Elderly (AMSTEL)," *Journal of Neurology, Neurosurgery, and Psychiatry* 85, no. 2 (February 2014): 135–42.

13. "Loneliness on the RISE: One in Eight People Have No Close Friends to Turn To," *Express*, March 1, 2017, http://www.express.co.uk/news/uk/773002/One-in-eight-people-faced -with-loneliness.

14. Kira Asatryan, "4 Disorders That May Thrive on Loneliness," *Psychology Today*, July 23, 2015, https://www.psychologytoday.com/us/blog/the-art-closeness/201507/4-disorders -may-thrive-loneliness.

15. E. E. Lee et al., "High Prevalence and Adverse Health Effects of Loneliness in Community-Dwelling Adults across the Lifespan: Role of Wisdom as a Protective Factor," *International Psychogeriatrics* (published online December 18, 2018): 1–16.

16. S. Korkmaz et al., "Frequency of Anemia in Chronic Psychiatry Patients," *Neuropsychiatric Disease and Treatment* 11 (October 22, 2015): 2737–41.

17. Joseph Mercola, "Iron: This Life-Saving Mineral Found to Actually Increase Senility in Many," *Mercola*, July 19, 2012, http://articles.mercola.com/sites/articles/archive/2012/07 /19/excess-iron-leads-to-alzheimers.aspx#_edn1.

    D. J. Hare et al., "Is Early-Life Iron Exposure Critical in Neurodegeneration?"

    A. C. Leskovjan et al., "Increased Brain Iron Coincides with Early Plaque Formation in a Mouse Model of Alzheimer's Disease," *Neuroimage* 55, no. 1 (March 1, 2011): 32–38.

18. C. C. Meltzer et al., "Serotonin in Aging, Late-Life Depression, and Alzheimer's Disease: The Emerging Role of Functional Imaging," *Neuropsychopharmacology* 18, no. 6 (June 1998): 407–30.

19. S. E. Hemby et al., "Neuron-Specific Age-Related Decreases in Dopamine Receptor Subtype mRNAs," *Journal of Comparative Neurology* 456, no. 2 (February 3, 2003): 176–83.

    Jean-Claude Dreher et al., "Age-Related Changes in Midbrain Dopaminergic Regulation of the Human Reward System," *Proceedings of the National Academy of Sciences of the United States of America* 105, no. 39 (September 30, 2008): 15,106–11.

20. Thomas McNeill and Michael Jakowec, "Neurotransmitters: GABA and Glutamate," *Medicine Encyclopedia* (2019), http://medicine.jrank.org/pages/1225/Neurotransmitters -GABA-glutamate.html.

21. J. L. Muir, "Acetylcholine, Aging, and Alzheimer's Disease," *Pharmacology, Biochemistry, and Behavior* 56, no. 4 (April 1997): 687–96.

22. John Hiscock, "Judi Dench Interview: 'Retirement Is a Rude Word,'" *Telegraph*, February 21, 2015, https://www.telegraph.co.uk/culture/film/film-news/11420407/Judi-Dench -interview-second-exotic-marigold-hotel.html.

23. S. Samman et al., "Green Tea or Rosemary Extract Added to Foods Reduces Nonheme-Iron Absorption," *American Journal of Clinical Nutrition* 73, no. 3 (March 2001): 607–12.

24. Y. Jiao et al., "Iron Chelation in the Biological Activity of Curcumin," *Free Radical Biology and Medicine* 40, no. 7 (April 1, 2006): 1152–60.

25. Sonja Hilbrand et al., "Caregiving within and beyond the Family Is Associated with Lower Mortality for the Caregiver: A Prospective Study," *Evolution and Human Behavior* 38, no. 3 (May 2017): 397–403.

26. M. C. Carlson et al., "Impact of the Baltimore Experience Corps Trial on Cortical and Hippocampal Volumes," *Alzheimer's and Dementia* 11, no. 11 (November 2015): 1340–48.

27. O. Dean et al., "N-acetylcysteine in Psychiatry: Current Therapeutic Evidence and Potential Mechanisms of Action," *Journal of Psychiatry and Neuroscience* 36, no. 2 (March 2011): 78–86.

28. Ibid.

29. J. C. Adair et al., "Controlled Trial of N-acetylcysteine for Patients with Probable Alzheimer's Disease," *Neurology* 57, no. 8 (October 23, 2001): 1515–17.

   W. R. Shankle et al., "CerefolinNAC Therapy of Hyperhomocysteinemia Delays Cortical and White Matter Atrophy in Alzheimer's Disease and Cerebrovascular Disease," *Journal of Alzheimer's Disease* 54, no. 3 (October 4, 2016): 1073–84.

30. Wei Zheng et al., "Huperzine A for Treatment of Cognitive Impairment in Major Depressive Disorder: A Systematic Review of Randomized Controlled Trials," *Shanghai Archives of Psychiatry* 28, no. 2 (April 25, 2016): 64–71.

31. Wei Zheng et al., "Adjunctive Huperzine A for Cognitive Deficits in Schizophrenia: A Systematic Review and Meta-Analysis," *Human Psychopharmacology* 31, no. 4 (July 2016): 286–95.

32. B. S. Wang et al., "Efficacy and Safety of Natural Acetylcholinesterase Inhibitor Huperzine A in the Treatment of Alzheimer's Disease: An Updated Meta-Analysis," *Journal of Neural Transmission* 116, no. 4 (April 2009): 457–65.

33. H. A. Hausenblas et al., "Saffron (Crocus sativus L.) and Major Depressive Disorder: A Meta-Analysis of Randomized Clinical Trials," *Journal of Integrative Medicine* 11, no. 6 (November 2013): 377–83.

34. M. A. Papandreou et al., "Inhibitory Activity on Amyloid-Beta Aggregation and Antioxidant Properties of Crocus sativus Stigmas Extract and Its Crocin Constituents," *Journal of Agricultural and Food Chemistry* 54, no. 23 (November 15, 2006): 8762–68.

35. Shinji Soeda et al., "Neuroprotective Activities of Saffron and Crocin" in *The Benefits of Natural Products for Neurogenerative Diseases: Advances in Neurobiology*, vol. 12, eds. M. Mohamed Essa, Akbar Mohammed, and Gilles Guillemin (New York: Springer, 2016), 275–92.

36. M. Tsolaki et al., "Efficacy and Safety of Crocus sativus L. in Patients with Mild Cognitive Impairment: One Year Single-Blind Randomized, with Parallel Groups, Clinical Trial," *Journal of Alzheimer's Disease* 54, no. 1 (July 2016): 129–33.

   S. Akhondzadeh et al., "A 22-Week, Multicenter, Randomized, Double-Blind Controlled Trial of Crocus sativus in the Treatment of Mild-to-Moderate Alzheimer's Disease," *Psychopharmacology* 207, no. 4 (January 2010): 637–43.

   S. Akhondzadeh et al., "Saffron in the Treatment of Patients with Mild to Moderate Alzheimer's Disease: A 16-Week, Randomized and Placebo-Controlled Trial," *Journal of Clinical Pharmacy and Therapeutics* 35, no. 5 (October 2010): 581–88.

   M. Farokhnia et al., "Comparing the Efficacy and Safety of Crocus sativus L. with Memantine in Patients with Moderate to Severe Alzheimer's Disease: A Double-Blind Randomized Clinical Trial," *Human Psychopharmacology* 29, no. 4 (July 2014): 351–59.

37. E. Tamaddonfard et al., "Crocin Improved Learning and Memory Impairments in Streptozotocin-Induced Diabetic Rats," *Iranian Journal of Basic Medical Sciences* 16, no. 1 (January 2013): 91–100.

38. G. D. Geromichalos et al., "Saffron as a Source of Novel Acetylcholinesterase Inhibitors: Molecular Docking and In Vitro Enzymatic Studies," *Journal of Agricultural and Food Chemistry* 60, no. 24 (June 2012): 6131–38.

39. Sabrina Morelli et al., "Neuronal Membrane Bioreactor as a Tool for Testing Crocin Neuroprotective Effect in Alzheimer's Disease," *Chemical Engineering Journal* 305 (December 2016): 69–78.

   M. Rashedinia et al., "Protective Effect of Crocin on Crolein-Induced Tau Phosphorylation in the Rat Brain," *Acta Neurobiologiae Experimentalis* 75, no. 2 (2015): 208–19.

40. N. T. Tildesley et al., "Salvia lavandulaefolia (Spanish Sage) Enhances Memory in Healthy Young Volunteers," *Pharmacology Biochemistry and Behavior* 75, no. 3 (June 2003): 669–74.

   A. B. Scholey et al., "An Extract of Salvia (Sage) with Anticholinesterase Properties Improves Memory and Attention in Healthy Older Volunteers," *Psychopharmacology* 198, no. 1 (May 2008): 127–39.

   D. O. Kennedy et al., "Monoterpenoid Extract of Sage (Salvia lavandulaefolia) with Cholinesterase Inhibiting Properties Improves Cognitive Performance and Mood in Healthy Adults," *Journal of Psychopharmacology* 25, no. 8 (August 2011): 1088–100.

41. Mohsen Hamidpour et al., "Chemistry, Pharmacology, and Medicinal Property of Sage (*Salvia*) to Prevent and Cure Illnesses Such as Obesity, Diabetes, Depression, Dementia, Lupus, Autism, Heart Disease, and Cancer," *Journal of Traditional and Complementary Medicine* 4, no. 2 (2014): 82–88.

42. J. Hellhammer et al., "Effects of Soy Lecithin Phosphatidic Acid and Phosphatidylserine Complex (PAS) on the Endocrine and Psychological Responses to Mental Stress," *Stress* 7, no. 2 (June 2004): 119–26.

43. S. Hirayama et al., "The Effect of Phosphatidylserine Administration on Memory and Symptoms of Attention-Deficit Hyperactivity Disorder: A Randomised, Double-Blind, Placebo-Controlled Clinical Trial," *Journal of Human Nutrition and Dietetics* (April 2014): 27 Suppl 2: 284–91.

   I. Manor et al., "The Effect of Phosphatidylserine Containing Omega3 Fatty-Acids on Attention-Deficit Hyperactivity Disorder Symptoms in Children: A Double-Blind Placebo-Controlled Trial, Followed by an Open-Label Extension," *European Psychiatry* 27, no. 5 (July 2012): 335–42.

44. Marcus Herdener et al., "Musical Training Induces Functional Plasticity in Human Hippocampus," *Journal of Neuroscience* 30, no. 4 (January 2010): 1377–84.

   B. R. Zendel et al., "Neuroplastic Effects of Music Lessons on Hippocampal Volume in Children with Congenital Hypothyroidism," *Neuroreport* 24, no. 17 (December 4, 2013): 947–50.

   M. S. Oechslin et al., "Hippocampal Volume Predicts Fluid Intelligence in Musically Trained People," *Hippocampus* 23, no. 7 (July 2013): 552–58.

CHAPTER 7: I IS FOR INFLAMMATION

1. G. Fond, "Inflammation in Psychiatric Disorders," *European Psychiatry* 29, no. 8 (November 2014): 551–52.

   A. H. Miller et al., "Therapeutic Implications of Brain-Immune Interactions: Treatment in Translation," *Neuropsychopharmacology* 42, no. 1 (January 2017): 334–59.

2. J. C. Felger et al., "Inflammation Is Associated with Decreased Functional Connectivity within Corticostriatal Reward Circuitry in Depression," *Molecular Psychiatry* 21, no. 10 (October 2016): 1358–65.

3. L. Brundin et al., "Role of Inflammation in Suicide: From Mechanisms to Treatment," *Neuropsychopharmacology* 42, no. 1 (January 2017): 271–83.

4. George M. Slavich et al., "Neural Sensitivity to Social Rejection Is Associated with Inflammatory Responses to Social Stress," *Proceedings of the National Academy of Sciences of the United States of America* 107, no. 33 (August 17, 2010): 14817–22.

5. C. L. Raison et al., "A Randomized Controlled Trial of the Tumor Necrosis Factor Antagonist Infliximab for Treatment-Resistant Depression: The Role of Baseline Inflammatory Biomarkers," *JAMA Psychiatry* 70, no. 1 (January 2013): 31–41.

6. O. Köhler et al., "Inflammation and Depression: Combined Use of Selective Serotonin Reuptake Inhibitors and NSAIDs or Paracetamol and Psychiatric Outcomes," *Brain and Behavior* 5, no. 8 (August 2015): e00338, doi: 10.1002/brb3.338.

R. L. Iyengar et al., "NSAIDs Are Associated with Lower Depression Scores in Patients with Osteoarthritis," *American Journal of Medicine* 126, no. 11 (November 2013): 1017. e11-8.

7. P. H. Wirtz and R. von Känel, "Psychological Stress, Inflammation, and Coronary Heart Disease," *Current Cardiology Reports* 19, no. 11 (September 2017): 111.

8. K. Lukaschek et al., "Cognitive Impairment Is Associated with a Low Omega-3 Index in the Elderly: Results from the KORA-Age Study," *Dementia and Geriatric Cognitive Disorders* 42, nos. 3–4 (2016): 236–45.

9. Megan Clapp et al., "Gut Microbiota's Effect on Mental Health: The Gut-Brain Axis," *Clinical Practice* 7, no. 4 (September 15, 2017): 987.

10. Jennifer Lea Reynolds, "Is There a Connection between Gut Health and ADHD?" *U.S. News & World Report*, September 8, 2017, https://health.usnews.com/health-care /patient-advice/articles/2017-09-08/is-there-a-connection-between-gut-health -and-adhd.

11. C. Jiang et al., "The Gut Microbiota and Alzheimer's Disease," *Journal of Alzheimer's Disease* 58, no. 1 (2017): 1–15, doi: 10.3233/JAD-161141.

C. A. Köhler et al., "The Gut-Brain Axis, Including the Microbiome, Leaky Gut and Bacterial Translocation: Mechanisms and Pathophysiological Role in Alzheimer's Disease," *Current Pharmaceutical Design* 22, no. 40 (2016): 6152–66.

12. Qinghui Mu et al., "Leaky Gut as a Danger Signal for Autoimmune Diseases," *Frontiers in Immunology* 8 (May 23, 2017): 598.

13. Iman Salem et al., "The Gut Microbiome as a Major Regulator of the Gut-Skin Axis," *Frontiers in Microbiology* 9 (July 10, 2018): 1459.

14. A. C. Logan and M. Katzman, "Major Depressive Disorder: Probiotics May Be an Adjuvant Therapy," *Medical Hypotheses* 64, no. 3 (2005): 533–38.

15. A. Kato-Kataoka et al., "Fermented Milk Containing Lactobacillus casei Strain Shirota Prevents the Onset of Physical Symptoms in Medical Students under Academic Examination Stress," *Beneficial Microbes* 7, no. 2 (2016): 153–56.

16. Y. Wang et al., "Effects of Alcohol on Intestinal Epithelial Barrier Permeability and Expression of Tight Junction-Associated Proteins," *Molecular Medicine Reports* 9, no. 6 (June 2014): 2352–56.

17. L. Möhle et al., "Ly6C(hi) Monocytes Provide a Link between Antibiotic-Induced Changes in Gut Microbiota and Adult Hippocampal Neurogenesis," *Cell Reports* 15, no. 9 (May 31, 2016): 1945–56.

18. T. A. Mori and L. J. Beilin, "Omega-3 Fatty Acids and Inflammation," *Current Atherosclerosis Reports* 6, no. 6 (November 2004): 461–67.

D. Moertl et al., "Dose-Dependent Effects of Omega-3-Polyunsaturated Fatty Acids on Systolic Left Ventricular Function, Endothelial Function, and Markers of Inflammation in Chronic Heart Failure of Nonischemic Origin: A Double-Blind, Placebo-Controlled, 3-Arm Study," *American Heart Journal* 161, no. 5 (May 2011): 915.e1-9, doi: 10.1016/j. ahj.2011.02.011.

J. G. Devassy et al., "Omega-3 Polyunsaturated Fatty Acids and Oxylipins in Neuroinflammation and Management of Alzheimer Disease," *Advances in Nutrition* 7, no. 5 (September 15, 2016): 905–16.

19. "Smoking, High Blood Pressure and Being Overweight Top Three Preventable Causes of Death in the U.S.," Harvard School of Public Health, April 27, 2009, www.hsph.harvard .edu/news/press-releases/smoking-high-blood-pressure-overweight-preventable -causes-death-us/.

20. E. Messamore et al., "Polyunsaturated Fatty Acids and Recurrent Mood Disorders: Phenomenology, Mechanisms, and Clinical Application," *Progress in Lipid Research* 66 (April 2017): 1–13, doi: 10.1016/j.plipres.2017.01.001.

J. Sarris et al., "Omega-3 for Bipolar Disorder: Meta-Analyses of Use in Mania and Bipolar Depression," *Journal of Clinical Psychiatry* 73, no. 1 (January 2012): 81–86, doi: 10.4088/JCP.10r06710.

R. J. Mocking et al., "Meta-Analysis and Meta-Regression of Omega-3 Polyunsaturated Fatty Acid Supplementation for Major Depressive Disorder," *Translational Psychiatry* 6, (March 15, 2016).

21. J. R. Hibbeln and R. V. Gow, "The Potential for Military Diets to Reduce Depression, Suicide, and Impulsive Aggression: A Review of Current Evidence for Omega-3 and Omega-6 Fatty Acids," *Military Medicine* 179, supplement 11 (November 2014): 117–28.

M. Huan et al., "Suicide Attempt and n-3 Fatty Acid Levels in Red Blood Cells: A Case Control Study in China," *Biological Psychiatry* 56, no. 7 (October 1, 2004): 490–96.

M. E. Sublette et al., "Omega-3 Polyunsaturated Essential Fatty Acid Status as a Predictor of Future Suicide Risk," *American Journal of Psychiatry* 163, no. 6 (June 2006): 1100–1102.

M. D. Lewis et al., "Suicide Deaths of Active-Duty US Military and Omega-3 Fatty-Acid Status: A Case-Control Comparison," *Journal of Clinical Psychiatry* 72, no. 12 (December 2011): 1585–90.

22. C. M. Milte et al., "Increased Erythrocyte Eicosapentaenoic Acid and Docosahexaenoic Acid Are Associated with Improved Attention and Behavior in Children with ADHD in a Randomized Controlled Three-Way Crossover Trial," *Journal of Attention Disorders* 19, no. 11 (November 2015): 954–64.

M. H. Bloch and A. Qawasmi, "Omega-3 Fatty Acid Supplementation for the Treatment of Children with Attention-Deficit/Hyperactivity Disorder Symptomatology: Systematic Review and Meta-Analysis," *Journal of the American Academy of Child and Adolescent Psychiatry* 50, no. 10 (October 2011): 991–1000.

23. Y. Zhang et al., "Intakes of Fish and Polyunsaturated Fatty Acids and Mild-to-Severe Cognitive Impairment Risks: A Dose-Response Meta-Analysis of 21 Cohort Studies," *American Journal of Clinical Nutrition* 103, no. 2 (February 2016): 330–40.

T. A. D'Ascoli et al., "Association between Serum Long-Chain Omega-3 Polyunsaturated Fatty Acids and Cognitive Performance in Elderly Men and Women: The Kuopio Ischaemic Heart Disease Risk Factor Study," *European Journal of Clinical Nutrition* 70, no. 8 (August 2016): 970–75.

24. C. Couet et al., "Effect of Dietary Fish Oil on Body Fat Mass and Basal Fat Oxidation in Healthy Adults," *International Journal of Obesity and Related Metabolic Disorders* 21, no. 8 (August 1997): 637–43.

J. D. Buckley and P. R. Howe, "Anti-Obesity Effects of Long-Chain Omega-3 Polyunsaturated Fatty Acids," *Obesity Reviews* 10, no. 6 (November 2009): 648–59.

25. C. von Schacky, "The Omega-3 Index as a Risk Factor for Cardiovascular Diseases," *Prostaglandins & Other Lipid Mediators* 96, nos. 1–4 (November 2011): 94–98.

S. P. Whelton et al., "Meta-Analysis of Observational Studies on Fish Intake and Coronary Heart Disease, *American Journal of Cardiology* 93, no. 9 (May 1, 2004): 1119–23.

26. Daniel G. Amen et al., "Quantitative Erythrocyte Omega-3 EPA Plus DHA Levels Are Related to Higher Regional Cerebral Blood Flow on Brain SPECT," *Journal of Alzheimer's Disease* 58, no. 4 (2017): 1189–99.

27. Daniel G. Amen, *Memory Rescue* (Carol Stream, IL: Tyndale, 2017), 101.

28. R. J. Mocking et al., "Meta-Analysis and Meta-Regression of Omega-3 Polyunsaturated Fatty Acid Supplementation for Major Depressive Disorder."

29. L. A. Colangelo et al., "Higher Dietary Intake of Long-Chain Omega-3 Polyunsaturated Fatty Acids Is Inversely Associated with Depressive Symptoms in Women," *Nutrition* 25, no. 10 (October 2009): 1011–19.

30. Giuseppe Grosso et al., "Omega-3 Fatty Acids and Depression: Scientific Evidence and Biological Mechanisms," *Oxidative Medicine and Cellular Longevity* (March 18, 2014).

31. E. Derbyshire, "Do Omega-3/6 Fatty Acids Have a Therapeutic Role in Children and Young People with ADHD?" *Journal of Lipids* (2017).

32. G. P. Amminger et al., "Long-Chain Omega-3 Fatty Acids for Indicated Prevention of Psychotic Disorders: A Randomized, Placebo-Controlled Trial," *Archives of General Psychiatry* 67, no. 2 (February 2010): 146–54.

33. M. K. Jha et al., "Can C-Reactive Protein Inform Antidepressant Medication Selection in Depressed Outpatients? Findings from the CO-MED Trial," *Psychoneuroendocrinology* 78 (April 2017): 105–13.

34. G. Douaud et al., "Preventing Alzheimer's Disease-Related Gray Matter Atrophy by B-Vitamin Treatment," *Proceedings of the National Academy of Sciences of the United States of America* 110, no. 23 (June 4, 2013): 9523–28.

35. J. A. Gil-Montoya et al., "Is Periodontitis a Risk Factor for Cognitive Impairment and Dementia? A Case-Control Study," *Journal of Periodontology* 86, no. 2 (February 2015): 244–53.

    J. Luo et al., "Association between Tooth Loss and Cognitive Function among 3063 Chinese Older Adults: A Community-Based Study," *PLOS One* 10, no. 3 (March 24, 2015).

36. Z. Asemi et al., "Effects of Daily Consumption of Probiotic Yoghurt on Inflammatory Factors in Pregnant Women: A Randomized Controlled Trial," *Pakistan Journal of Biological Sciences* 14, no. 8 (April 15, 2011): 476–82.

    L. Valentini et al., "Impact of Personalized Diet and Probiotic Supplementation on Inflammation, Nutritional Parameters and Intestinal Microbiota—The 'RISTOMED Project': Randomized Controlled Trial in Healthy Older People," *Clinical Nutrition* 34, no. 4 (August 2015): 593–602.

    S. K. Hegazy and M. M. El-Bedewy, "Effect of Probiotics on Pro-Inflammatory Cytokines and NF-kappaB Activation in Ulcerative Colitis," *World Journal of Gastroenterology* 16, no. 33 (September 7, 2010): 4145–51.

    E. J. Giamarellos-Bourboulis et al., "Pro- and Synbiotics to Control Inflammation and Infection in Patients with Multiple Injuries," *Journal of Trauma* 67, no. 4 (October 2009): 815–21.

    D. Viramontes-Hörner et al., "Effect of a Symbiotic Gel (Lactobacillus acidophilus + Bifidobacterium lactis + Inulin) on Presence and Severity of Gastrointestinal Symptoms in Hemodialysis Patients," *Journal of Renal Nutrition* 25, no. 3 (May 2015): 284–91.

    J. Villar-García et al., "Effect of Probiotics (Saccharomyces boulardii) on Microbial Translocation and Inflammation in HIV-Treated Patients: A Double-Blind, Randomized, Placebo-Controlled Trial," *Journal of Acquired Immune Deficiency Syndromes* 68, no. 3 (March 1, 2015): 256–63.

    A. Toiviainen et al., "Impact of Orally Administered Lozenges with Lactobacillus rhamnosus GG and Bifidobacterium animalis Subsp. Lactis BB-12 on the Number of Salivary Mutans Streptococci, Amount of Plaque, Gingival Inflammation and the Oral Microbiome in Healthy Adults," *Clinical Oral Investigations* 19, no. 1 (January 2015): 77–83.

    S. J. Spaiser et al., "Lactobacillus gasseri KS-13, Bifidobacterium bifidum G9-1, and Bifidobacterium longum MM-2 Ingestion Induces a Less Inflammatory Cytokine Profile and a Potentially Beneficial Shift in Gut Microbiota in Older Adults: A Randomized, Double-Blind, Placebo-Controlled, Crossover Study," *Journal of the American College of Nutrition* 34, no. 6 (2015): 459–69.

    A. K. Szkaradkiewicz et al., "Effect of Oral Administration Involving a Probiotic Strain of Lactobacillus reuteri on Pro-Inflammatory Cytokine Response in Patients with Chronic Periodontitis," *Archivum Immunologiae et Therapiae Experimentalis (Warszawa)* 62, no. 6 (December 2014): 495–500.

    Z. H. Liu, "The Effects of Perioperative Probiotic Treatment on Serum Zonulin Concentration and Subsequent Postoperative Infectious Complications after Colorectal Cancer Surgery: A Double-Center and Double-Blind Randomized Clinical Trial," *American Journal of Clinical Nutrition* 97, no. 1 (January 2013): 117–26.

37. H. Rajkumar et al., "Effect of Probiotic Lactobacillus salivarius UBL S22 and Prebiotic Fructo-oligosaccharide on Serum Lipids, Inflammatory Markers, Insulin Sensitivity, and Gut Bacteria in Healthy Young Volunteers: A Randomized Controlled Single-Blind Pilot

Study," *Journal of Cardiovascular Pharmacolology and Therapeutics* 20, no. 3 (May 2015): 289–98.

38. S. Ghosh et al., "The Beneficial Role of Curcumin on Inflammation, Diabetes and Neurodegenerative Disease: A Recent Update," *Food and Chemical Toxicology* 83 (September 2015): 111–24.

39. J Mildenberger et al. "N-3 PUFAs Induce Inflammatory Tolerance by Formation of KEAP1-Containing SQSTM1/p62-bodies and Activation of NFE2L2," *Autophagy* 13, no. 10 (August 2017): 1664–78.

40. J. K. Kiecolt-Glaser et al., "Omega-3 Supplementation Lowers Inflammation and Anxiety in Medical Students: A Randomized Controlled Trial," *Brain, Behavior, and Immunity* 25, no. 8 (November 2011): 1725–34.

41. R. J. Mocking et al., "Meta-Analysis and Meta-Regression of Omega-3 Polyunsaturated Fatty Acid Supplementation for Major Depressive Disorder."

42. Mandy Oaklander, "5 Surprising Ways to Help Your Memory," Time.com, June 10, 2015, time.com/3915030/boost-memory-exercise/.

   P. A. Jackson et al., "DHA-Rich Oil Modulates the Cerebral Haemodynamic Response to Cognitive Tasks in Healthy Young Adults: A Near IR Spectroscopy Pilot Study," *British Journal of Nutrition* 107, no. 8 (April 2012): 1093–98.

   T. J. Song et al., "Low Levels of Plasma Omega 3-Polyunsaturated Fatty Acids Are Associated with Cerebral Small Vessel Diseases in Acute Ischemic Stroke Patients," *Nutrition Research* 35, no. 5 (May 2015): 368–74.

43. N. Hamazaki-Fujita et al., "Polyunsaturated Fatty Acids and Blood Circulation in the Forebrain during a Mental Arithmetic Task," *Brain Research* (June 23, 2011): 38–45.

44. E. L. Boespflug et al., "Fish Oil Supplementation Increases Event-Related Posterior Cingulate Activation in Older Adults with Subjective Memory Impairment," *Journal of Nutrition, Health and Aging* 20, no. 2 (February 2016): 161–69.

45. A. V. Witte et al., "Long-Chain Omega-3 Fatty Acids Improve Brain Function and Structure in Older Adults," *Cerebral Cortex* 24, no. 11 (November 2014): 3059–68.

46. F. Jernerén et al., "Brain Atrophy in Cognitively Impaired Elderly: The Importance of Long-Chain ω-3 Fatty Acids and B Vitamin Status in a Randomized Controlled Trial," *American Journal of Clinical Nutrition* 102, no. 1 (July 2015): 215–21.

CHAPTER 8: G IS FOR GENETICS

1. Daniel G. Amen and Tana Amen, *The Brain Warrior's Way* (New York: New American Library, 2016), 31.

2. Rosaline J. Neuman et al., "Latent Class Analysis of ADHD and Comorbid Symptoms in a Population Sample of Adolescent Female Twins," *Journal of Child Psychology and Psychiatry* 42, no. 7 (October 2001): 933–42.

   Cori Bargmann, "Overview of Genes and Behavior," YouTube, November 1, 2013, www.youtube.com/watch?v=4qhrnOP8euI&feature=youtu.be.

3. Joshua Wolf Shenk, *Lincoln's Melancholy* (New York: Houghton Mifflin, 2005), 80.

4. Brian G. Dias and Kerry J. Ressler, "Parental Olfactory Experience Influences Behavior and Neural Structure in Subsequent Generations," *Nature Neuroscience* 17, no. 1 (2014): 89–96.

5. Katharina Gapp et al., "Early Life Stress in Fathers Improves Behavioural Flexibility in Their Offspring," *Nature Communications* 5, no. 5466 (2014).

6. Michael J. Gandal et al., "Shared Molecular Neuropathology across Major Psychiatric Disorders Parallels Polygenic Overlap," *Science* 359, no. 6376 (February 9, 2018)): 693–97, doi: 10.1126/science.aad6469.

   D. B. Hancock et al., "Genome-Wide Association Study across European and African American Ancestries Identifies a SNP in DNMT3B Contributing to Nicotine Dependence," *Molecular Psychiatry* 23, no. 9 (September 2018): 1911–19.

7. U. Amstutz et al., "Recommendations for HLA-B*15:02 and HLA-A*31:01 Genetic Testing to Reduce the Risk of Carbamazepine-Induced Hypersensitivity Reactions," *Epilepsia* 55, no. 4 (April 2014): 496–506. doi: 10.1111/epi.12564.

8. M. X. Tang et al., "Effect of Age, Ethnicity, and Head Injury on the Association between APOE Genotypes and Alzheimer's Disease," *Annals of New York Academy of Sciences* 802 (December 16, 1996): 6–15.

9. S. T. Cheng, "Cognitive Reserve and the Prevention of Dementia: The Role of Physical and Cognitive Activities," *Current Psychiatry Reports* 18, no. 9 (September 2016): 85, doi:10.1007/s11920-016-0721-2.

CHAPTER 9: H IS FOR HEAD TRAUMA

1. Joe Namuth, interview by Howard Stern, "How Joe Namath Reversed His Own Brain Damage Caused by Football," *The Howard Stern Show*, June 24, 2019, www.youtube .com/watch?v=s7nxU3QadlA&feature=youtu.be.

2. "Traumatic Brain Injury and Concussion," Centers for Disease Control and Prevention, March 3, 2019, www.cdc.gov/traumaticbraininjury/get_the_facts.html.

3. Blue Cross Blue Shield, "The Health of America Report: The Steep Rise in Concussion Diagnoses in the U.S.," September 27, 2016, https://www.bcbs.com/the-health-of -america/reports/the-steep-rise-concussion-diagnoses-the-us.

4. Daniel G. Amen, *Memory Rescue* (Carol Stream, IL: Tyndale, 2017), 124–25.

5. Alana Semuels, "The White Flight from Football," *Atlantic*, February 1, 2019, www.theatlantic.com/health/archive/2019/02/football-white-flight-racial-divide/581623/.

6. "DoD Worldwide Numbers for TBI," Defense and Veterans Brain Injury Center, July 7, 2019, http://dvbic.dcoe.mil/dod-worldwide-numbers-tbi.

7. A. L. Zaninotto et al., "Updates and Current Perspectives of Psychiatric Assessments after Traumatic Brain Injury: A Systematic Review," *Frontiers in Psychiatry* 7 (June 14, 2016): 95.

8. R. J. Schachar et al., "Mental Health Implications of Traumatic Brain Injury (TBI) in Children and Youth," *Journal of Canadian Academy of Child and Adolescent Psychiatry* 24, no. 2, (Fall 2015) : 100–108.

9. Daryl and Daniel C. Fujii, "Psychotic Disorder Due to Traumatic Brain Injury: Analysis of Case Studies in the Literature," *Journal of Neuropsychiatry and Clinical Neurosciences* 24, no. 3 (Summer 2012): 278–89.

10. G. J. McHugo et al., "The Prevalence of Traumatic Brain Injury among People With Co-Occurring Mental Health and Substance Use Disorders," *Journal of Head Trauma Rehabilitation* 32, no. 3 (May/June 2017) : E65–E74.

11. Jessica L. Mackelprang et al., "Adverse Outcomes among Homeless Adolescents and Young Adults Who Report a History of Traumatic Brain Injury," *American Journal of Public Health* 104, no. 10 (October 2014): 1986–92.

12. Ibid.

13. Schachar et al., "Mental Health Implications of Traumatic Brain Injury (TBI)."

14. R. Lajiness-O'Neill et al., "Memory and Learning in Pediatric Traumatic Brain Injury: A Review and Examination of Moderators of Outcome," *Applied Neuropsychology* 17, no. 2 (April 2010): 83–92.

15. G. J. McHugo et al., "The Prevalence of Traumatic Brain Injury among People with Co-Occurring Mental Health and Substance Use Disorders," *Journal of Head Trauma Rehabilitation* 32, no. 3 (May/June 2017): E65–E74.

16. R. C. Gardner et al., "Dementia Risk after Traumatic Brain Injury vs Nonbrain Trauma: The Role of Age and Severity," *JAMA Neurology* 17, no. 12 (December 2014): 1490–97.

17. V. Rao et al., "Aggression after Traumatic Brain Injury: Prevalence and Correlates," *Journal of Neuropsychiatry and Clinical Neurosciences* 21, no. 4 (2009): 420–29.

18. J. Topolovec-Vranic et al., "Traumatic Brain Injury among People Who Are Homeless: A Systematic Review," *BMC Public Health* 12 (December 2012): 1059.

19. Mackelprang, "Adverse Outcomes among Homeless Adolescents," 1986–92.

20. P. J. Schechter and R. I. Henkin, "Abnormalities of Taste and Smell after Head Trauma," *Journal of Neurology, Neurosurgery, and Psychiatry* 35, no. 7 (1974): 802–10.

21. "One in Four Prisoners Have Suffered Traumatic Brain Injury, Study Finds," *Glasgow Live*, January 18, 2019, www.glasgowlive.co.uk/news/glasgow-news/ one-four-prisoners-suffered-traumatic-15695721.

22. Brian Im et al., "TBI and Incarceration," *American Psychological Association*, December 2014, www.apa.org/pi/disability/resources/publications/newsletter/2014/12/incarceration.

23. Jennifer Bronson et al., "Veterans in Prison and Jail, 2011–2012," *Bureau of Justice Statistics*, December 7, 2015, https://www.bjs.gov/index.cfm?ty=pbdetail&iid=5479.

24. I ask all my patients these questions and referenced them in *Memory Rescue*, 134.

25. Daniel F. Mackay et al., "Neurodegenerative Disease Mortality among Former Professional Soccer Players," *New England Journal of Medicine* (October 21, 2019), https:// doi:10.1056/NEJMoa1908483.

26. "Fighting in Ice Hockey," Wikipedia, June 12, 2019, en.wikipedia.org/wiki/Fighting_in _ice_hockey.

27. H. Ling et al., "Mixed Pathologies Including Chronic Traumatic Encephalopathy Account for Dementia in Retired Association Football (Soccer) Players," *Acta Neuropathologica* 133, no. 3 (March 2017): 337–352.

28. T. Surmeli et al., "Quantitative EEG Neurometric Analysis-Guided Neurofeedback Treatment in Postconcussion Syndrome (PCS): Forty Cases. How Is Neurometric Analysis Important for the Treatment of PCS and as a Biomarker?" *Clinical EEG and Neuroscience* 48, no. 3 (June 27, 2016): 217–30.

29. E. J. Cheon et al., "The Efficacy of Neurofeedback in Patients with Major Depressive Disorder: An Open Labeled Prospective Study," *Applied Psychophysiology and Biofeedback* 41, no. 1 (March 2016): 103–10.

30. V. Meisel et al., "Neurofeedback and Standard Pharmacological Intervention in ADHD: A Randomized Controlled Trial with Six-month Follow-up," *Biological Psychology* 94, no. 1 (September 2013): 12–21.

31. J. Kopřivová et al., "Prediction of Treatment Response and the Effect of Independent Component Neurofeedback in Obsessive-Compulsive Disorder: A Randomized, Sham-Controlled, Double-Blind Study," *Neuropsychobiology* 67, no. 4 (2013): 210–23.

32. R. Rostami and F. Dehghani-Arani, "Neurofeedback Training as a New Method in Treatment of Crystal Methamphetamine Dependent Patients: A Preliminary Study," *Applied Psychophysiological Biofeedback* 40, no. 3 (September 2015): 151–61.

33. J. Guez et al., "Influence of Electroencephalography Neurofeedback Training on Episodic Memory: A Randomized, Sham-Controlled, Double-Blind Study," *Memory* 23, no. 5 (2015): 683–94.

    S. Xiong et al., "Working Memory Training Using EEG Neurofeedback in Normal Young Adults," *Bio-Medical Materials and Engineering* 24, no. 6 (2014): 3637–44.

    J. R. Wang and S. Hsieh, "Neurofeedback Training Improves Attention and Working Memory Performance," *Clinical Neurophysiology* 124, no. 12 (December 2013): 2406–20.

34. S. E. Kober et al., "Specific Effects of EEG Based Neurofeedback Training on Memory Functions in Post-Stroke Victims," *Journal of NeuroEngineering and Rehabilitation* 12 (December 2015): 107.

35. P. Kubik et al., "Neurofeedback Therapy Influence on Clinical Status and Some EEG Parameters in Children with Localized Epilepsy," *Przegl Lek* 73, no. 3 (2016): 157–60.

36. M. P. Jensen et al. "Use of Neurofeedback to Enhance Response to Hypnotic Analgesia in Individuals with Multiple Sclerosis," *International Journal of Clinical and Experimental Hypnosis* 64, no 1 (2016): 1–23.

37. A. Azarpaikan et al., "Neurofeedback and Physical Balance in Parkinson's Patients," *Gait & Posture* 40, no. 1 (2014): 177–81.

38. Michael D. Lewis, *When Brains Collide: What Every Athlete and Parent Should Know about the Prevention and Treatment of Concussions and Head Injuries* (n.p.: Lioncrest Publishing, 2016).

CHAPTER 10: T̲ IS FOR TOXINS

1. Ian H. Stanley et al., "A Systematic Review of Suicidal Thoughts and Behaviors among Police Officers, Firefighters, EMTs, and Paramedics," *Clinical Psychology Review* 44 (March 2016): 25–44.

   Samuel B. Harvey et al., "The Mental Health of Fire-Fighters: An Examination of the Impact of Repeated Trauma Exposure," *Australian and New Zealand Journal of Psychiatry* 50, no. 7 (July 2016): 649–58.

2. Melanie A. Hom et al., "Mental Health Service Use among Firefighters with Suicidal Thoughts and Behaviors," *Psychiatric Services* 67, no. 6 (June 1, 2016): 688–91.

3. Yasser Iturria-Medina et al., "Early Role of Vascular Dysregulation on Late-Onset Alzheimer's Disease Based on Multifactorial Data-Driven Analysis," *Nature Communications* 7 (June 21, 2016): 11934.

4. Eric Emerson et al., "Risk of Exposure to Air Pollution among British Children with and without Intellectual Disabilities," *Journal of Intellectual Disability Research* 63, no. 2 (February 2019): 161–67.

5. Tesifon Parrón et al., "Association between Environmental Exposure to Pesticides and Neurodegenerative Diseases," *Toxicology and Applied Pharmacology* 256, no. 3 (November 1, 2011): 379–85.

6. "Don't Pucker Up: Lead in Lipstick," Campaign for Safe Cosmetics, October 12, 2007, http://www.safecosmetics.org/about-us/media/news-coverage/dont-pucker-up-lead-in-lipstick/.

7. This quiz also appears in Daniel G. Amen, *Memory Rescue* (Carol Stream, IL: Tyndale, 2017).

8. Gabriella Gobbi et al., "Association of Cannabis Use in Adolescence and Risk of Depression, Anxiety, and Suicidality in Young Adulthood: A Systematic Review and Meta-analysis," *JAMA Psychiatry* 76, no. 4 (April 2019), 426–34.

9. Amen, *Memory Rescue*, 145–46.

10. Ibid., 144–45.

11. Curt T. DellaValle et al., "Dietary Nitrate and Nitrite Intake and Risk of Colorectal Cancer in the Shanghai Women's Health Study," *International Journal of Cancer* 134, no. 12 (June 15, 2014): 2917–26.

12. Kim Harley, "The Health Costs of Beauty: EDCs in Personal Care Products and the HERMOSA Study," Collaborative on Health and the Environment, March 22, 2016, www.healthandenvironment.org/partnership_calls/18271.

    Suzanne M. de la Monte et al., "Epidemilogical Trends Strongly Suggest Exposures as Etiologic Agents in the Pathogenesis of Sporadic Alzheimer's Disease, Diabetes Mellitus, and Non-Alcoholic Steatohepatitis," *Journal of Alzheimer's Disease* 17, no. 3 (2009): 519–29.

13. Céline Gasnier et al., "Glyphosate-Based Herbicides Are Toxic and Endocrine Disruptors in Human Cell Lines," *Toxicology* 262, no. 3 (August 21, 2009): 184–91.

14. Luoping Zhang et al., "Exposure to Glyphosate-Based Herbicides and Risk for Non-Hodgkin Lymphoma: A Meta-analysis and Supporting Evidence," *Mutation Research/Reviews in Mutation Research* 781 (July–September 2019): 186–206.

15. Ki-Su Kim et al., "Associations between Organochlorine Pesticides and Cognition in U.S. Elders: National Health and Nutrition Examination Survey 1999–2002," *Environment International* 75 (February 2015): 87–92.

16. Kaarin J. Anstey et al., "Alcohol Consumption as a Risk Factor for Dementia and Cognitive Decline: Meta-analysis of Prospective Studies," *American Journal of Geriatric Psychiatry* 17, no. 7 (July 2009): 542–55.

Ruth Peters et al., "Alcohol, Dementia and Cognitive Decline in the Elderly: A Systematic Review," *Age and Ageing* 37, no. 5 (September 2008): 505–12.

Edward Neafsey and Michael A. Collins, "Moderate Alcohol Consumption and Cognitive Risk," *Neuropsychiatric Disease and Treatment* 7 (2011): 465–84.

17. Jingzhong Ding et al., "Alcohol Intake and Cerebral Abnormalities on Magnetic Resonance Imaging in a Community-Based Population of Middle-Aged Adults: The Atherosclerosis Risk in Communities (ARIC) Study," *Stroke* 35, no. 1 (January 2004): 16–21.

18. George F. Koob, "Neurobiology of Addiction: Toward the Development of New Therapies," *Annals of the New York Academy of Sciences* 909 (2000): 170–85.

19. Elizabeth P. Handing et al., "Midlife Alcohol Consumption and Risk of Dementia over 43 Years of Follow-Up: A Population-Based Study from the Swedish Twin Registry," *Journals of Gerontology: Series A* 70, no. 10 (October 2015): 1248–54.

20. Jennie Connor, "Alcohol Consumption as a Cause of Cancer," *Addiction* 112, no. 2 (February 2017): 222–28.

21. Zach Walsh et al., "Medical Cannabis and Mental Health: A Guided Systematic Review," *Clinical Psychology Review* 51 (February 2017): 15–29.

22. Daniel G. Amen et al., "Discriminative Properties of Hippocampal Hypoperfusion in Marijuana Users Compared to Healthy Controls: Implications for Marijuana Administration in Alzheimer's Dementia," *Journal of Alzheimer's Disease* 56, no. 1 (2017): 261–73.

23. Gobbi et al., "Association of Cannabis Use in Adolescence," 426–34.

24. Marta Di Forti et al., "The Contribution of Cannabis Use to Variation in the Incidence of Psychotic Disorder across Europe (EU-GEI): A Multicentre Case-Control Study," *Lancet Psychiatry* 6, no. 5 (May 2019): 427–36.

25. Judith Prochaska et al., "Tobacco Use among Individuals with Schizophrenia: What Role Has the Tobacco Industry Played?" *Schizophrenia Bulletin* 34, no. 3 (May 2008): 555–67. Used with permission,

26. Prochaska et al., "Tobacco Use among Individuals with Schizophrenia," 555–67.

27. "Tobacco Use among Adults with Mental Illness and Substance Use Disorders," Centers for Disease Control and Prevention, last reviewed January 14, 2019, https://www.cdc.gov /tobacco/disparities/mental-illness-substance-use/index.htm.

28. "Teens Using Vaping Devices in Record Numbers," National Institute on Drug Abuse, December 17, 2018, https://www.drugabuse.gov/news-events/news-releases/2018/12 /teens-using-vaping-devices-in-record-numbers.

29. "Surgeon General's Advisory on E-cigarette Use among Youth," Office of the US Surgeon General, 2018, https://e-cigarettes.surgeongeneral.gov/documents/surgeon-generals -advisory-on-e-cigarette-use-among-youth-2018.pdf.

30. Amen, *Memory Rescue*, 152.

31. World Health Organization, "Fumonisins," Food Safety Digest series, Department of Food Safety and Zoonoses, February 2018, https://www.who.int/foodsafety/FSDigest _Fumonisins_EN.pdf.

32. Silvia W. Gratz, Neil Havis, and Fiona Burnett, "*Fusarium* Mycotoxin Contamination in the Human Food Chain," *New Food*, September 1, 2015, https://www.newfoodmagazine .com/article/19318/fusarium-mycotoxin-contamination-in-the-human-food-chain/.

33. "About Aspergillosis," Centers for Disease Control and Prevention, last reviewed January 2, 2019, https://www.cdc.gov/fungal/diseases/aspergillosis/definition.html.

34. Susan P. McCormick et al., "Trichothecenes: From Simple to Complex Mycotoxins," *Toxins* 3, no. 7 (July 2011): 802–14.

35. Amen, *Memory Rescue*, 152–53.

36. James S. Brown Jr., "Introduction: An Update on Psychiatric Effects of Toxic Exposures," *Psychiatric Times* 33, no. 9 (October 1, 2016).

37. Amanda Habermann, "Lead Poisoning's Harmful Impact on Physical and Mental Health," Sovereign Health, February 20, 2016, https://www.sovhealth.com/health-and-wellness/lead-poisonings-harmful-impact-on-physical-and-mental-health/.

38. Brown, "Update on Psychiatric Effects of Toxic Exposures."

39. Maryse F. Bouchard et al., "Blood Lead Levels and Major Depressive Disorder, Panic Disorder, and Generalized Anxiety Disorder in US Young Adults," *Archives of General Psychiatry* 66, no. 12 (December 2009): 1313–19.

40. "Don't Pucker Up," Campaign for Safe Cosmetics.

41. Sa Liu, Sally Katharine Hammond, and Ann Rojas-Cheatham, "Concentrations and Potential Health Risks of Metals in Lip Products," *Environmental Health Perspectives* 121, no. 6 (June 2013): 705–10.

42. Amen, *Memory Rescue*, 153.

43. Edward A. Bittner, Yun Yue, and Zhongcong Xie, "Brief Review: Anesthetic Neurotoxicity in the Elderly, Cognitive Dysfunction and Alzheimer's Disease," *Canadian Journal of Anesthesia* 58, no. 2 (February 2011): 216–23.

    Chia-Wen Chen et al., "Increased Risk of Dementia in People with Previous Exposure to General Anesthesia: A Nationwide Population-Based Case-Control Study," *Alzheimer's and Dementia* 10, no. 2 (March 2014): 196–204.

44. Barynia Backeljauw et al., "Cognition and Brain Structure following Early Childhood Surgery with Anesthesia," *Pediatrics* 136, no. 1 (July 2015): e1–12.

45. N. Efimova et al., "Changes in Cerebral Blood Flow and Cognitive Function in Patients Undergoing Coronary Bypass Surgery with Cardiopulmonary Bypass," *Kardiologiia* 55, no. 6 (June 2015): 40–46.

46. University of Rochester Medical Center, "Chemotherapy's Damage to the Brain Detailed," ScienceDaily, April 22, 2008, https://www.sciencedaily.com/releases/2008/04/080422103947.htm.

47. Harley, "Health Costs of Beauty."

48. A. Guttmann, "Advertising Spending in the Perfumes, Cosmetics, and Other Toilet Preparations Industry in the United States from 2010 to 2019 (in Million U.S. Dollars)," Statista, last edited November 29, 2018, https://www.statista.com/statistics/470467/perfumes-cosmetics-and-other-toilet-preparations-industry-ad-spend-usa/.

49. Stacy Malkan, "Johnson & Johnson Is Just the Tip of the Toxic Iceberg," *Time*, March 2, 2016, https://time.com/4239561/johnson-and-johnson-toxic-ingredients/.

50. Gina L. LoSasso, Lisa J. Rapport, and Bradley Axelrod, "Neuropsychological Symptoms Associated with Low-Level Exposure to Solvents and (Meth)Acrylates among Nail Technicians," *Neuropsychiatry, Neuropsychology, and Behavioral Neurology* 14, no. 3 (July–September 2001): 183–89.

51. Masahiro Kawahara and Midori Kato-Negishi, "Link between Aluminum and the Pathogenesis of Alzheimer's Disease: The Integration of the Aluminum and Amyloid Cascade Hypotheses," *International Journal of Alzheimer's Disease* 2011 (March 8, 2011): 276393.

    Samantha Davenward et al., "Silicon-Rich Mineral Water as a Non-invasive Test of the 'Aluminum Hypothesis' in Alzheimer's Disease," *Journal of Alzheimer's Disease* 33, no. 2 (2013): 423–30.

    S. Maya et al., "Multifaceted Effects of Aluminium in Neurodegenerative Diseases: A Review," *Biomedicine and Pharmacotherapy* 83 (October 2016): 746–54.

    Trond Peder Flaten, "Aluminium as a Risk Factor in Alzheimer's Disease, with Emphasis on Drinking Water," *Brain Research Bulletin* 55, no. 2 (May 15, 2001): 187–96.

52. Michael Fenech, Armen Nersesyan, and Siegfried Knasmueller, "A Systematic Review of the Association between Occupational Exposure to Formaldehyde and Effects on Chromosomal DNA Damage Measured Using the Cytokinesis-Block Micronucleus Assay in Lymphocytes," *Mutation Research/Reviews in Mutation Research* 770, part A (October–December 2016): 46–57.

53. Ann Pontén and Magnus Bruze, "Formaldehyde," *Dermatitis* 26, no. 1 (January/February 2015): 3–6.

54. Philippa D. Darbre and Philip W. Harvey, "Parabens Can Enable Hallmarks and Characteristics of Cancer in Human Breast Epithelial Cells: A Review of the Literature with Reference to New Exposure Data and Regulatory Status," *Journal of Applied Toxicology* 34, no. 9 (September 2014): 925–38.

55. Pinar Erkekoglu and Belma Kocer-Gumusel, "Genotoxicity of Phthalates," *Toxicology Mechanisms and Methods* 24, no. 9 (December 2014): 616–26.

56. Pam Factor-Litvak et al., "Persistent Associations between Maternal Prenatal Exposure to Phthalates on Child IQ at Age 7 Years," *PLOS One* 9, no. 12 (December 10, 2014): e114003.

57. Catherine A. Smith and Matthew R. Holahan, "Reduced Hippocampal Dendritic Spine Density and BDNF Expression following Acute Postnatal Exposure to Di(2-Ethylhexyl) Phthalate in Male Long Evans Rats," *PLOS One* 9, no. 10 (October 8, 2014): e109522.

58. Carcinogenic Potency Project, "Ethylene Glycol," U.S. National Library of Medicine, last updated October 3, 2007, https://toxnet.nlm.nih.gov/cpdb/chempages/ETHYLENE%20 GLYCOL.html.

59. Allyson E. Kennedy et al., "E-cigarette Aerosol Exposure Can Cause Craniofacial Defects in *Xenopus laevis* Embryos and Mammalian Neural Crest Cells," *PLOS One* 12, no. 9 (September 28, 2017): e0185729.

60. "Five Things to Know about Triclosan," U.S. Food and Drug Administration, last reviewed May 16, 2019, https://www.fda.gov/ForConsumers/ConsumerUpdates/ucm205999.htm.

Marta Axelstad et al., "Triclosan Exposure Reduces Thyroxine Levels in Pregnant and Lactating Rat Dams and in Directly Exposed Offspring," *Food and Chemical Toxicology* 59 (September 2013): 534–40.

61. Alyson L. Yee and Jack A. Gilbert, "MICROBIOME. Is Triclosan Harming Your Microbiome?" *Science* 353, no. 6297 (July 22, 2016): 348–49.

62. Kang-sheng Liu et al., "Neurotoxicity and Biomarkers of Lead Exposure: A Review," *Chinese Medical Sciences Journal* 28, no. 3 (September 2013): 178–88.

63. Duke University, "Children Carry Evidence of Toxins from Home Flooring and Furniture," EurekAlert! American Association for the Advancement of Science (Heather M. Stapleton et al., "Children's Exposure to Chemicals Emitted from the Home Environment," presented at AAAS annual meeting, February 17, 2019), https://eurekalert .org/pub_releases/2019-02/du-cce021419.php.

64. Joseph Pizzorno, *The Toxin Solution: How Hidden Poisons in the Air, Water, Food, and Products We Use Are Destroying Our Health—And What We Can Do to Fix It* (New York: HarperOne, 2018).

65. Petra M. Gaum et al., "Prevalence and Incidence Rates of Mental Syndromes after Occupational Exposure to Polychlorinated Biphenyls," *International Journal of Hygiene and Environmental Health* 217, no. 7 (May 27, 2014): 765–74.

66. Dongren Yang et al., "Developmental Exposure to Polychlorinated Biphenyls Interferes with Experience-Dependent Dendritic Plasticity and Ryanodine Receptor Expression in Weanling Rats," *Environmental Health Perspectives* 117, no. 3 (March 2009): 426–35.

Montserrat Samsó et al., "Coordinated Movement of Cytoplasmic and Transmembrane Domains of RyR1 upon Gating," *PLOS Biology* 7, no. 4 (April 2009): e1000085.

67. Lynda Ann Frassetto, Ralph Curtis Morris Jr., and Antonio Sebastian, "Effect of Age on Blood Acid-Base Composition in Adult Humans: Role of Age-Related Renal Functional Decline," *American Journal of Physiology—Renal Physiology* 271, no. 6 (December 1996): F1114–22.

68. Alena Hall, "What Happened after One Family Went Organic for Just Two Weeks," *HuffPost Life*, May 14, 2015, https://www.huffpost.com/entry/the-organic-effect_n _7244000.

69. Cynthia L. Curl, Richard A. Fenske, and Kai Elgethun, "Organophosphorus Pesticide

Exposure of Urban and Suburban Preschool Children with Organic and Conventional Diets," *Environmental Health Perspectives* 111, no. 3 (March 2003): 377–82.

70. Wahyu Wulaningsih et al., "Investigating Nutrition and Lifestyle Factors as Determinants of Abdominal Obesity: An Environment-Wide Study," *International Journal of Obesity* 41, no. 2 (February 2017): 340–47.

71. Sharon P. G. Fowler, "Low-Calorie Sweetener Use and Energy Balance: Results from Experimental Studies in Animals, and Large-Scale Prospective Studies in Humans," *Physiology and Behavior* 164, part B (October 1, 2016): 517–23.

72. Moreno Paolini et al., "Aspartame, a Bittersweet Pill," *Carcinogenesis* 38, no. 12 (December 2017): 1249–50.

    Morando Soffritti et al., "The Carcinogenic Effects of Aspartame: The Urgent Need for Regulatory Re-evaluation," *American Journal of Industrial Medicine* 57, no. 4 (April 2014): 383–97.

73. Jodi E. Nettleton, Raylene A. Reimer, and Jane Shearer, "Reshaping the Gut Microbiota: Impact of Low Calorie Sweeteners and the Link to Insulin Resistance?" *Physiology and Behavior* 164, part B (October 1, 2016): 488–93.

    Jotham Suez et al., "Artificial Sweeteners Induce Glucose Intolerance by Altering the Gut Microbiota," *Nature* 514, no. 7521 (October 9, 2014): 181–86.

74. Amen, *Memory Rescue*, 160.

75. Ibid., 160–61.

76. Sarah Yang, "Teen Girls See Big Drop in Chemical Exposure with Switch in Cosmetics," *Berkeley News*, March 7, 2016, https://news.berkeley.edu/2016/03/07/cosmetics-chemicals/.

77. Dana Edwin King, Arch G. Mainous, and Carol A. Lambourne, "Trends in Dietary Fiber Intake in the United States, 1999–2008," *Journal of the Academy of Nutrition and Dietetics* 112, no. 5 (May 2012): 642–48.

78. Robert J. Flanagan and T. J. Meridith, "Use of N-acetylcysteine in Clinical Toxicology," *American Journal of Medicine* 91, no. 3, suppl. 3 (September 30, 1991): S131–39.

79. Reinhold Kirchhoff et al., "Increase in Choleresis by Means of Artichoke Extract," *Phytomedicine* 1, no. 2 (September 1994): 107–15.

80. Suzan M. Mansour et al., "*Ginkgo Biloba* Extract (EGb 761) Normalizes Hypertension in 2K, 1C Hypertensive Rats: Role of Antioxidant Mechanisms, ACE Inhibiting Activity and Improvement of Endothelial Dysfunction," *Phytomedicine* 18, nos. 8–9 (June 15, 2011): 641–47.

81. Kültiğin Cavuşoğlu et al., "Protective Effect of *Ginkgo Biloba* L. Leaf Extract against Glyphosate Toxicity in Swiss Albino Mice," *Journal of Medicinal Food* 14, no. 10 (October 2011): 1263–72.

82. Shi-Sheng Zhou et al., "The Skin Function: A Factor of Anti-Metabolic Syndrome," *Diabetology and Metabolic Syndrome* 4, no. 1 (April 26, 2012): 15.

83. Margaret E. Sears, Kathleen J. Kerr, and Riina I. Bray, "Arsenic, Cadmium, Lead, and Mercury in Sweat: A Systematic Review," *Journal of Environmental and Public Health* 2012 (2012): 184745.

    Stephen J. Genuis et al., "Blood, Urine, and Sweat (BUS) Study: Monitoring and Elimination of Bioaccumulated Toxic Elements," *Archives of Environmental Contamination and Toxicology* 61, no. 2 (August 2011): 344–57.

84. Margaret E. Sears and Stephen J. Genuis, "Environmental Determinants of Chronic Disease and Medical Approaches: Recognition, Avoidance, Supportive Therapy, and Detoxification," *Journal of Environmental and Public Health* 2012 (2012): 356798.

85. H. Lew and A. Quintanilha, "Effects of Endurance Training and Exercise on Tissue Antioxidative Capacity and Acetaminophen Detoxification," *European Journal of Drug Metabolism and Pharmacokinetics* 16, no. 1 (January–March 1991): 59–68.

    Chandan K. Sen, "Glutathione Homeostasis in Response to Exercise Training and Nutritional Supplements," *Molecular and Cellular Biochemistry* 196, nos. 1–2 (June 1999): 31–42.

86. Margaret O. Murphy et al., "Exercise Protects against PCB-Induced Inflammation and Associated Cardiovascular Risk Factors," *Environmental Science and Pollution Research* 23, no. 3 (February 2016): 2201–11.

87. Stephen J. Genuis et al., "Human Elimination of Phthalate Compounds: Blood, Urine, and Sweat (BUS) Study," *Scientific World Journal* 2012 (2012): 615068.

88. Stephen J. Genuis et al., "Human Excretion of Bisphenol A: Blood, Urine, and Sweat (BUS) Study," *Journal of Environmental and Public Health* 2012 (2012): 185731.

89. Kaye H. Kilburn, Raphael H. Warsaw, and Megan G. Shields, "Neurobehavioral Dysfunction in Firemen Exposed to Polychlorinated Biphenyls (PCBs): Possible Improvement after Detoxification," *Archives of Environmental Health* 44, no. 6 (1989): 345–50.

90. Tanjaniina Laukkanen et al., "Sauna Bathing Is Inversely Associated with Dementia and Alzheimer's Disease in Middle-Aged Finnish Men," *Age and Ageing* 46, no. 2 (March 1, 2017): 245–49.

91. Tanjaniina Laukkanen et al., "Association between Sauna Bathing and Fatal Cardiovascular and All-Cause Mortality Events," *JAMA Internal Medicine* 175, no. 4 (April 2015): 542–48.

92. Kelli F. Koltyn et al., "Changes in Mood State following Whole-Body Hyperthermia," *International Journal of Hyperthermia* 8, no. 3 (May/June 1992): 305–7.

93. K. Kukkonen-Harjula and K. Kauppinen, "How the Sauna Affects the Endocrine System," *Annals of Clinical Research* 20, no. 4 (1988): 262–66.

    D. Jezová et al., "Rise in Plasma Beta-endorphin and ACTH in Response to Hyperthermia in Sauna," *Hormone and Metabolic Research* 17, no. 12 (December 1985): 693–94.

94. K. Kukkonen-Harjula et al., "Haemodynamic and Hormonal Responses to Heat Exposure in a Finnish Sauna Bath," *European Journal of Applied Physiology and Occupational Physiology* 58, no. 5 (1989): 543–50.

95. Satoshi Kokura et al., "Whole Body Hyperthermia Improves Obesity-Induced Insulin Resistance in Diabetic Mice," *International Journal of Hyperthermia* 23, no. 3 (May 2007): 259–65.

96. Laukkanen et al., Association between "Sauna Bathing and Fatal Cardiovascular and All-Cause Mortality Events," 542–48.

CHAPTER 11: M IS FOR MIND STORMS

1. Ronald C. Kessler et al., "Prevalence, Severity, and Comorbidity of 12-Month *DSM-IV* Disorders in the National Comorbidity Survey Replication," *Archives of General Psychiatry* 62, no. 6 (June 2005): 617–27.

2. Jack Dreyfus, *A Remarkable Medicine Has Been Overlooked* (New York: Dreyfus Medical Foundation, 1992).

3. Emil Kraepelin and A. Ross Diefendorf, *Clinical Psychiatry* (New York: Macmillan, 1907; Delmar, NY: Scholars' Facsimiles and Reprints, 1981).

4. Luke Plunkett, "The Banned *Pokémon* Episode That Gave Children Seizures," Kotaku, October 20, 2015, https://kotaku.com/the-banned-pokemon-episode-that-gave-children-seizures-5757570.

5. Ibid.

6. Kirsty Martin et al., "Ketogenic Diet and Other Dietary Treatments for Epilepsy," *Cochrane Database of Systematic Reviews*, no. 2 (February 9, 2016): CD001903.

7. Emmanuelle C. Bostock, Kenneth C. Kirby, and Bruce V. Taylor, "The Current Status of the Ketogenic Diet in Psychiatry," *Frontiers in Psychiatry* 8 (March 20, 2017): 43.

    Elisa Brietzke et al., "Ketogenic Diet as a Metabolic Therapy for Mood Disorders: Evidence and Developments," *Neuroscience and Biobehavioral Reviews* 94 (November 2018): 11–16.

    James R. Phelps, Susan V. Siemers, and Rif S. El-Mallakh, "The Ketogenic Diet for Type II Bipolar Disorder," *Neurocase* 19, no. 5 (2013): 423–26.

8. Laura R. Saslow et al., "An Online Intervention Comparing a Very Low-Carbohydrate Ketogenic Diet and Lifestyle Recommendations versus a Plate Method Diet in Overweight Individuals with Type 2 Diabetes: A Randomized Controlled Trial," *Journal of Medical Internet Research* 19, no. 2 (February 13, 2017): e36.

9. Antonio Paoli et al., "Nutrition and Acne: Therapeutic Potential of Ketogenic Diets," *Skin Pharmacology and Physiology* 25, no. 3 (2012): 111–17.

10. Daniela D. Weber, Sepideh Aminzadeh-Gohari, and Barbara Kofler, "Ketogenic Diet in Cancer Therapy," *Aging* 10, no. 2 (February 11, 2018): 164–65.

11. Javad Anjom-Shoae et al., "The Association between Dietary Intake of Magnesium and Psychiatric Disorders among Iranian Adults: A Cross-Sectional Study," *British Journal of Nutrition* 120, no. 6 (September 2018): 693–702.

12. Alan W. Yuen and Josemir Sander, "Can Magnesium Supplementation Reduce Seizures in People with Epilepsy? A Hypothesis," *Epilepsy Research* 100, nos. 1–2 (June 2012): 152–56.

13. Etienne Pouteau et al., "Superiority of Magnesium and Vitamin B6 over Magnesium Alone on Severe Stress in Healthy Adults with Low Magnesemia: A Randomized, Single-Blind Clinical Trial," *PLOS One* 13, no. 12 (December 18, 2018): e0208454.

14. Anna E. Kirkland, Gabrielle L. Sarlo, and Kathleen F. Holton, "The Role of Magnesium in Neurological Disorders," *Nutrients* 10, no. 6 (June 6, 2018): e730.

    Emily K. Tarleton et al., "Role of Magnesium Supplementation in the Treatment of Depression: A Randomized Clinical Trial," *PLOS One* 12, no. 6 (June 27, 2017): e0180067.

15. Evert Boonstra et al., "Neurotransmitters as Food Supplements: The Effects of GABA on Brain and Behavior," *Frontiers in Psychology* 6 (2015): 1520.

16. A. M. Abdou et al., "Relaxation and Immunity Enhancement Effects of Gamma-aminobutyric Acid (GABA) Administration in Humans," *BioFactors* 26, no. 3 (2006): 201–8.

CHAPTER 12: I IS FOR IMMUNITY AND INFECTIONS

1. Daniel G. Amen, *Memory Rescue* (Carol Stream, IL: Tyndale, 2017), 185–86.

2. Ibid.

3. "HIV/AIDS and Mental Health," National Institute of Mental Health, last revised November 2016, https://www.nimh.nih.gov/health/topics/hiv-aids/index.shtml.

4. Nian-Sheng Tzeng et al., "Increased Risk of Psychiatric Disorders in Allergic Diseases: A Nationwide, Population-Based, Cohort Study," *Frontiers in Psychiatry* 9 (April 24, 2018): 133.

5. Yi-Hao Peng et al., "Adult Asthma Increases Dementia Risk: A Nationwide Cohort Study," *Journal of Epidemiology and Community Health* 69, no. 2 (February 2015): 123–28.

    Minna Rusanen et al., "Chronic Obstructive Pulmonary Disease and Asthma and the Risk of Mild Cognitive Impairment and Dementia: A Population Based CAIDE Study," *Current Alzheimer Research* 10, no. 5 (June 2013): 549–55.

6. Ora Nakash et al., "Comorbidity of Common Mental Disorders with Cancer and Their Treatment Gap: Findings from the World Mental Health Surveys," *Psycho-Oncology* 23, no. 1 (January 2014): 40–51.

7. William F. Pirl, "Evidence Report on the Occurrence, Assessment, and Treatment of Depression in Cancer Patients," *JNCI Monographs* 2004, no. 32 (July 2004): 32–39.

8. "Women & Autoimmunity," American Autoimmune Related Diseases Association, accessed August 15, 2019, https://www.aarda.org/who-we-help/patients/women-and-autoimmunity/.

9. Marc Malkin, "Lady Gaga Opens Up about Her 'Mental Health Crisis,'" *Variety*, November 9, 2018, https://variety.com/2018/scene/news/lady-gaga-mental-health-struggles-1203023093/.

10. Michael E. Benros et al., "Autoimmune Diseases and Severe Infections as Risk Factors for Mood Disorders: A Nationwide Study," *JAMA Psychiatry* 70, no. 8 (August 2013): 812–20.

Gianluca Bagnato et al., "Comparation of Levels of Anxiety and Depression in Patients with Autoimmune and Chronic-Degenerative Rheumatic: Preliminary Data," *Reumatismo* (Italian) 58, no. 3 (July–September 2006): 206–11.

11. William W. Eaton et al., "Association of Schizophrenia and Autoimmune Diseases: Linkage of Danish National Registers," *American Journal of Psychiatry* 163, no. 3 (March 2006): 521–28.

12. Joshua D. Rosenblat and Roger S. McIntyre, "Bipolar Disorder and Immune Dysfunction: Epidemiological Findings, Proposed Pathophysiology and Clinical Implications," *Brain Sciences* 7, no. 11 (October 30, 2017): e144.

13. Philip Rising Nielsen, Michael Eriksen Benros, and Søren Dalsgaard, "Associations between Autoimmune Diseases and Attention-Deficit/Hyperactivity Disorder: A Nationwide Study," *Journal of the American Academy of Child and Adolescent Psychiatry* 56, no. 3 (March 2017): 234–40.e1.

14. Clare J. Wotton and Michael J. Goldacre, "Associations between Specific Autoimmune Diseases and Subsequent Dementia: Retrospective Record-Linkage Cohort Study, UK," *Journal of Epidemiology and Community Health* 71, no. 6 (June 2017): 576–83.

15. Amen, *Memory Rescue*, 188.

16. Ole Köhler-Forsberg et al., "A Nationwide Study in Denmark of the Association between Treated Infections and the Subsequent Risk of Treated Mental Disorders in Children and Adolescents," *JAMA Psychiatry* 76, no. 3 (March 2019): 271–79.

17. Michael E. Benros et al., "Autoimmune Diseases and Severe Infections as Risk Factors for Mood Disorders: A Nationwide Study," *JAMA Psychiatry* 70, no. 8 (August 2013): 812–20.

18. Amen, *Memory Rescue*, 189.

19. R. A. Underhill, "Myalgic Encephalomyelitis, Chronic Fatigue Syndrome: An Infectious Disease," *Medical Hypotheses* 85, no. 6 (December 2015): 765–73.

20. Z. Marinković and S. Dukić, "Historical and Medical Review of Syphilis-Afflicted Army Leaders, Rulers and Statesmen," *Medicinski Pregled* 64, nos. 7–8 (July/August 2011): 423–27.

21. Lucas Lonardoni Crozatti et al., "Atypical Behavioral and Psychiatric Symptoms: Neurosyphilis Should Always Be Considered," *Autopsy Case Reports* 5, no. 3 (July–September 2015): 43–47.

22. Ruth F. Itzhaki et al., "Microbes and Alzheimer's Disease," *Journal of Alzheimer's Disease* 51, no. 4 (2016): 979–84.

23. James S. Brown Jr., "Geographic Correlation of Schizophrenia to Ticks and Tick-Borne Encephalitis," *Schizophrenia Bulletin* 20, no. 4 (1994): 755–75; used with permission.

24. Ying Qiang Xiang et al., "Adjunctive Minocycline for Schizophrenia: A Meta-analysis of Randomized Controlled Trials," *European Neuropsychopharmacology* 27, no. 1 (January 2017): 8–18.

25. Amen, *Memory Rescue*, 192.

26. "Toxoplasmosis Frequently Asked Questions (FAQs)," Centers for Disease Control and Prevention, last reviewed September 28, 2018, https://www.cdc.gov/parasites /toxoplasmosis/gen_info/faqs.html.

27. Claudia Del Grande et al., "Is *Toxoplasma gondii* a Trigger of Bipolar Disorder?" *Pathogens* 6, no. 1 (March 2017): e3.

28. Jaana Suvisaari et al., "*Toxoplasma gondii* Infection and Common Mental Disorders in the Finnish General Population," *Journal of Affective Disorders* 223 (December 1, 2017): 20–25.

29. C. J. Carter, "Toxoplasmosis and Polygenic Disease Susceptibility Genes: Extensive *Toxoplasma gondii* Host/Pathogen Interactome Enrichment in Nine Psychiatric or Neurological Disorders," *Journal of Pathogens* 2013 (2013): 965046.

30. Ed Yong, "Zombie Roaches and Other Parasite Tales," TED Talk, March 2014, video, 13:02, https://www.ted.com/talks/ed_yong_suicidal_wasps_zombie_roaches_and_other _tales_of_parasites.

31. "What Is PANS?" Moleculera Labs, accessed August 16, 2019, https://www.moleculeralabs .com/what-is-pans/

32. O. Köhler et al., "Infections and Exposure to Anti-infective Agents and the Risk of Severe Mental Disorders: A Nationwide Study," *Acta Psychiatrica Scandinavica* 135, no. 2 (February 2017): 97–105.

33. Emily G. Severance et al., "*Candida albicans* Exposures, Sex Specificity and Cognitive Deficits in Schizophrenia and Bipolar Disorder," *npj Schizophrenia* 2 (May 4, 2016): 16018.

34. Emily Severance, quoted at "Yeast Infection Linked to Mental Illness," Johns Hopkins Medicine, May 4, 2016, https://www.hopkinsmedicine.org/news/media/releases/yeast _infection_linked_to_mental_illness.

35. Yifan Wu et al., "Microglia and Amyloid Precursor Protein Coordinate Control of Transient *Candida* Cerebritis with Memory Deficits," *Nature Communications* 10, no. 1 (January 4, 2019): 58.

36. Adit A. Ginde, Mark C. Liu, and Carlos A. Camargo Jr., "Demographic Differences and Trends of Vitamin D Insufficiency in the US Population, 1988–2004," *Archives of Internal Medicine* 169, no. 6 (March 23, 2009): 626–32.

37. Amen, *Memory Rescue*, 194.

38. Frederic Blanc et al., "Lyme Neuroborreliosis and Dementia," *Journal of Alzheimer's Disease* 41, no. 4 (2014): 1087–93.

39. Justin C. McArthur, "HIV Dementia: An Evolving Disease," *Journal of Neuroimmunology* 157, nos. 1–2 (December 2004): 3–10.

40. Judith Miklossy, "Historic Evidence to Support a Causal Relationship between Spirochetal Infections and Alzheimer's Disease," *Frontiers in Aging Neuroscience* 7 (April 16, 2015): 46.

41. Steven A. Harris and Elizabeth A. Harris, "Herpes Simplex Virus Type 1 and Other Pathogens Are Key Causative Factors in Sporadic Alzheimer's Disease," *Journal of Alzheimer's Disease* 48, no. 2 (2015): 319–53.

    Ariah J. Steel and Guy D. Eslick, "Herpes Viruses Increase the Risk of Alzheimer's Disease: A Meta-Analysis," *Journal of Alzheimer's Disease* 47, no. 2 (2015): 351–64.

42. Lisa L. Barnes et al., "Cytomegalovirus Infection and Risk of Alzheimer Disease in Older Black and White Individuals," *Journal of Infectious Diseases* 211, no. 2 (January 15, 2015): 230–37.

43. S. M. Shim et al., "Elevated Epstein-Barr Virus Antibody Level Is Associated with Cognitive Decline in the Korean Elderly," *Journal of Alzheimer's Disease* 55, no. 1 (2017): 293–301.

44. Mahmoud Mahami-Oskouei et al., "Toxoplasmosis and Alzheimer: Can *Toxoplasma gondii* Really Be Introduced as a Risk Factor in Etiology of Alzheimer?" *Parasitology Research* 115, no. 8 (August 2016): 3169–74.

45. Tali Shindler-Itskovitch et al., "A Systematic Review and Meta-Analysis of the Association between *Helicobacterpylori* Infection and Dementia," *Journal of Alzheimer's Disease* 52, no. 4 (2016): 1431–42.

46. Priya Maheshwari and Guy D. Eslick, "Bacterial Infection and Alzheimer's Disease: A Meta-analysis," *Journal of Alzheimer's Disease* 43, no. 3 (2015): 957–66.

47. Brunetta Porcelli et al., "Association between Stressful Life Events and Autoimmune Diseases: A Systematic Review and Meta-analysis of Retrospective Case-Control Studies," *Autoimmunity Reviews* 15, no. 4 (April 2016): 325–34.

    A. Matos-Santos et al., "Relationship between the Number and Impact of Stressful Life Events and the Onset of Graves' Disease and Toxic Nodular Goitre," *Clinical Endocrinology* (Oxford) 55, no. 1 (July 2001): 15–19.

    David C. Mohr et al., "Association between Stressful Life Events and Exacerbation in Multiple Sclerosis: A Meta-analysis," *BMJ* 328 (March 27, 2004): 731.

48. Lee S. Berk et al., "Modulation of Neuroimmune Parameters during the Eustress of Humor-Associated Mirthful Laughter," *Alternative Therapies in Health and Medicine* 7, no. 2 (March 2001): 62–72, 74–76.

Kyung Hee Ryu, Hye Sook Shin, and Eun Young Yang, "Effects of Laughter Therapy on Immune Responses in Postpartum Women," *Journal of Alternative and Complementary Medicine* 21, no. 12 (December 2015): 781–88.

Norman Cousins, "Anatomy of an Illness (as Perceived by the Patient)," *New England Journal of Medicine* 295, no. 26 (December 23, 1976): 1458–63.

49. S. P. Wasser, "Medicinal Mushrooms as a Source of Antitumor and Immunomodulating Polysaccharides," *Applied Microbiology and Biotechnology* 60, no. 3 (November 2002): 258–74.

50. Peter Roupas et al., "The Role of Edible Mushrooms in Health: Evaluation of the Evidence," *Journal of Functional Foods* 4, no. 4 (October 2012): 687–709.

Seema Patel and Arun Goyal, "Recent Developments in Mushrooms as Anti-cancer Therapeutics: A Review," *3 Biotech* 2, no. 1 (March 2012): 1–15.

Lu Ren, Conrad Perera, and Yacine Hemar, "Antitumor Activity of Mushroom Polysaccharides: A Review," *Food and Function* 3, no. 11 (November 2012): 1118–30.

Dhanushka Gunawardena et al., "Anti-inflammatory Effects of Five Commercially Available Mushroom Species Determined in Lipopolysaccharide and Interferon-γ Activated Murine Macrophages," *Food Chemistry* 148 (April 1, 2014): 92–96.

51. Mayumi Nagano et al., "Reduction of Depression and Anxiety by 4 Weeks *Hericium erinaceus* Intake," *Biomedical Research* 31, no. 4 (August 2010): 231–37.

52. Koichiro Mori et al., "Improving Effects of the Mushroom Yamabushitake (*Hericium erinaceus*) on Mild Cognitive Impairment: A Double-Blind Placebo-Controlled Clinical Trial," *Phytotherapy Research* 23, no. 3 (March 2009): 367–72.

53. Xiaoshuang Dai et al., "Consuming *Lentinula edodes* (Shiitake) Mushrooms Daily Improves Human Immunity: A Randomized Dietary Intervention in Healthy Young Adults," *Journal of the American College of Nutrition* 34, no. 6 (2015): 478–87.

Mary Jo Feeney et al., "Mushrooms and Health Summit Proceedings," *Journal of Nutrition* 144, no. 7 (July 2014): 1128S–36S.

J. M. Gaullier et al., "Supplementation with a Soluble β-glucan Exported from Shiitake Medicinal Mushroom, *Lentinus edodes* (Berk.) Singer Mycelium: A Crossover, Placebo-Controlled Study in Healthy Elderly," *International Journal of Medicinal Mushrooms* 13, no. 4 (2011): 319–26.

54. B. S. Sanodiya et al., "*Ganoderma lucidum*: A Potent Pharmacological Macrofungus," *Current Pharmaceutical Biotechnology* 10, no. 8 (December 2009): 717–42.

Hong Zhao et al., "Spore Powder of *Ganoderma lucidum* Improves Cancer-Related Fatigue in Breast Cancer Patients Undergoing Endocrine Therapy: A Pilot Clinical Trial," *Evidence-Based Complementary and Alternative Medicine* 2012 (2012): 809614.

55. Xing-Tai Li et al., "Protective Effects on Mitochondria and Anti-aging Activity of Polysaccharides from Cultivated Fruiting Bodies of *Cordyceps militaris*," *American Journal of Chinese Medicine* 38, no. 6 (2010): 1093–106.

56. Amen, *Memory Rescue*, 197.

57. Susan S. Percival, "Aged Garlic Extract Modifies Human Immunity," *Journal of Nutrition* 146, no. 2 (February 2016): 433S–36S.

Craig S. Charron et al., "A Single Meal Containing Raw, Crushed Garlic Influences Expression of Immunity- and Cancer-Related Genes in Whole Blood of Humans," *Journal of Nutrition* 145, no. 11 (November 2015): 2448–55.

58. Cheryl A. Rowe et al., "Regular Consumption of Concord Grape Juice Benefits Human Immunity," *Journal of Medicinal Food* 14, nos. 1–2 (January/February 2011): 69–78.

Susan J. Zunino, "Type 2 Diabetes and Glycemic Response to Grapes or Grape Products," *Journal of Nutrition* 139, no. 9 (September 2009): 1794S–1800S.

M. P. Nantz et al., "Immunity and Antioxidant Capacity in Humans Is Enhanced by Consumption of a Dried, Encapsulated Fruit and Vegetable Juice Concentrate," *Journal of Nutrition* 136, no. 10 (October 2006): 2606–610.

59. Marlies Karsch-Völk et al., "Echinacea for Preventing and Treating the Common Cold," *Cochrane Database of Systematic Reviews*, no. 2 (February 20, 2014): CD000530.

Keith I. Block and Mark N. Mead, "Immune System Effects of Echinacea, Ginseng, and Astragalus: A Review," *Integrative Cancer Therapies* 2, no. 3 (September 2003): 247–67.

60. Angélica T. Vieira, Mauro M. Teixeira, and Flaviano S. Martins, "The Role of Probiotics and Prebiotics in Inducing Gut Immunity," *Frontiers in Immunology* 4 (December 12, 2013): 445.

Rohit Sharma et al., "Dietary Supplementation of Milk Fermented with Probiotic *Lactobacillus fermentum* Enhances Systemic Immune Response and Antioxidant Capacity in Aging Mice," *Nutrition Research* (New York) 34, no. 11 (November 2014): 968–81.

61. Chad Robertson, "The Link between Vitamin C and Optimal Immunity," *Life Extension* magazine, November 2015, https://www.lifeextension.com/magazine/2015/11/the-link-between-vitamin-c-and-optimal-immunity/page-01.

M. de la Fuente et al., "Immune Function in Aged Women Is Improved by Ingestion of Vitamins C and E," *Canadian Journal of Physiology and Pharmacology* 76, no. 4 (1998): 373–80.

62. J. Rodrigo Mora, Makoto Iwata, and Ulrich H. von Andrian, "Vitamin Effects on the Immune System: Vitamins A and D Take Centre Stage," *Nature Reviews Immunology* 8, no. 9 (September 2008): 685–98.

Cynthia Aranow, "Vitamin D and the Immune System," *Journal of Investigative Medicine* 59, no. 6 (August 2011): 881–86.

Oregon State University, "Key Feature of Immune System Survived in Humans, Other Primates for 60 Million Years," EurekAlert! American Association for the Advancement of Science, August 18, 2009, https://www.eurekalert.org/pub_releases/2009-08/osu-kfo081809.php.

Mitsuyoshi Urashima et al., "Randomized Trial of Vitamin D Supplementation to Prevent Seasonal Influenza A in Schoolchildren," *American Journal of Clinical Nutrition* 91, no. 5 (May 2010): 1255–60.

63. Satoru Moriguchi and Mikako Muraga, "Vitamin E and Immunity," *Vitamins and Hormones* 59 (2000): 305–36.

64. Junaidah B. Barnett et al., "Effect of Zinc Supplementation on Serum Zinc Concentration and T cell Proliferation in Nursing Home Elderly: A Randomized, Double-Blind, Placebo-Controlled Trial," *American Journal of Clinical Nutrition* 103, no. 3 (March 2016): 942–51.

Laura Kahmann et al., "Effect of Improved Zinc Status on T helper Cell Activation and TH1/TH2 Ratio in Healthy Elderly Individuals," *Biogerontology* 7, nos. 5–6 (October–December 2006): 429–35.

Ananda S. Prasad et al., "Effect of Zinc Supplementation on Incidence of Infections and Hospital Admissions in Sickle Cell Disease (SCD)," *American Journal of Hematology* 61, no. 3 (July 1999): 194–202.

65. Jorge Correale, María Célica Ysrraelit, and María Inés Gaitán, "Immunomodulatory Effects of Vitamin D in Multiple Sclerosis," *Brain* 132, part 5 (May 2009): 1146–60.

66. See "835 Abstracts with Vitamin D Research," Vitamin D, GreenMedInfo, accessed August 16, 2019, https://www.greenmedinfo.com/substance/vitamin-d.

67. Herbert W. Harris et al., "Vitamin D Deficiency and Psychiatric Illness," *Current Psychiatry* 12, no. 4 (April 2013): 18–27.

68. Paul Knekt et al., "Serum 25-hydroxyvitamin D Concentration and Risk of Dementia," *Epidemiology* (Cambridge, MA) 25, no. 6 (November 2014): 799–804.

69. Rathish Nair and Arun Maseeh, "Vitamin D: The 'Sunshine' Vitamin," *Journal of Pharmacology and Pharmacotherapeutics* 3, no. 2 (April–June 2012): 118–26.

70. R. Jorde et al., "Effects of Vitamin D Supplementation on Symptoms of Depression in Overweight and Obese Subjects: Randomized Double Blind Trial," *Journal of Internal Medicine* 264, no. 6 (December 2008): 599–609.

71. Albina Nowak et al., "Effect of Vitamin D3 on Self-Perceived Fatigue: A Double-Blind Randomized Placebo-Controlled Trial," *Medicine (Baltimore)* 95, no. 52 (December 2016): e5353.

72. Adit A. Ginde, Mark C. Liu, and Carlos A. Camargo Jr., "Demographic Differences and Trends of Vitamin D Insufficiency in the US Population, 1988–2004," *Archives of Internal Medicine* 169, no. 6 (2009): 626–32.

73. Amen, *Memory Rescue*, 198–99.

74. E. Sohl et al., "The Impact of Medication on Vitamin D Status in Older Individuals," *European Journal of Endocrinology* 166, no. 3 (March 2012): 477–85.

75. Phillip A. Engen et al., "The Gastrointestinal Microbiome: Alcohol Effects on the Composition of Intestinal Microbiota," *Alcohol Research: Current Reviews* 37, no. 2 (2015): 223–36.

CHAPTER 13: N IS FOR NEUROHORMONE ISSUES

1. Mark L. Gordon, *Traumatic Brain Injury: A Clinical Approach to Diagnosis and Treatment* (Los Angeles: Millennium Health Centers, 2016).

2. Mark L. Gordon, "ISNR Keynote Speaker Mark L. Gordon 2015," Andrew Marr, December 25, 2016, video, 1:00:12, https://www.youtube.com/watch?v=Q_Uu-soMavQ&feature =youtu.be.

3. J. McGaffee, M. A. Barnes, and S. Lippmann, "Psychiatric Presentations of Hypothyroidism," *American Family Physician* 23, no. 5 (May 1, 1981): 129–33.

4. Thomas W. Heinrich and Garth Grahm, "Hypothyroidism Presenting as Psychosis: Myxedema Madness Revisited," *Primary Care Companion to the Journal of Clinical Psychiatry* 5, no. 6 (December 2003): 260–66.

5. P. C. Whybrow, A. J. Prange Jr., and C. R. Treadway, "Mental Changes Accompanying Thyroid Gland Dysfunction: A Reappraisal Using Objective Psychological Measurement," *Archives of General Psychiatry* 20, no. 1 (1969): 48–63.

6. Thomas D. Geracioti Jr., "Identifying Hypothyroidism's Psychiatric Presentations," *Current Psychiatry* 5, no. 11 (November 2006): 98–117.

   Nadine Correia Santos et al., "Revisiting Thyroid Hormones in Schizophrenia," *Journal of Thyroid Research* 2012 (2012): 569147.

7. Jeffrey Garber, et al., "Clinical Practice Guidelines for Hypothyroidism in Adults: Cosponsored by the American Association of Clinical Endocrinologists and the American Thyroid Association," *Endocrine Practice* 18, no. 6 (November 2012): 988–1028.

8. Daniel G. Amen, *Unleash the Power of the Female Brain* (New York: Harmony Books, 2013), 122.

9. Heinrich and Grahm, "Hypothyroidism Presenting as Psychosis," 260–66.

10. John J. Haggerty Jr., Dwight L. Evans, Arthur J. Prange Jr., "Organic Brain Syndrome Associated with Marginal Hypothyroidism," *American Journal of Psychiatry* 143, no. 6 (June 1986): 785–86.

11. Amen, *Unleash the Power*, 124.

12. "Hyperthyroidism (Overactive Thyroid)," National Institute of Diabetes and Digestive and Kidney Diseases, August 2016, https://www.niddk.nih.gov/health-information/endocrine -diseases/hyperthyroidism.

13. "Thyroid Deficiency and Mental Health," Harvard Health Publishing, Harvard Medical School, May 2007, http://www.health.harvard.edu/diseases-and-conditions/thyroid -deficiency-and-mental-health.

   Mirella P. Hage and Sami T. Azar, "The Link between Thyroid Function and Depression," *Journal of Thyroid Research* 2012 (2012): 590648.

14. G. Marian et al., "Hyperthyroidism—Cause of Depression and Psychosis: A Case Report," *Journal of Medicine and Life* 2, no. 4 (October–December 2009): 440–42.

15. Amen, *Unleash the Power*, 123.

16. S. Chetty et al., "Stress and Glucocorticoids Promote Oligodendrogenesis in the Adult Hippocampus," *Molecular Psychiatry* 19, no. 12 (December 2014): 1275–83.

17. Ibid.

18. Camilla A. M. Glad et al., "Reduced DNA Methylation and Psychopathology following Endogenous Hypercortisolism—A Genome-Wide Study," *Scientific Reports* 7 (2017): 44445.

19. Paul Ardayfio and Kwang-Soo Kim, "Anxiogenic-Like Effect of Chronic Corticosterone in the Light–Dark Emergence Task in Mice," *Behavioral Neuroscience* 120, no. 2 (2006): 249–56.

20. Sarah Khan and Rafeeq Alam Khan, "Chronic Stress Leads to Anxiety and Depression," *Annals of Psychiatry and Mental Health* 5, no. 1 (January 2017): 1091.

21. Daniel G. Amen, *Memory Rescue* (Carol Stream, IL: Tyndale, 2017), 208.

22. Amen, *Unleash the Power*, 131.

23. Amen, *Memory Rescue*, 210.

24. Claudia Barth, Arno Villringer, and Julia Sacher, "Sex Hormones Affect Neurotransmitters and Shape the Adult Female Brain during Hormonal Transition Periods," *Frontiers in Neuroscience* 9 (2015): 37.

25. Linda A. Bean, Lara Ianov, and Thomas C. Foster, "Estrogen Receptors, the Hippocampus, and Memory," *Neuroscientist* 20, no. 5 (October 2014): 534–45.

26. Laila Adly et al., "Serum Concentrations of Estrogens, Sex Hormone-Binding Globulin, and Androgens and Risk of Breast Cancer in Postmenopausal Women," *International Journal of Cancer* 119, no. 10 (November 15, 2006): 2402–7.

27. Silvia Deandrea et al., "Alcohol and Breast Cancer Risk Defined by Estrogen and Progesterone Receptor Status: A Case-Control Study," *Cancer Epidemiology, Biomarkers and Prevention* 17, no. 8 (August 2008): 2025–28.

28. Samantha S. Solden et al., "Immune Modulation in Multiple Sclerosis Patients Treated with the Pregnancy Hormone Estriol," *Journal of Immunology* 171, no. 11 (December 1, 2003): 6267–74.

29. Amen, *Unleash the Power*, 95–96.

30. Ibid., 102.

31. Loyola University Health System, "Increased Stroke Risk from Birth Control Pills, Review Finds," ScienceDaily, October 27, 2009, https://www.sciencedaily.com/releases/2009/10/091026152820.htm.

32. Belinda A. Pletzer and Hubert H. Kerschbaum, "50 Years of Hormonal Contraception—Time to Find Out, What It Does to Our Brain," *Frontiers in Neuroscience* 8 (August 21, 2014): 256.

33. Charlotte Weissel Skovlund et al., "Association of Hormonal Contraception with Depression," *JAMA Psychiatry* 73, no. 11 (November 2016): 1154–62.

34. G. B. Slap, "Oral Contraceptives and Depression: Impact, Prevalence and Cause," *Journal of Adolescent Health Care* 2, no. 11 (September 1981): 53–64.

35. William V. Williams, "Hormonal Contraception and the Development of Autoimmunity: A Review of the Literature," *Linacre Quarterly* 84, no. 3 (August 2017): 275–95.

36. Johannes Hertel et al., "Evidence for Stress-Like Alterations in the HPA-Axis in Women Taking Oral Contraceptives," *Scientific Reports* 7, no. 1 (October 26, 2017): 14111.

37. Y. Zimmerman et al., "The Effect of Combined Oral Contraception on Testosterone Levels in Healthy Women: A Systematic Review and Meta-analysis," *Human Reproduction Update* 20, no. 1 (January/February 2014): 76–105.

38. Claudia Panzer et al., "Impact of Oral Contraceptives on Sex Hormone-Binding Globulin and Androgen Levels: A Retrospective Study in Women with Sexual Dysfunction," *Journal of Sexual Medicine* 3, no. 1 (January 2006): 104–13.

39. Hamed Khalili, "Risk of Inflammatory Bowel Disease with Oral Contraceptives and Menopausal Hormone Therapy: Current Evidence and Future Directions," *Drug Safety* 39, no. 3 (March 2016): 193–97.

40. Amen, *Unleash the Power*, 115.

41. Carlo Pergola et al., "Testosterone Suppresses Phospholipase D, Causing Sex Differences in Leukotriene Biosynthesis in Human Monocytes," *FASEB Journal* 25, no. 10 (October 2011): 3377–87.

    Amen, *Unleash the Power*, 106.

42. Linnea Hergot Berglund et al., "Testosterone Levels and Psychological Health Status in Men from a General Population: The Tromsø Study," *Aging Male* 14, no. 1 (March 2011): 37–41.

43. Amen, *Memory Rescue*, 216.

44. Amen, *Unleash the Power*, 127–28.

45. Lu Sun et al., "Meta-Analysis Suggests That Smoking Is Associated with an Increased Risk of Early Natural Menopause," *Menopause (New York)* 19, no. 2 (February 2012): 126–32.

46. Ana M. Fernández-Alonso et al., "Obesity Is Related to Increased Menopausal Symptoms among Spanish Women," *Menopause International* 16, no. 3 (September 2010): 105–10.

47. Reini W. Bretveld et al., "Pesticide Exposure: The Hormonal Function of the Female Reproductive System Disrupted?" *Reproductive Biology and Endocrinology* 4 (May 31, 2006): 30.

48. Amen, *Memory Rescue*, 220.

49. Amen, *Unleash the Power*, 99.

50. Thomas T. Y. Wang et al., "Estrogen Receptor Alpha as a Target for Indole-3-Carbinol," *Journal of Nutritional Biochemistry* 17, no. 10 (October 2006): 659–64.

51. Gregory A. Reed et al., "A Phase I Study of Indole-3-Carbinol in Women: Tolerability and Effects," *Cancer Epidemiology, Biomarkers and Prevention* 14, no. 8 (2005): 1953–60.

52. E. Sherwood Brown et al., "A Randomized, Double-Blind, Placebo-Controlled Trial of Pregnenolone for Bipolar Depression," *Neuropsychopharmacology* 39, no. 12 (November 2014): 2867–73.

53. C. E. Marx et al., "Pregnenolone as a Novel Therapeutic Candidate in Schizophrenia: Emerging Preclinical and Clinical Evidence," *Neuroscience* 191 (September 15, 2011): 78–90.

54. Nicole Ducharme et al., "Brain Distribution and Behavioral Effects of Progesterone and Pregnenolone after Intranasal or Intravenous Administration," *European Journal of Pharmacology* 641, nos. 2–3 (September 1, 2010): 128–34.

55. Amen, *Unleash the Power*, 99.

56. Amen, *Memory Rescue*, 221.

CHAPTER 14: D IS FOR DIABESITY

1. Cyrus A. Raji et al., "Brain Structure and Obesity," *Human Brain Mapping* 31, no. 3 (March 2010): 353–64.

2. Andy Menke et al., "Prevalence of and Trends in Diabetes among Adults in the United States, 1988–2012," *JAMA* 314, no. 10 (2015): 1021–29.

3. "Adult Obesity Facts," Overweight and Obesity, Centers for Disease Control and Prevention, last reviewed August 13, 2018, https://www.cdc.gov/obesity/data/adult.html.

4. Gregory E. Simon et al., "Association between Obesity and Psychiatric Disorders in the US Adult Population," *Archives of General Psychiatry* 63, no. 7 (July 2006): 824–30.

    Nancy M. Petry et al., "Overweight and Obesity Are Associated with Psychiatric Disorders: Results from the National Epidemiologic Survey on Alcohol and Related Conditions," *Psychosomatic Medicine* 70, no. 3 (April 2008): 288–97.

5. H. C. M. Byrd, C. Curtin, and S. E. Anderson, "Attention-Deficit/Hyperactivity Disorder and Obesity in US Males and Females, Age 8–15 Years: National Health and Nutrition Examination Survey 2001–2004," *Pediatric Obesity* 8, no. 6 (December 2013): 445–53.

6. Michael Hinck, "How Obesity Can Affect Your Teen's Self Esteem," Health Beat, Jamaica Hospital Medical Center, September 26, 2014, https://jamaicahospital.org/newsletter/how-obesity-can-affect-your-teens-self-esteem/.

7. Zhang Xue-Yan et al., "Obese Chinese Primary-School Students and Low Self-Esteem: A Cross-Sectional Study," *Iranian Journal of Pediatrics* 26, no. 4 (August 2016): e3777.

8. Kenneth M. Carpenter et al., "Relationships between Obesity and *DSM-IV* Major Depressive Disorder, Suicide Ideation, and Suicide Attempts: Results from a General Population Study," *American Journal of Public Health* 90, no. 2 (2000): 251–57.

9. Cyrus A. Raji et al., "Brain Structure and Obesity," *Human Brain Mapping* 31, no. 3 (March 2010): 353–64.

   Kristen C. Willeumier, Derek V. Taylor, and Daniel G. Amen, "Elevated BMI Is Associated with Decreased Blood Flow in the Prefrontal Cortex Using SPECT Imaging in Healthy Adults," *Obesity* (Silver Spring, MD) 19, no. 5 (May 2011): 1095–97.

   Mark Hamer, G. David Batty, "Association of Body Mass Index and Waist-to-Hip Ratio with Brain Structure," *Neurology* 92, no. 6 (February 2019): e594–600.

10. Alan R. Schwartz et al., "Obesity and Obstructive Sleep Apnea: Pathogenic Mechanisms and Therapeutic Approaches," *Proceedings of the American Thoracic Society* 5, no. 2 (2008): 185–92.

11. J. M. Zanoveli et al., "Depression Associated with Diabetes: From Pathophysiology to Treatment," *Current Diabetes Reviews* 12, no. 3 (2016): 165–78.

    A. M. Castellano-Guerrero et al., "Prevalence and Predictors of Depression and Anxiety in Adult Patients with Type 1 Diabetes in Tertiary Care Setting," *Acta Diabetologica* 55, no. 9 (September 2018): 943–53.

12. Hirokatsu Niwa et al., "Clinical Analysis of Cognitive Function in Diabetic Patients by MMSE and SPECT," *Diabetes Research and Clinical Practice* 72, no. 2 (May 2006): 142–47.

    J. F. Jimenez-Bonilla et al., "Assessment of Cerebral Blood Flow in Diabetic Patients with No Clinical History of Neurological Disease," *Nuclear Medicine Communications* 17, no. 9 (September 1996): 790–94.

13. F. Pasquier et al., "Diabetes Mellitus and Dementia," *Diabetes and Metabolism* 32, no. 5, part 1 (November 2006): 403–14.

    Kapil Gudala et al., "Diabetes Mellitus and Risk of Dementia: A Meta-analysis of Prospective Observational Studies," *Journal of Diabetes Investigation* 4, no. 6 (November 2013): 640–50.

14. Ewa Racicka and Anita Brynska, "Eating Disorders in Children and Adolescents with Type 1 and Type 2 Diabetes: Prevalance, Risk Factors, Warning Signs," *Psychiatria Polska* 49, no. 5 (2015): 1017–24.

15. Syudo Yamasaki et al., "Maternal Diabetes in Early Pregnancy, and Psychotic Experiences and Depressive Symptoms in 10-Year-Old Offspring: A Population-Based Birth Cohort Study," *Schizophrenia Research* 206 (April 2019): 52–57.

16. Monique Aucoin and Sukriti Bhardwaj, "Generalized Anxiety Disorder and Hypoglycemia Symptoms Improved with Diet Modification," *Case Reports in Psychiatry* 2016 (2016): 7165425.

17. Ibid.

18. Malcolm Peet, "International Variations in the Outcome of Schizophrenia and the Prevalence of Depression in Relation to National Dietary Practices: An Ecological Analysis," *British Journal of Psychiatry* 184, no. 5 (May 2004): 404–8.

19. "Type 1 Diabetes Low Blood Sugar Symptoms," JDRF, accessed August 19, 2019, https://www.jdrf.org/t1d-resources/about/symptoms/low-blood-sugar/.

20. Peter Bongiorno, "Is There a Blood Sugar Monster Lurking within You?" *Psychology Today*, November 13, 2014, https://www.psychologytoday.com/us/blog/inner-source/201311/is-there-blood-sugar-monster-lurking-within-you.

21. Belinda S. Lennerz et al., "Effects of Dietary Glycemic Index on Brain Regions Related to

Reward and Craving in Men," *American Journal of Clinical Nutrition* 98, no. 3 (September 2013): 641–47.

22. "Type 1 Diabetes," JDRF.

23. Chris E. Zwilling et al., "Nutrient Biomarker Patterns, Cognitive Function, and fMRI Measures of Network Efficiency in the Aging Brain," *NeuroImage* 188 (March 2019): 239–51.

24. E. Duron and Olivier Hanon, "Vascular Risk Factors, Cognitive Decline, and Dementia," *Vascular Health and Risk Management* 4, no. 2 (2008): 363–81.

25. Rachel A. Whitmer, "The Epidemiology of Adiposity and Dementia," *Current Alzheimer Research* 4, no. 2 (April 2007): 117–22.

Duron and Hanon, "Vascular Risk Factors."

26. Jaakko Tuomilehto et al., "Prevention of Type 2 Diabetes Mellitus by Changes in Lifestyle among Subjects with Impaired Glucose Tolerance," *New England Journal of Medicine* 344, no. 18 (May 3, 2001): 1343–50.

27. Julie C. Antvorskov et al., "Association between Maternal Gluten Intake and Type 1 Diabetes in Offspring: National Prospective Cohort Study in Denmark," *BMJ* 362 (September 19, 2018): k3547.

28. Daniel G. Amen and Tana Amen, *The Brain Warrior's Way* (New York: New American Library, 2016), 1, 28.

29. Associated Press, "450 Sheep Jump to Their Deaths in Turkey," *USA Today*, July 8, 2005, http://usatoday30.usatoday.com/news/offbeat/2005-07-08-sheep-suicide_x.htm.

30. Daniel G. Amen, *Memory Rescue* (Carol Stream, IL: Tyndale, 2017), 235–36.

31. Andrew Reynolds et al., "Carbohydrate Quality and Human Health: A Series of Systematic Reviews and Meta-analyses," *Lancet* 393, no. 10170 (February 2, 2019): 434–45.

32. Cornell University, "Weighing Yourself Daily Can Tip the Scale in Your Favor," ScienceDaily, June 17, 2015, https://www.sciencedaily.com/releases/2015/06/150617134622.htm.

33. Chun-Ju Chiang et al., "Midlife Risk Factors for Subtypes of Dementia: A Nested Case-Control Study in Taiwan," *American Journal of Geriatric Psychiatry* 15, no. 9 (September 2007): 762–71.

Heidi White et al., "Weight Change in Alzheimer's Disease," *Journal of the American Geriatrics Society* 44, no. 3 (March 1996): 265–72.

34. Eric J. Shiroma et al., "Strength Training and the Risk of Type 2 Diabetes and Cardiovascular Disease," *Medicine and Science in Sports and Exercise* 49, no. 1 (January 2017): 40–46.

35. Frank B. Hu et al., "Walking Compared with Vigorous Physical Activity and Risk of Type 2 Diabetes in Women: A Prospective Study," *JAMA* 282, no. 15 (1999): 1433–39.

36. Carl J. Caspersen and Janet E. Fulton, "Epidemiology of Walking and Type 2 Diabetes," *Medicine and Science in Sports and Exercise* 40, suppl. 7 (July 2008): S519–S528.

37. Amen, *Memory Rescue*, 236.

38. Ibid.

39. Artemis P. Simopoulos, "Dietary Omega-3 Fatty Acid Deficiency and High Fructose Intake in the Development of Metabolic Syndrome, Brain Metabolic Abnormalities, and Non-alcoholic Fatty Liver Disease," *Nutrients* 5, no. 8 (July 26, 2013): 2901–23.

40. Luc Djoussé et al., "Plasma Omega-3 Fatty Acids and Incident Diabetes in Older Adults," *American Journal of Clinical Nutrition* 94, no. 2 (August 2011): 527–33.

41. Shokouh Sarbolouki et al., "Eicosapentaenoic Acid Improves Insulin Sensitivity and Blood Sugar in Overweight Type 2 Diabetic Mellitus Patients: A Double-Blind Randomized Clinical Trial," *Singapore Medical Journal* 54, no. 7 (2013): 387–90.

42. Kimberly A. Brownley et al., "A Double-Blind, Randomized Pilot Trial of Chromium Picolinate for Binge Eating Disorder: Results of the Binge Eating and Chromium (BEACh) Study," *Journal of Psychosomatic Research* 75, no. 1 (July 2013): 36–42.

43. N. Suksomboon, N. Poolsup, and A. Yuwanakorn, "Systematic Review and Meta-analysis of the Efficacy and Safety of Chromium Supplementation in Diabetes," *Journal of Clinical Pharmacy and Therapeutics* 39, no. 3 (2014): 292–306.

  H. Rabinovitz et al., "Effect of Chromium Supplementation on Blood Glucose and Lipid Levels in Type 2 Diabetes Mellitus Elderly Patients," *International Journal for Vitamin and Nutrition Research* 74, no. 3 (2004): 178–82.

44. Amen, *Memory Rescue*, 237.

45. Ting Lu et al., "Cinnamon Extract Improves Fasting Blood Glucose and Glycosylated Hemoglobin in Chinese Patients with Type 2 Diabetes," *Nutrition Research* (New York) 32, no. 6 (June 2012): 408–12.

  Paul A. Davis and Wallace Yokoyama, "Cinnamon Intake Lowers Fasting Blood Glucose: Meta-Analysis," *Journal of Medicinal Food* 14, no. 9 (September 2011): 884–89.

  Ashley Magistrelli and Jo Carol Chezem, "Effect of Ground Cinnamon on Postprandial Blood Glucose Concentration in Normal-Weight and Obese Adults," *Journal of the Academy of Nutrition and Dietetics* 112, no. 11 (November 2012): 1806–9.

  Ashley N. Hoehn and Amy L. Stockert, "The Effects of *Cinnamomum cassia* on Blood Glucose Values Are Greater Than Those of Dietary Changes Alone," *Nutrition and Metabolic Insights* 5 (2012): 77–83.

46. Mark L. Wahlqvist et al., "Cinnamon Users with Prediabetes Have a Better Fasting Working Memory: A Cross-Sectional Function Study," *Nutrition Research* (New York) 36, no. 4 (April 2016): 305–10.

47. Robert Krikorian et al., "Improved Cognitive-Cerebral Function in Older Adults with Chromium Supplementation," *Nutritional Neuroscience* 13, no. 3 (2010): 116–22.

CHAPTER 15: S IS FOR SLEEP

1. "Sleep and Sleep Disorder Statistics," American Sleep Association, accessed August 20, 2019, https://www.sleepassociation.org/about-sleep/sleep-statistics/.

2. Ibid.

3. "Sleep and Mental Health," Harvard Health Publishing, Harvard Medical School, updated March 18, 2019, http://www.health.harvard.edu/newsletter_article/sleep-and -mental-health.

4. "Sleep Disorders: The Connection between Sleep and Mental Health," National Alliance on Mental Illness, accessed August 20, 2019, https://www.nami.org/Learn-More/Mental -Health-Conditions/Related-Conditions/sleep-disorders.

5. David Nutt, Sue Wilson, and Louise Paterson, "Sleep Disorders as Core Symptoms of Depression," *Dialogues in Clinical Neuroscience* 10, no. 3 (September 2008): 329–36.

6. Alexandra K. Gold and Louisa G. Sylvia, "The Role of Sleep in Bipolar Disorder," *Nature and Science of Sleep* 8 (June 29, 2016): 207–14.

7. "Sleep and Mental Health," Harvard Health Publishing.

8. Samuele Cortese et al., "Sleep and Alertness in Children with Attention-Deficit/ Hyperactivity Disorder: A Systematic Review of the Literature," *Sleep* 29, no. 4 (2006): 504–11.

9. Kristine Yaffe et al., "Sleep-Disordered Breathing, Hypoxia, and Risk of Mild Cognitive Impairment and Dementia in Older Women," *JAMA* 306, no. 6 (2011): 613–19.

  Yo-El S. Ju, Brendan P. Lucey, and David M. Holtzman, "Sleep and Alzheimer Disease Pathology—A Bidirectional Relationship," *Nature Reviews Neurology* 10, no. 2 (February 2014): 115–19.

  Wei-Pin Chang et al., "Sleep Apnea and the Risk of Dementia: A Population-Based 5-Year Follow-Up Study in Taiwan," *PLOS One* 8 (October 24, 2013): e78655.

  Roxanne Sterniczuk et al., "Sleep Disturbance Is Associated with Incident Dementia and Mortality," *Current Alzheimer Research* 10, no. 7 (September 2013): 767–75.

10. Tori Rodriguez, "Teenagers Who Don't Get Enough Sleep at Higher Risk for Mental Health

Problems," Scientific American, July 1, 2015, https://www.scientificamerican.com/article
/teenagers-who-don-t-get-enough-sleep-at-higher-risk-for-mental-health-problems/.

11. R. Morgan Griffin, "The Health Risks of Shift Work," WebMD, March 25, 2010,
https://www.webmd.com/sleep-disorders/features/shift-work.

12. B. C. Tefft, "Acute Sleep Deprivation and Risk of Motor Vehicle Crash Involvement," AAA
Foundation for Traffic Safety, December 2016, https://aaafoundation.org/acute-sleep
-deprivation-risk-motor-vehicle-crash-involvement/.

13. Gregory Belenky et al., "The Effects of Sleep Deprivation on Performance during
Continuous Combat Operations," in *Food Components to Enhance Performance: An
Evaluation of Potential Performance-Enhancing Food Components for Operational Rations*,
Institute of Medicine (US) Committee on Military Nutrition Research, ed. Bernadette
M. Marriott (Washington, DC: National Academies Press, 1994), https://www.ncbi.nlm
.nih.gov/books/NBK209071/.

14. Daniel F. Kripke, Robert D. Langer, and Lawrence E. Kline, "Hypnotics' Association with
Mortality or Cancer: A Matched Cohort Study," *BMJ Open* 2, no. 1 (February 27, 2012):
e000850.

15. "Serious Ambien Side Effects: Memory, Depression, and More," American Addiction
Centers, last updated July 25, 2019, https://americanaddictioncenters.org/ambien
-treatment/side-effects.

16. Daniel G. Amen, *Memory Rescue* (Carol Stream, IL: Tyndale, 2017), 248.

17. Daniel G. Amen and Tana Amen, *The Brain Warrior's Way* (New York: New American
Library, 2016), 203.

18. Ibid., 205.

19. Ibid., 203.

20. László Harmat, Johanna Takács, and Róbert Bódizs, "Music Improves Sleep Quality
in Students," *Journal of Advanced Nursing* 62, no. 3 (May 2008): 327–35.

21. Amen and Amen, *Brain Warrior's Way*, 205.

22. Ibid.

23. Namni Goel, Hyungsoo Kim, and Raymund P. Lao, "An Olfactory Stimulus Modifies
Nighttime Sleep in Young Men and Women," *Chronobiology International* 22, no. 5 (2005):
889–904.

Mark Hardy, Michael D. Kirk-Smith, and David D. Stretch, "Replacement of Drug
Treatment for Insomnia by Ambient Odour," *Lancet* 346, no. 8976 (September 9, 1995):
701.

CHAPTER 16: MIND MEDS VERSUS NUTRACEUTICALS

1. Dnyanraj Choudhary, Sauvik Bhattacharyya, and Kedar Joshi, "Body Weight Management
in Adults under Chronic Stress through Treatment with Ashwagandha Root Extract:
A Double-Blind, Randomized, Placebo-Controlled Trial," *Journal of Evidence-Based
Complementary and Alternative Medicine* 22, no. 1 (January 2017): 96–106.

K. Chandrasekhar, Jyoti Kapoor, and Sridhar Anishetty, "A Prospective, Randomized
Double-Blind, Placebo-Controlled Study of Safety and Efficacy of a High-Concentration
Full-Spectrum Extract of Ashwagandha Root in Reducing Stress and Anxiety in Adults,"
Indian Journal of Psychological Medicine 34, no. 3 (July–September, 2012): 255–62.

Morgan A. Pratte et al., "An Alternative Treatment for Anxiety: A Systematic Review
of Human Trial Results Reported for the Ayurvedic Herb Ashwagandha (*Withania
somnifera*)," *Journal of Alternative and Complementary Medicine* 20, no. 12 (December
2014): 901–8.

Chittaranjan Andrade et al., "A Double-Blind, Placebo-Controlled Evaluation of the
Anxiolytic Efficacy of an Ethanolic Extract of *Withania somnifera*," *Indian Journal of
Psychiatry* 42, no. 3 (July–September 2000): 295–301.

2. Seyedeh Pardis Jahanbakhsh et al., "Evaluation of the Efficacy of *Withania somnifera*
(Ashwagandha) Root Extract in Patients with Obsessive-Compulsive Disorder: A

Randomized Double-Blind Placebo-Controlled Trial," *Complementary Therapies in Medicine* 27 (August 2016): 25–29.

3. Shinsuke Hidese et al., "Effects of Chronic L-theanine Administration in Patients with Major Depressive Disorder: An Open-Label Study," *Acta Neuropsychiatrica* 29, no. 2 (April 2017): 72–79.

   David J. White et al., "Anti-Stress, Behavioural and Magnetoencephalography Effects of an L-Theanine-Based Nutrient Drink: A Randomised, Double-Blind, Placebo-Controlled, Crossover Trial," *Nutrients* 8, no. 1 (January 19, 2016): e53.

   Keiko Unno et al., "Anti-stress Effect of Theanine on Students during Pharmacy Practice: Positive Correlation among Salivary α-amylase Activity, Trait Anxiety and Subjective Stress," *Pharmacology Biochemistry and Behavior* 111 (October 2013): 128–35.

   Ai Yoto et al., "Effects of L-theanine or Caffeine Intake on Changes in Blood Pressure under Physical and Psychological Stresses," *Journal of Physiological Anthropology* 31, no. 1 (October 29, 2012): 28.

   Michael S. Ritsner et al., "L-Theanine Relieves Positive, Activation, and Anxiety Symptoms in Patients with Schizophrenia and Schizoaffective Disorder: An 8-Week, Randomized, Double-Blind, Placebo-Controlled, 2-Center Study," *Journal of Clinical Psychiatry* 72, no. 1 (January 2011): 34–42.

   Kristy Lu et al., "The Acute Effects of L-theanine in Comparison with Alprazolam on Anticipatory Anxiety in Humans," *Human Psychopharmacology* 19, no. 7 (October 2004): 457–65.

   K. Kimura et al. "L-Theanine Reduces Psychological and Physiological Stress Responses," *Biological Psychology* 74, no. 1 (January 2007): 39–45.

4. Pamela Barbadoro et al., "Fish Oil Supplementation Reduces Cortisol Basal Levels and Perceived Stress: A Randomized, Placebo-Controlled Trial in Abstinent Alcoholics," *Molecular Nutrition and Food Research* 57, no. 6 (June 2013): 1110–14.

   Laure Buydens-Branchey, Marc Branchey, and Joseph R. Hibbeln, "Associations between Increases in Plasma n-3 Polyunsaturated Fatty Acids following Supplementation and Decreases in Anger and Anxiety in Substance Abusers," *Progress in Neuro-Psychopharmacology and Biological Psychiatry* 32, no. 2 (February 15, 2008): 568–75.

   Delbert G. Robinson et al., "A Potential Role for Adjunctive Omega-3 Polyunsaturated Fatty Acids for Depression and Anxiety Symptoms in Recent Onset Psychosis: Results from a 16 Week Randomized Placebo-Controlled Trial for Participants Concurrently Treated with Risperidone," *Schizophrenia Research* 204 (February 2019): 295–303.

   Janice K. Kiecolt-Glaser et al., "Omega-3 Supplementation Lowers Inflammation and Anxiety in Medical Students: A Randomized Controlled Trial," *Brain, Behavior, and Immunity* 25, no. 8 (November 2011): 1725–34.

   Felice N. Jacka et al., "Dietary Intake of Fish and PUFA, and Clinical Depressive and Anxiety Disorders in Women," *British Journal of Nutrition* 109, no. 11 (June 2013): 2059–66.

   Kenta Matsumura et al., "Effects of Omega-3 Polyunsaturated Fatty Acids on Psychophysiological Symptoms of Post-Traumatic Stress Disorder in Accident Survivors: A Randomized, Double-Blind, Placebo-Controlled Trial," *Journal of Affective Disorders* 224 (December 15, 2017): 27–31.

   Kuan-Pin Su et al., "Association of Use of Omega-3 Polyunsaturated Fatty Acids with Changes in Severity of Anxiety Symptoms: A Systematic Review and Meta-analysis," *JAMA Network Open* 1, no. 5 (September 14, 2018): e182327.

5. Joseph Levine, "Controlled Trials of Inositol in Psychiatry," *European Neuropsychopharmacology* 7, no. 2 (May 1997): 147–55.

6. P. D. Carey et al., "Single Photon Emission Computed Tomography (SPECT) in Obsessive-Compulsive Disorder before and after Treatment with Inositol," *Metabolic Brain Disease* 19, nos. 1–2 (June 2004): 125–34.

7. Alex Palatnik et al., "Double-Blind, Controlled, Crossover Trial of Inositol versus Fluvoxamine for the Treatment of Panic Disorder," *Journal of Clinical Psychopharmacology* 21, no. 3 (June 2001): 335–39.

8. Adham M. Abdou et al., "Relaxation and Immunity Enhancement Effects of γ-Aminobutyric Acid (GABA) Administration in Humans," *Biofactors* 26, no. 3 (2006): 201–8.

9. Neil Bernard Boyle, Clare Lawton, and Louise Dye, "The Effects of Magnesium Supplementation on Subjective Anxiety and Stress–A Systematic Review," *Nutrients* 9, no. 5 (April 26, 2017): e429.

Emily K. Tarleton et al., "Role of Magnesium Supplementation in the Treatment of Depression: A Randomized Clinical Trial," *PLOS One* 12, no. 6 (June 27, 2017): e0180067.

Miriam C. de Souza et al., "A Synergistic Effect of a Daily Supplement for 1 Month of 200 mg Magnesium Plus 50 mg Vitamin B6 for the Relief of Anxiety-Related Premenstrual Symptoms: A Randomized, Double-Blind, Crossover Study," *Journal of Women's Health and Gender-Based Medicine* 9, no. 2 (2000): 131–39.

Gordana Kovacevic et al., "A 6-Month Follow-Up of Disability, Quality of Life, and Depressive and Anxiety Symptoms in Pediatric Migraine with Magnesium Prophylaxis," *Magnesium Research* 30, no. 4 (October–December 2017): 133–41.

10. Etienne Pouteau et al., "Superiority of Magnesium and Vitamin B6 over Magnesium Alone on Severe Stress in Healthy Adults with Low Magnesemia: A Randomized, Single-Blind Clinical Trial," *PLOS One* 13, no. 12 (December 18, 2018): e0208454.

11. Alireza Milajerdi et al., "The Effects of Alcoholic Extract of Saffron (*Crocus satious* L.) on Mild to Moderate Comorbid Depression-Anxiety, Sleep Quality, and Life Satisfaction in Type 2 Diabetes Mellitus: A Double-Blind, Randomized and Placebo-Controlled Clinical Trial," *Complementary Therapies in Medicine* 41 (December 2018): 196–202.

Adrian L. Lopresti et al., "Affron, a Standardised Extract from Saffron (*Crocus sativus* L.) for the Treatment of Youth Anxiety and Depressive Symptoms: A Randomised, Double-Blind, Placebo-Controlled Study," *Journal of Affective Disorders* 232 (May 2018): 349–57.

Mohsen Mazidi et al., "A Double-Blind, Randomized and Placebo-Controlled Trial of Saffron (*Crocus sativus* L.) in the Treatment of Anxiety and Depression," *Journal of Complementary and Integrative Medicine* 13, no. 2 (2016): 195–99.

Sophia Esalatmanesh et al., "Comparison of Saffron and Fluvoxamine in the Treatment of Mild to Moderate Obsessive-Compulsive Disorder: A Double Blind Randomized Clinical Trial," *Iranian Journal of Psychiatry* 12, no. 3 (July 2017): 154–62.

12. Jerome Sarris, "Herbal Medicines in the Treatment of Psychiatric Disorders: 10-Year Updated Review," *Phytotherapy Research* 32, no. 7 (July 2018): 1147–62.

Liliane-Poconé Dantas et al., "Effects of *Passiflora incarnata* and Midazolam for Control of Anxiety in Patients Undergoing Dental Extraction," *Medicina Oral Patologia Oral y Cirugia Bucal* 22, no. 1 (January 2017): e95–101.

13. Benjamin J. Malcolm and Kimberly Tallian, "Essential Oil of Lavender in Anxiety Disorders: Ready for Prime Time?" *Mental Health Clinician* 7, no. 4 (July 2017): 147–55.

A. Henneman et al., "Lavender Oil Supplementation for the Management of Anxiety Disorder," *Medical Case Reports and Reviews* 1, no. 2 (June 8, 2018): 1–5.

14. René S. Kahn et al., "Effect of a Serotonin Precursor and Uptake Inhibitor in Anxiety Disorders; a Double-Blind Comparison of 5-Hydroxytryptophan, Clomipramine and Placebo," *International Clinical Psychopharmacology* 2, no. 1 (January 1987): 33–45.

Koen Schruers et al., "Acute L-5-Hydroxytryptophan Administration Inhibits Carbon Dioxide-Induced Panic in Panic Disorder Patients," *Psychiatry Research* 113, no. 3 (December 30, 2002): 237–43.

E. Emanuele et al., "An Open-Label Trial of L-5-Hydroxytryptophan in Subjects with Romantic Stress," *Neuroendocrinology Letters* 31, no. 5 (2010): 663–66.

15. Sara-Jayne Long and David Benton, "Effects of Vitamin and Mineral Supplementation on Stress, Mild Psychiatric Symptoms, and Mood in Nonclinical Samples: A Meta-Analysis," *Psychosomatic Medicine* 75, no. 2 (February/March 2013): 144–53.

Julia J. Rucklidge et al., "Shaken but Unstirred? Effects of Micronutrients on Stress and Trauma after an Earthquake: RCT Evidence Comparing Formulas and Doses," *Human Psychopharmacology* 27, no. 5 (September 2012): 440–54.

Bonnie J. Kaplan et al., "A Randomised Trial of Nutrient Supplements to Minimise Psychological Stress after a Natural Disaster," *Psychiatry Research* 228, no. 3 (August 30, 2015): 373–79.

Julia Rucklidge et al., "Micronutrients Reduce Stress and Anxiety in Adults with Attention-Deficit/Hyperactivity Disorder following a 7.1 Earthquake," *Psychiatry Research* 189, no. 2 (September 30, 2011): 281–87.

16. Daniel L. C. Costa et al., "Randomized, Double-Blind, Placebo-Controlled Trial of *N*-Acetylcysteine Augmentation for Treatment-Resistant Obsessive-Compulsive Disorder," *Journal of Clinical Psychiatry* 78, no. 7 (July 2017): e766–73.

Hamid Afshar et al., "*N*-Acetylcysteine Add-On Treatment in Refractory Obsessive-Compulsive Disorder: A Randomized, Double-Blind, Placebo-Controlled Trial," *Journal of Clinical Psychopharmacology* 32, no. 6 (December 2012): 797–803.

17. Sudie E. Back et al., "A Double-Blind, Randomized, Controlled Pilot Trial of *N*-Acetylcysteine in Veterans with Posttraumatic Stress Disorder and Substance Use Disorders," *Journal of Clinical Psychiatry* 77, no. 11 (November 2016): e1439–46.

18. Jennifer McKean et al., "Probiotics and Subclinical Psychological Symptoms in Healthy Participants: A Systematic Review and Meta-Analysis," *Journal of Alternative and Complementary Medicine* 23, no. 4 (April 2017): 249–58.

A. P. Allen et al., "*Bifidobacterium longum* 1714 as a Translational Psychobiotic: Modulation of Stress, Electrophysiology and Neurocognition in Healthy Volunteers," *Translational Psychiatry* 6, no. 11 (November 1, 2016): e939.

M. Takada et al., "Probiotic *Lactobacillus casei* Strain Shirota Relieves Stress-Associated Symptoms by Modulating the Gut–Brain Interaction in Human and Animal Models," *Neurogastroenterology and Motility* 28, no. 7 (July 2016): 1027–36.

Ali Akbar Mohammadi et al., "The Effects of Probiotics on Mental Health and Hypothalamic–Pituitary–Adrenal Axis: A Randomized, Double-Blind, Placebo-Controlled Trial in Petrochemical Workers," *Nutritional Neuroscience* 19, no. 9 (2016): 387–95.

Hui Yang et al., "Probiotics Reduce Psychological Stress in Patients before Laryngeal Cancer Surgery," *Asia-Pacific Journal of Clinical Oncology* 12, no. 1 (March 2016): e92–96.

Michaël Messaoudi et al., "Beneficial Psychological Effects of a Probiotic Formulation (*Lactobacillus helveticus* R0052 and *Bifidobacterium longum* R0175) in Healthy Human Volunteers," *Gut Microbes* 2, no. 4 (July/August 2011): 256–61.

19. Mark Cropley, Adrian P. Banks, and Julia Boyle, "The Effects of *Rhodiola rosea* L. Extract on Anxiety, Stress, Cognition and Other Mood Symptoms," *Phytotherapy Research* 29, no. 12 (December 2015): 1934–39.

Alexander Bystritsky, Lauren Kerwin, and Jamie D. Feusner, "A Pilot Study of *Rhodiola rosea* (Rhodax) for Generalized Anxiety Disorder (GAD)," *Journal of Alternative and Complementary Medicine* 14, no. 2 (March 2008): 175–80.

D. Edwards, A. Heufelder, and A. Zimmermann, "Therapeutic Effects and Safety of Rhodiola rosea Extract WS 1375 in Subjects with Life-Stress Symptoms—Results of an Open-Label Study," *Phytotherapy Research* 26, no. 8 (August 2012): 1220–25.

20. H. Woelk et al., "*Ginkgo biloba* Special Extract EGb 761 in Generalized Anxiety Disorder and Adjustment Disorder with Anxious Mood: A Randomized, Double-Blind, Placebo-Controlled Trial," *Journal of Psychiatric Research* 41, no. 6 (September 2007): 472–80.

21. Shawn M. Talbott, Julie A. Talbott, and Mike Pugh, "Effect of *Magnolia officinalis* and *Phellodendron amurense* (Relora) on Cortisol and Psychological Mood State in Moderately Stressed Subjects," *Journal of the International Society of Sports Nutrition* 10 (August 7, 2013): 37.

Douglas S. Kalman et al., "Effect of a Proprietary *Magnolia* and *Phellodendron* Extract on Stress Levels in Healthy Women: A Pilot, Double-Blind, Placebo-Controlled Clinical Trial," *Nutrition Journal* 7 (April 21, 2008): 11.

22. Zabun Nahar et al., "Comparative Analysis of Serum Manganese, Zinc, Calcium, Copper and Magnesium Level in Panic Disorder Patients," *Biological Trace Element Research* 133, no. 3 (March 2010): 284–90.

23. Jane Pei-Chen Chang et al., "Omega-3 Polyunsaturated Fatty Acids in Youths with Attention Deficit Hyperactivity Disorder: A Systematic Review and Meta-Analysis of Clinical Trials and Biological Studies," *Neuropsychopharmacology* 43, no. 3 (February 2018): 534–45.

    E. Derbyshire, "Do Omega-3/6 Fatty Acids Have a Therapeutic Role in Children and Young People with ADHD?" *Journal of Lipids* 2017 (2017): 6285218.

    Dienke J. Bos et al., "Reduced Symptoms of Inattention after Dietary Omega-3 Fatty Acid Supplementation in Boys with and without Attention Deficit/Hyperactivity Disorder," *Neuropsychopharmacology* 40, no. 10 (September 2015): 2298–306.

    Catherine M. Milte et al., "Increased Erythrocyte Eicosapentaenoic Acid and Docosahexaenoic Acid Are Associated with Improved Attention and Behavior in Children with ADHD in a Randomized Controlled Three-Way Crossover Trial," *Journal of Attention Disorders* 19, no. 11 (November 2015): 954–64.

    M. Hariri et al., "Effect of n-3 Supplementation on Hyperactivity, Oxidative Stress and Inflammatory Mediators in Children with Attention-Deficit-Hyperactivity Disorder," *Malaysian Journal of Nutrition* 18, no. 3 (December 2012): 329–35.

    Per A. Gustafsson et al., "EPA Supplementation Improves Teacher-Rated Behaviour and Oppositional Symptoms in Children with ADHD," *Acta Paediatrica* 99, no. 10 (October 2010): 1540–49.

24. S. Hirayama et al., "The Effect of Phosphatidylserine Administration on Memory and Symptoms of Attention-Deficit Hyperactivity Disorder: A Randomised, Double-Blind, Placebo-Controlled Clinical Trial," *Journal of Human Nutrition and Dietetics* 27, suppl. 2 (April 2014): 284–91.

    I. Manor et al., "The Effect of Phosphatidylserine Containing Omega3 Fatty-Acids on Attention-Deficit Hyperactivity Disorder Symptoms in Children: A Double-Blind Placebo-Controlled Trial, Followed by an Open-Label Extension," *European Psychiatry* 27, no. 5 (July 2012): 335–42.

25. L. Eugene Arnold et al., "Zinc for Attention-Deficit/Hyperactivity Disorder: Placebo-Controlled Double-Blind Pilot Trial Alone and Combined with Amphetamine," *Journal of Child and Adolescent Psychopharmacology* 21, no. 1 (February 2011): 1–19.

    Yasemin Üçkardeş et al., "Effects of Zinc Supplementation on Parent and Teacher Behaviour Rating Scores in Low Socioeconomic Level Turkish Primary School Children," *Acta Paediatrica* 98, no. 4 (April 2009): 731–36.

    Mustafa Bilici et al., "Double-Blind, Placebo-Controlled Study of Zinc Sulfate in the Treatment of Attention Deficit Hyperactivity Disorder," *Progress in Neuro-Psychopharmacology and Biological Psychiatry* 28, no. 1 (January 2004): 181–90.

26. R. Luzzi et al., "Pycnogenol Supplementation Improves Cognitive Function, Attention and Mental Performance in Students," *Panminerva Medica* 53, no. 3, suppl. 1 (September 2011): 75–82.

    Zuzana Chovanová et al., "Effect of Polyphenolic Extract, Pycnogenol, on the Level of 8Oxoguanine in Children Suffering from Attention Deficit/Hyperactivity Disorder," *Free Radical Research* 40, no. 9 (2006): 1003–10.

    Jana Trebatická et al., "Treatment of ADHD with French Maritime Pine Bark Extract, Pycnogenol," *European Child and Adolescent Psychiatry* 15, no. 6 (September 2006): 329–35.

27. Farida El Baza et al., "Magnesium Supplementation in Children with Attention Deficit Hyperactivity Disorder," *Egyptian Journal of Medical Human Genetics* 17, no. 1 (January 2016): 63–70.

    M. Mousain-Bosc et al., "Improvement of Neurobehavioral Disorders in Children Supplemented with Magnesium-Vitamin B6," *Magnesium Research* 19, no. 1 (March 2006): 46–52.

Michael Huss, Andreas Völp, and Manuela Stauss-Grabo, "Supplementation of Polyunsaturated Fatty Acids, Magnesium and Zinc in Children Seeking Medical Advice for Attention-Deficit/Hyperactivity Problems—An Observational Cohort Study," *Lipids in Health and Disease* 9 (September 24, 2010): 105.

28. Erik M. G. Olsson, Bo von Schéele, and Alexander G. Panossian, "A Randomised, Double-Blind, Placebo-Controlled, Parallel-Group Study of the Standardised Extract SHR-5 of the Roots of *Rhodiola rosea* in the Treatment of Subjects with Stress-Related Fatigue," *Planta Medica* 75, no. 2 (2009): 105–12.

V. Darbinyan et al., "*Rhodiola rosea* in Stress Induced Fatigue—A Double Blind Cross-Over Study of a Standardized Extract SHR-5 with a Repeated Low-Dose Regimen on the Mental Performance of Healthy Physicians during Night Duty," *Phytomedicine* 7, no. 5 (October 2000): 365–71.

V. Fintelmann and J. Gruenwald, "Efficacy and Tolerability of a *Rhodiola rosea* Extract in Adults with Physical and Cognitive Deficiencies," *Advances in Therapy* 24, no. 4 (July/August 2007): 929–39.

V. A. Shevtsov et al., "A Randomized Trial of Two Different Doses of a SHR-5 *Rhodiola rosea* Extract versus Placebo and Control of Capacity for Mental Work," *Phytomedicine* 10, nos. 2–3 (2003): 95–105.

A. A. Spasov et al., "A Double-Blind, Placebo-Controlled Pilot Study of the Stimulating and Adaptogenic Effect of *Rhodiola rosea* SHR-5 Extract on the Fatigue of Students Caused by Stress during an Examination Period with a Repeated Low-Dose Regimen," *Phytomedicine* 7, no. 2 (April 2000): 85–89.

A. A. Spasov, V. B. Mandrikov, and I. A. Mironova, "The Effect of the Preparation Rodakson on the Psychophysiological and Physical Adaptation of Students to an Academic Load," *Eksperimental'naia i Klinicheskaia Farmakologiia* 63, no. 1 (January/February 2000): 76–78.

29. Hae-Jin Ko et al., "Effects of Korean Red Ginseng Extract on Behavior in Children with Symptoms of Inattention and Hyperactivity/Impulsivity: A Double-Blind Randomized Placebo-Controlled Trial," *Journal of Child and Adolescent Psychopharmacology* 24, no. 9 (November 2014): 501–8.

Hyeong-Geug Kim et al., "Antifatigue Effects of *Panax ginseng* C.A. Meyer: A Randomised, Double-Blind, Placebo-Controlled Trial," *PLOS One* 8, no. 4 (April 17, 2013): e61271.

D. O. Kennedy, A. B. Scholey, and K. A. Wesnes, "Dose Dependent Changes in Cognitive Performance and Mood following Acute Administration of *Ginseng* to Healthy Young Volunteers," *Nutritional Neuroscience* 4, no. 4 (2001): 295–310.

30. Dnyanraj Choudhary, Sauvik Bhattacharyya, and Sekhar Bose, "Efficacy and Safety of Ashwagandha (*Withania somnifera* (L.) Dunal) Root Extract in Improving Memory and Cognitive Functions," *Journal of Dietary Supplements* 14, no. 6 (2017): 599–612.

Bakhtiar Choudhary, A. Shetty, and Deepak G. Langade, "Efficacy of Ashwagandha (*Withania somnifera* [L.] Dunal) in Improving Cardiorespiratory Endurance in Healthy Athletic Adults," *Ayu* 36, no. 1 (January–March 2015): 63–68.

31. S. Borgwardt et al., "Neural Effects of Green Tea Extract on Dorsolateral Prefrontal Cortex," *European Journal of Clinical Nutrition* 66, no. 11 (November 2012): 1187–92.

32. Julia J. Rucklidge et al., "Vitamin-Mineral Treatment Improves Aggression and Emotional Regulation in Children with ADHD: A Fully Blinded, Randomized, Placebo-Controlled Trial," *Journal of Child Psychology and Psychiatry* 59, no. 3 (March 2018): 232–46.

33. U. P. Dave et al., "An Open-Label Study to Elucidate the Effects of Standardized *Bacopa monnieri* Extract in the Management of Symptoms of Attention-Deficit Hyperactivity Disorder in Children," *Advances in Mind-Body Medicine* 28, no. 2 (Spring 2014): 10–15.

34. Kobra Tahmasebi et al., "Association of Mood Disorders with Serum Zinc Concentrations in Adolescent Female Students," *Biological Trace Element Research* 178, no. 2 (August 2017): 180–88.

35. David Mischoulon et al., "A Double-Blind, Randomized Controlled Trial of Ethyl-Eicosapentaenoate for Major Depressive Disorder," *Journal of Clinical Psychiatry* 70, no. 12 (December 2009): 1636–44.

Julian G. Martins, "EPA but Not DHA Appears to Be Responsible for the Efficacy of Omega-3 Long Chain Polyunsaturated Fatty Acid Supplementation in Depression: Evidence from a Meta-Analysis of Randomized Controlled Trials," *Journal of the American College of Nutrition* 28, no. 5 (2009): 525–42.

François Lespérance et al., "The Efficacy of Omega-3 Supplementation for Major Depression: A Randomized Controlled Trial," *Journal of Clinical Psychiatry* 72, no. 8 (August 2011): 1054–62.

Mariangela Rondanelli et al., "Long Chain Omega 3 Polyunsaturated Fatty Acids Supplementation in the Treatment of Elderly Depression: Effects on Depressive Symptoms, on Phospholipids Fatty Acids Profile and on Health-Related Quality of Life," *Journal of Nutrition, Health and Aging* 15, no. 1 (2011): 37–44.

Mehri Jamilian et al., "The Effects of Omega-3 and Vitamin E Co-supplementation on Parameters of Mental Health and Gene Expression Related to Insulin and Inflammation in Subjects with Polycystic Ovary Syndrome," *Journal of Affective Disorders* 229 (March 15, 2018): 41–47.

M. Elizabeth Sublette et al., "Meta-Analysis of the Effects of Eicosapentaenoic Acid (EPA) in Clinical Trials in Depression," *Journal of Clinical Psychiatry* 72, no. 12 (December 2011): 1577–84.

Maciej Haberka et al., "Effects of n-3 Polyunsaturated Fatty Acids on Depressive Symptoms, Anxiety and Emotional State in Patients with Acute Myocardial Infarction," *Pharmacological Reports* 65, no. 1 (2013): 59–68.

36. Klaus Linde, Michael M. Berner, Levente Kriston, "St John's Wort for Major Depression," *Cochrane Database of Systematic Reviews* no. 4 (October 8, 2008): CD000448.

Maurizio Fava et al., "A Double-Blind, Randomized Trial of St John's Wort, Fluoxetine, and Placebo in Major Depressive Disorder," *Journal of Clinical Psychopharmacology* 25, no. 5 (October 2005): 441–47.

Jerome Sarris et al., "Conditional Probability of Response or Nonresponse of Placebo Compared with Antidepressants or St John's Wort in Major Depressive Disorder," *Journal of Clinical Psychopharmacology* 33, no. 6 (December 2013): 827–30.

37. Xiangying Yang et al., "Comparative Efficacy and Safety of *Crocus sativus* L. for Treating Mild to Moderate Major Depressive Disorder in Adults: A Meta-analysis of Randomized Controlled Trials," *Neuropsychiatric Disease and Treatment* 2018, no. 14 (May 21, 2018): 1297–305.

Graham Kell et al., "Affron a Novel Saffron Extract (*Crocus sativus* L.) Improves Mood in Healthy Adults over 4 Weeks in a Double-Blind, Parallel, Randomized, Placebo-Controlled Clinical Trial," *Complementary Therapies in Medicine* 33 (August 2017): 58–64.

Lopresti et al., "Affron, a Standardised Extract," 349–57.

Gholamali Jelodar et al., "Saffron Improved Depression and Reduced Homocysteine Level in Patients with Major Depression: A Randomized, Double-Blind Study," *Avicenna Journal of Phytomedicine* 8, no. 1 (January/February 2018): 43–50.

38. A. L. Williams et al., "S-Adenosylmethionine (SAMe) as Treatment for Depression: A Systematic Review," *Clinical and Investigative Medicine* 28, no. 3 (June 2005): 132–39.

Jerome Sarris et al., "S-Adenosyl Methionine (SAMe) versus Escitalopram and Placebo in Major Depression RCT: Efficacy and Effects of Histamine and Carnitine as Moderators of Response," *Journal of Affective Disorders* 164 (August 1, 2014): 76–81.

George I. Papakostas et al., "S-Adenosyl Methionine (SAMe) Augmentation of Serotonin Reuptake Inhibitors for Antidepressant Nonresponders with Major Depressive Disorder: A Double-Blind, Randomized Clinical Trial," *American Journal of Psychiatry* 167, no. 8 (August 2010): 942–48.

R. Andrew Shippy et al., "S-Adenosylmethionine (SAM-e) for the Treatment of Depression in People Living with HIV/AIDS," *BMC Psychiatry* 4 (November 11, 2004): 38.

K. M. Bell et al., "S-Adenosylmethionine Treatment of Depression: A Controlled Clinical Trial," *American Journal of Psychiatry* 145, no. 9 (September 1988): 1110–14.

P. Salmaggi et al., "Double-Blind, Placebo-Controlled Study of S-Adenosyl-*L*-Methionine in Depressed Postmenopausal Women," *Psychotherapy and Psychosomatics* 59, no. 1 (1993): 34–40.

K. M. Bell et al., "S-Adenosylmethionine Blood Levels in Major Depression: Changes with Drug Treatment," *Acta Neurologica Scandinavica* 89, no. S154 (May 1994): 15–18.

Roberto Delle Chiaie, Paolo Pancheri, and Pierluigi Scapicchio, "Efficacy and Tolerability of Oral and Intramuscular S-Adenosyl-L-Methionine 1,4-Butanedisulfonate (SAMe) in the Treatment of Major Depression: Comparison with Imipramine in 2 Multicenter Studies," *American Journal of Clinical Nutrition* 76, no. 5 (November 2002): 1172S–76S.

Anup Sharma et al., "S-Adenosylmethionine (SAMe) for Neuropsychiatric Disorders: A Clinician-Oriented Review of Research," *Journal of Clinical Psychiatry* 78, no. 6 (June 2017): e656–67.

39. Adrian L. Lopresti and Peter D. Drummond, "Efficacy of Curcumin, and a Saffron/Curcumin Combination for the Treatment of Major Depression: A Randomised, Double-Blind, Placebo-Controlled Study," *Journal of Affective Disorders* 207 (January 1, 2017): 188–96.

Jayesh Sanmukhani et al., "Efficacy and Safety of Curcumin in Major Depressive Disorder: A Randomized Controlled Trial," *Phytotherapy Research* 28, no. 4 (April 2014): 579–85.

Adrian L. Lopresti et al., "Curcumin for the Treatment of Major Depression: A Randomised, Double-Blind, Placebo Controlled Study," *Journal of Affective Disorders* 167 (October 1, 2014): 368–75.

Buranee Kanchanatawan et al., "Add-on Treatment with Curcumin Has Antidepressive Effects in Thai Patients with Major Depression: Results of a Randomized Double-Blind Placebo-Controlled Study," *Neurotoxicity Research* 33, no. 3 (April 2018): 621–33.

Jing-Jie Yu et al., "Chronic Supplementation of Curcumin Enhances the Efficacy of Antidepressants in Major Depressive Disorder: A Randomized, Double-Blind, Placebo-Controlled Pilot Study," *Journal of Clinical Psychopharmacology* 35, no. 4 (August 2015): 406–10.

40. Jun Lai et al., "The Efficacy of Zinc Supplementation in Depression: Systematic Review of Randomised Controlled Trials," *Journal of Affective Disorders* 136, nos. 1–2 (January 2012): e31–39.

Ann M. DiGirolamo et al., "Randomized Trial of the Effect of Zinc Supplementation on the Mental Health of School-Age Children in Guatemala," *American Journal of Clinical Nutrition* 92, no. 5 (November 2010): 1241–50.

Zahra Solati et al., "Zinc Monotherapy Increases Serum Brain-Derived Neurotrophic Factor (BDNF) Levels and Decreases Depressive Symptoms in Overweight or Obese Subjects: A Double-Blind, Randomized, Placebo-Controlled Trial," *Nutritional Neuroscience* 18, no. 4 (2015): 162–68.

Elham Ranjbar et al., "Effects of Zinc Supplementation on Efficacy of Antidepressant Therapy, Inflammatory Cytokines, and Brain-Derived Neurotrophic Factor in Patients with Major Depression," *Nutritional Neuroscience* 17, no. 2 (2014): 65–71.

Soheila Salari et al., "Zinc Sulphate: A Reasonable Choice for Depression Management in Patients with Multiple Sclerosis: A Randomized, Double-Blind, Placebo-Controlled Clinical Trial," *Pharmacological Reports* 67, no. 3 (June 2015): 606–9.

T. Sawada and K. Yokoi, "Effect of Zinc Supplementation on Mood States in Young Women: A Pilot Study," *European Journal of Clinical Nutrition* 64, no. 3 (March 2010): 331–33.

41. Afsaneh Rajizadeh et al., "Effect of Magnesium Supplementation on Depression Status in

Depressed Patients with Magnesium Deficiency: A Randomized, Double-Blind, Placebo-Controlled Trial," *Nutrition* 35 (March 2017): 56–60.

Tarleton et al., "Role of Magnesium Supplementation," e0180067.

42. Purushottam Jangid et al., "Comparative Study of Efficacy of L-5-Hydroxytryptophan and Fluoxetine in Patients Presenting with First Depressive Episode," *Asian Journal of Psychiatry* 6, no. 1 (February 2013): 29–34.

    Brent M. Kious et al., "An Open-Label Pilot Study of Combined Augmentation with Creatine Monohydrate and 5-Hydroxytryptophan for Selective Serotonin Reuptake Inhibitor–or Serotonin-Norepinephrine Reuptake Inhibitor–Resistant Depression in Adult Women," *Journal of Clinical Psychopharmacology* 37, no. 5 (October 2017): 578–83.

    J. J. Rousseau, "Effects of a Levo-5-Hydroxytryptophan-Dihydroergocristine Combination on Depression and Neuropsychic Performance: A Double-Blind Placebo-Controlled Clinical Trial in Elderly Patients," *Clinical Therapeutics* 9, no. 3 (1987): 267–72.

    J. Angst, B. Woggon, and J. Schoepf, "The Treatment of Depression with L-5-Hydroxytryptophan versus Imipramine. Results of Two Open and One Double-Blind Study," *Archiv für Psychiatrie Nervenkrankheiten* 224, no. 2 (October 11, 1977 [1970]): 175–86.

43. Jonathan E. Alpert et al., "Folinic Acid (Leucovorin) as an Adjunctive Treatment for SSRI-Refractory Depression," *Annals of Clinical Psychiatry* 14, no. 1 (March 2002): 33–38.

    George I. Papakostas et al., "L-Methylfolate as Adjunctive Therapy for SSRI-Resistant Major Depression: Results of Two Randomized, Double-Blind, Parallel-Sequential Trials," *American Journal of Psychiatry* 169, no. 12 (December 2012): 1267–74.

    George I. Papakostas et al., "Effect of Adjunctive L-Methylfolate 15 mg among Inadequate Responders to SSRIs in Depressed Patients Who Were Stratified by Biomarker Levels and Genotype: Results from a Randomized Clinical Trial," *Journal of Clinical Psychiatry* 75, no. 8 (August 2014): 855–63.

    John M. Zajecka et al., "Long-Term Efficacy, Safety, and Tolerability of L-Methylfolate Calcium 15 mg as Adjunctive Therapy with Selective Serotonin Reuptake Inhibitors: A 12-Month, Open-Label Study following a Placebo-Controlled Acute Study," *Journal of Clinical Psychiatry* 77, no. 5 (May 2016): 654–60.

44. Brisa S. Fernandes, et al., "N-Acetylcysteine in Depressive Symptoms and Functionality: A Systematic Review and Meta-Analysis," *Journal of Clinical Psychiatry* 77, no. 4 (April 2016): e457–66.

    Michael Berk et al., "N-Acetyl Cysteine for Depressive Symptoms in Bipolar Disorder—A Double-Blind Randomized Placebo-Controlled Trial," *Biological Psychiatry* 64, no. 6 (September 15, 2008): 468–75.

    Kyoko Hasebe et al., "Adjunctive *N*-acetylcysteine in Depression: Exploration of Interleukin-6, C-Reactive Protein and Brain-Derived Neurotrophic Factor," *Acta Neuropsychiatrica* 29, no. 6 (December 2017): 337–46.

45. Michael Berk et al., "The Efficacy of Adjunctive *N*-Acetylcysteine in Major Depressive Disorder: A Double-Blind, Randomized, Placebo-Controlled Trial," *Journal of Clinical Psychiatry* 75, no. 6 (June 2014): 628–36.

46. M. Maggioni et al., "Effects of Phosphatidylserine Therapy in Geriatric Patients with Depressive Disorders," *Acta Psychiatrica Scandinavica* 81, no. 3 (March 1990): 265–70.

    Teruhisa Komori, "The Effects of Phosphatidylserine and Omega-3 Fatty Acid-Containing Supplement on Late Life Depression," *Mental Illness* 7, no. 1 (February 24, 2015): 5647.

    D. Benton et al., "The Influence of Phosphatidylserine on Mood and Heart Rate When Faced with an Acute Stressor," *Nutritional Neuroscience* 4, no. 3 (2001): 169–78.

47. Jun J. Mao et al., "*Rhodiola rosea* versus Sertraline for Major Depressive Disorder: A Randomized Placebo-Controlled Trial," *Phytomedicine* 22, no. 3 (March 15, 2015): 394–99.

    V. Darbinyan et al., "Clinical Trial of *Rhodiola rosea* L. Extract SHR-5 in the Treatment of Mild to Moderate Depression," *Nordic Journal of Psychiatry* 61, no. 5 (2007): 343–48.

48. Phuong H. Nguyen et al., "Impact of Preconceptional Micronutrient Supplementation on

Maternal Mental Health during Pregnancy and Postpartum: Results from a Randomized Controlled Trial in Vietnam," *BMC Women's Health* 17, no. 1 (June 17, 2017): 44.

49. Zahra Sepehrmanesh et al., "Vitamin D Supplementation Affects the Beck Depression Inventory, Insulin Resistance, and Biomarkers of Oxidative Stress in Patients with Major Depressive Disorder: A Randomized, Controlled Clinical Trial," *Journal of Nutrition* 146, no. 2 (February 2016): 243–48.

Farideh Vaziri et al., "A Randomized Controlled Trial of Vitamin D Supplementation on Perinatal Depression: in Iranian Pregnant Mothers," *BMC Pregnancy and Childbirth* 16 (August 20, 2016): 239.

Ying Wang et al., "Efficacy of High-Dose Supplementation with Oral Vitamin D3 on Depressive Symptoms in Dialysis Patients with Vitamin D3 Insufficiency: A Prospective, Randomized, Double-Blind Study," *Journal of Clinical Psychopharmacology* 36, no. 3 (June 2016): 229–35.

Nahereh Khoraminya et al., "Therapeutic Effects of Vitamin D as Adjunctive Therapy to Fluoxetine in Patients with Major Depressive Disorder," *Australian and New Zealand Journal of Psychiatry* 47, no. 3 (March 2013): 271–75.

R. Jorde et al., "Effects of Vitamin D Supplementation on Symptoms of Depression in Overweight and Obese Subjects: Randomized Double Blind Trial," *Journal of Internal Medicine* 264, no. 6 (December 2008): 599–609.

F. M. Gloth, W. Alam, and B. Hollis, "Vitamin D vs Broad Spectrum Phototherapy in the Treatment of Seasonal Affective Disorder," *Journal of Nutrition Health and Aging* 3, no. 1 (1999): 5–7.

Allen T. Lansdowne and Stephen C. Provost, "Vitamin D3 Enhances Mood in Healthy Subjects during Winter," *Psychopharmacology* (Berlin) 135, no. 4 (February 1998): 319–23.

50. Ghodarz Akkasheh et al., "Clinical and Metabolic Response to Probiotic Administration in Patients with Major Depressive Disorder: A Randomized, Double-Blind, Placebo-Controlled Trial," *Nutrition* 32, no. 3 (March 2016): 315–20.

Fariba Raygan et al., "The Effects of Vitamin D and Probiotic Co-supplementation on Mental Health Parameters and Metabolic Status in Type 2 Diabetic Patients with Coronary Heart Disease: A Randomized, Double-Blind, Placebo-Controlled Trial," *Progress in Neuro-Psychopharmacology and Biological Psychiatry* 84, part A (June 8, 2018): 50–55.

Michaël Messaoudi et al., "Beneficial Psychological Effects of a Probiotic Formulation (*Lactobacillus helveticus* R0052 and *Bifidobacterium longum* R0175) in Healthy Human Volunteers," *Gut Microbes* 2, no. 4 (July/August 2011): 256–61.

Ruixue Huang, Ke Wang, and Jianan Hu, "Effect of Probiotics on Depression: A Systematic Review and Meta-Analysis of Randomized Controlled Trials," *Nutrients* 8, no. 8 (August 6, 2016): e483.

Ebrahim Kouchaki et al., "Clinical and Metabolic Response to Probiotic Supplementation in Patients with Multiple Sclerosis: A Randomized, Double-Blind, Placebo-Controlled Trial," *Clinical Nutrition* 36, no. 5 (October 2017): 1245–49.

Guo-Lin Mi et al., "Effectiveness of *Lactobacillus reuteri* in Infantile Colic and Colicky Induced Maternal Depression: A Prospective Single Blind Randomized Trial," *Antonie van Leeuwenhoek* 107, no. 6 (June 2015): 1547–53.

Laura Steenbergen et al., "A Randomized Controlled Trial to Test the Effect of Multispecies Probiotics on Cognitive Reactivity to Sad Mood," *Brain, Behavior, and Immunity* 48 (August 2015): 258–64.

51. Chun-Xiao Dai et al., "Role of *Ginkgo biloba* Extract as an Adjunctive Treatment of Elderly Patients with Depression and on the Expression of Serum S100B," *Medicine* (Baltimore) 97, no. 39 (September 2018): e12421.

Oleksandr Napryeyenko and Irina Borzenko for the GINDEM-NP Study Group, "*Ginkgo biloba* Special Extract in Dementia with Neuropsychiatric Features. A Randomised, Placebo-Controlled, Double-Blind Clinical Trial," *Arzneimittelforschung* 57, no. 1 (2007): 4–11.

52. Jerome Sarris et al., "Is S-Adenosyl Methionine (SAMe) for Depression Only Effective in Males? A Re-Analysis of Data from a Randomized Clinical Trial," *Pharmacopsychiatry* 48, nos. 4–5 (July 2015): 141–44.

53. Hesitha Abeysundera and Ramandeep Gill, "Possible SAMe-Induced Mania," *BMJ Case Reports* 2018 (June 27, 2018): bcr-2018-224338.

54. Papakostas et al., "L-Methylfolate as Adjunctive Therapy," 1267–74.

55. Mauro Porcu et al., "Effects of Adjunctive *N*-acetylcysteine on Depressive Symptoms: Modulation by Baseline High-Sensitivity C-Reactive Protein," *Psychiatry Research* 263 (May 2018): 268–74.

56. R. F. Santos et al., "Cognitive Performance, SPECT, and Blood Viscosity in Elderly Non-demented People Using *Ginkgo biloba*," *Pharmacopsychiatry* 36, no. 4 (July 2003): 127–33.

    Meng-Shan Tan, Jin-Tai Yu, Chen-Chen Tan et al. "Efficacy and Adverse Effects of *Ginkgo biloba* for Cognitive Impairment and Dementia: A Systematic Review and Meta-Analysis," *Journal of Alzheimer's Disease* 43, no. 2 (2015): 589–603.

    S. I. Gavrilova et al., "Efficacy and Safety of *Ginkgo biloba* Extract EGb 761 in Mild Cognitive Impairment with Neuropsychiatric Symptoms: A Randomized, Placebo-Controlled, Double-Blind, Multi-Center Trial," *International Journal of Geriatric Psychiatry* 29, no. 10 (October 2014): 1087–95.

    Horst Herrschaft et al., "*Ginkgo biloba* Extract EGb 761 in Dementia with Neuropsychiatric Features: A Randomised, Placebo-Controlled Trial to Confirm the Efficacy and Safety of a Daily Dose of 240 mg," *Journal of Psychiatric Research* 46, no. 6 (June 2012): 716–23.

    Ralf Ihl et al., "Efficacy and Safety of a Once-Daily Formulation of *Ginkgo biloba* Extract EGb 761 in Dementia with Neuropsychiatric Features: A Randomized Controlled Trial," *International Journal of Geriatric Psychiatry* 26, no. 11 (November 2011): 1186–94.

    Napryeyenko et al., "*Ginkgo biloba* Special Extract in Dementia," 4–11.

    Albert Attia et al., "Phase II Study of *Ginkgo biloba* in Irradiated Brain Tumor Patients: Effect on Cognitive Function, Quality of Life, and Mood," *Journal of Neuro-Oncology* 109, no. 2 (September 2012): 357–63.

    R. Kaschel, "Specific Memory Effects of Ginkgo biloba Extract EGb 761 in Middle-Aged Healthy Volunteers," *Phytomedicine* 18, no. 14 (November 15, 2011): 1202–7.

57. P. J. Delwaide et al., "Double-Blind Randomized Controlled Study of Phosphatidylserine in Senile Demented Patients," *Acta Neurologica Scandinavica* 73, no. 2 (February 1987): 136–40.

    T. H. Crook et al., "Effects of Phosphatidylserine in Age-Associated Memory Impairment," *Neurology* 41, no. 5 (May 1991): 644–49.

    T. Cenacchi et al., "Cognitive Decline in the Elderly: A Double-Blind, Placebo-Controlled Multicenter Study on Efficacy of Phosphatidylserine Administration," *Aging* (Milano) 5, no. 2 (April 1993): 123–33.

    Akito Kato-Kataoka et al., "Soybean-Derived Phosphatidylserine Improves Memory Function of the Elderly Japanese Subjects with Memory Complaints," *Journal of Clinical Biochemistry and Nutrition* 47, no. 3 (November 2010): 246–55.

    V. Vakhapova et al., "Phosphatidylserine Containing Omega-3 Fatty Acids May Improve Memory Abilities in Non-Demented Elderly with Memory Complaints: A Double-Blind Placebo-Controlled Trial," *Dementia and Geriatric Cognitive Disorders* 29, no. 5 (June 2010): 467–74.

58. L. Parnetti et al., "Multicentre Study of *l*-alpha-Glyceryl-Phosphorylcholine vs ST200 among Patients with Probable Senile Dementia of Alzheimer's Type," *Drugs and Aging* 3, no. 2 (March 1993): 159–64.

    R. Di Perri et al., "A Multicentre Trial to Evaluate the Efficacy and Tolerability of alpha-Glycerylphosphorylcholine versus Cytosine Diphosphocholine in Patients with Vascular Dementia," *Journal of International Medical Research* 19, no. 4 (July/August 1991): 330–41.

    Maria de Jesus Moreno Moreno, "Cognitive Improvement in Mild to Moderate Alzheimer's Dementia after Treatment with the Acetylcholine Precursor Choline

Alfoscerate: A Multicenter, Double-Blind, Randomized, Placebo-Controlled Trial," *Clinical Therapeutics* 25, no. 1 (January 2003): 178–93.

Francesco Amenta et al., "The ASCOMALVA (Association between the Cholinesterase Inhibitor Donepezil and the Cholinergic Precursor Choline Alphoscerate in Alzheimer's Disease) Trial: Interim Results after Two Years of Treatment," *Journal of Alzheimer's Disease* 42, no. s3 (2014): S281–88.

59. Nadine Külzow et al., "Impact of Omega-3 Fatty Acid Supplementation on Memory Functions in Healthy Older Adults," *Journal of Alzheimer's Disease* 51, no. 3 (2016): 713–25.

Claudie Hooper et al., "Cognitive Changes with Omega-3 Polyunsaturated Fatty Acids in Non-Demented Older Adults with Low Omega-3 Index," *Journal of Nutrition, Health and Aging* 21, no. 9 (2017): 988–93.

Hussein N. Yassine et al., "Association of Docosahexaenoic Acid Supplementation with Alzheimer Disease Stage in Apolipoprotein E ε4 Carriers: A Review," *JAMA Neurology* 74, no. 3 (March 2017): 339–47.

Yacong Bo et al., "The *n*-3 Polyunsaturated Fatty Acids Supplementation Improved the Cognitive Function in the Chinese Elderly with Mild Cognitive Impairment: A Double-Blind Randomized Controlled Trial," *Nutrients* 9, no. 1 (January 10, 2017): e54.

Karin Yurko-Mauro, Dominik D. Alexander, and Mary E. Van Elswyk, "Docosahexaenoic Acid and Adult Memory: A Systematic Review and Meta-Analysis," *PLOS One* 10, no. 3 (March 18, 2015): e0120391.

Yan-Ping Zhang et al., "Effects of DHA Supplementation on Hippocampal Volume and Cognitive Function in Older Adults with Mild Cognitive Impairment: A 12-Month Randomized, Double-Blind, Placebo-Controlled Trial," *Journal of Alzheimer's Disease* 55, no. 2 (2017): 497–507.

60. Natalie A. Grima et al., "The Effects of Multivitamins on Cognitive Performance: A Systematic Review and Meta-Analysis," *Journal of Alzheimer's Disease* 29, no. 3 (2012): 561–69.

61. Zhi-Qiang Xu et al., "Treatment with Huperzine A Improves Cognition in Vascular Dementia Patients," *Cell Biochemistry and Biophysics* 62, no. 1 (January 2012): 55–58.

Z. Zhang et al., "Clinical Efficacy and Safety of Huperzine Alpha in Treatment of Mild to Moderate Alzheimer Disease, a Placebo-Controlled, Double-Blind, Randomized Trial," *Zhonghua Yi Xue Za Zhi* 82, no. 14 (July 25, 2002): 941–44.

Q. Q. Sun et al., "Huperzine-A Capsules Enhance Memory and Learning Performance in 34 Pairs of Matched Adolescent Students," *Zhongguo Yao Li Xue Bao* 20, no. 7 (July 1999): 601–3.

S. S. Xu et al., "Huperzine-A in Capsules and Tablets for Treating Patients with Alzheimer Disease," *Zhongguo Yao Li Xue Bao* 20, no. 6 (June 1999): 486–90.

S. S. Xu et al., "Efficacy of Tablet Huperzine-A on Memory, Cognition, and Behavior in Alzheimer's Disease," *Zhongguo Yao Li Xue Bao* 16, no. 5 (September 1995): 391–95.

R. W. Zhang et al., "Drug Evaluation of Huperzine A in the Treatment of Senile Memory Disorders," *Zhongguo Yao Li Xue Bao* 12, no. 3 (May 1991): 250–52.

62. Sangeeta Raghav et al., "Randomized Controlled Trial of Standardized *Bacopa monniera* Extract in Age-Associated Memory Impairment," *Indian Journal of Psychiatry* 48, no. 4 (October–December 2006): 238–42.

Luke A. Downey et al., "An Acute, Double-Blind, Placebo-Controlled Crossover Study of 320 mg and 640 mg Doses of a Special Extract of *Bacopa monnieri* (CDRI 08) on Sustained Cognitive Performance," *Phytotherapy Research* 27, no. 9 (September 2013): 1407–13.

Annette Morgan and John Stevens, "Does *Bacopa monnieri* Improve Memory Performance in Older Persons? Results of a Randomized, Placebo-Controlled, Double-Blind Trial," *Journal of Alternative and Complementary Medicine* 16, no. 7 (July 2010): 753–59.

Carlo Calabrese et al., "Effects of a Standardized *Bacopa monnieri* Extract on Cognitive

Performance, Anxiety, and Depression in the Elderly: A Randomized, Double-Blind, Placebo-Controlled Trial," *Journal of Alternative and Complementary Medicine* 14, no. 6 (July 2008): 707–13.

Steven Roodenrys et al., "Chronic Effects of Brahmi (Bacopa monnieri) on Human Memory," *Neuropsychopharmacology* 27, no. 2 (August 2002): 279–81.

63. Sara Neshatdoust et al., "High-Flavonoid Intake Induces Cognitive Improvements Linked to Changes in Serum Brain-Derived Neurotrophic Factor: Two Randomised, Controlled Trials," *Nutrition and Healthy Aging* 4, no. 1 (2016): 81–93.

Daniela Mastroiacovo et al., "Cocoa Flavanol Consumption Improves Cognitive Function, Blood Pressure Control, and Metabolic Profile in Elderly Subjects: The Cocoa, Cognition, and Aging (CoCoA) Study—a Randomized Controlled Trial," *American Journal of Clinical Nutrition* 101, no. 3 (March 2015): 538–48.

Giovambattista Desideri et al., "Benefits in Cognitive Function, Blood Pressure, and Insulin Resistance through Cocoa Flavanol Consumption in Elderly Subjects with Mild Cognitive Impairment: The Cocoa, Cognition, and Aging (CoCoA) Study," *Hypertension* 60, no. 3 (September 2012): 794–801.

64. J. Ryan et al., "An Examination of the Effects of the Antioxidant Pycnogenol on Cognitive Performance, Serum Lipid Profile, Endocrinological and Oxidative Stress Biomarkers in an Elderly Population," *Journal of Psychopharmacology* 22, no. 5 (2008): 553–62.

R. Luzzi et al., "Pycnogenol Supplementation Improves Cognitive Function, Attention and Mental Performance in Students," *Panminerva Medica* 53, no. 3, suppl. 1 (September 2011): 75–82.

65. S. Akhondzadeh et al., "Saffron in the Treatment of Patients with Mild to Moderate Alzheimer's Disease: A 16-Week, Randomized and Placebo-Controlled Trial," *Journal of Clinical Pharmacy and Therapeutics* 35, no. 5 (October 2010): 581–88.

Shahin Akhondzadeh, Sabat M. Shafiee, and M. H. Harirchian et al., "A 22-Week, Multicenter, Randomized, Double-Blind Controlled Trial of *Crocus sativus* in the Treatment of Mild-to-Moderate Alzheimer's Disease," *Psychopharmacology (Berlin)* 207, no. 4 (January 2010): 637–43.

66. Dnyanraj Choudhary, Sauvik Bhattacharyya, and Sekhar Bose, "Efficacy and Safety of Ashwagandha *(Withania somnifera* (L.) *Dunal)* Root Extract in Improving Memory and Cognitive Functions," *Journal of Dietary Supplements* 14, no. 6 (2017): 599–612.

K. N. Roy Chengappa et al., "Randomized Placebo-Controlled Adjunctive Study of an Extract of *Withania somnifera* for Cognitive Dysfunction in Bipolar Disorder," *Journal of Clinical Psychiatry* 74, no. 11 (November 2013): 1076–83.

67. Jacqueline A. Pettersen, "Does High Dose Vitamin D Supplementation Enhance Cognition?: A Randomized Trial in Healthy Adults," *Experimental Gerontology* 90 (April 2017): 90–97.

V. A. Andreeva et al., "Midlife Dietary Vitamin D Intake and Subsequent Performance in Different Cognitive Domains," *Annals of Nutrition and Metabolism* 65, no. 1 (October 2014): 81–89.

68. Hsien-Yuan Lane et al., "A Randomized, Double-Blind, Placebo-Controlled Comparison Study of Sarcosine (*N*-Methylglycine) and D-Serine Add-on Treatment for Schizophrenia," *International Journal of Neuropsychopharmacology* 13, no. 4 (May 2010): 451–60.

Hsien-Yuan Lane et al., "Sarcosine (N-Methylglycine) Treatment for Acute Schizophrenia: A Randomized, Double-Blind Study," *Biological Psychiatry* 63, no. 1 (January 1, 2008): 9–12.

Guochuan Tsai et al., "Glycine Transporter I Inhibitor, N-Methylglycine (Sarcosine), Added to Antipsychotics for the Treatment of Schizophrenia," *Biological Psychiatry* 55, no. 5 (March 1, 2004): 452–56.

Dominik Strzelecki, Olga Kałużyńska, and Adam Wysokiński, "BDNF Serum Levels in Schizophrenic Patients during Treatment Augmentation with Sarcosine (Results of the PULSAR Study)," *Psychiatry Research* 242 (August 30, 2016): 54–60.

Dominik Strzelecki, Małgorzata Urban-Kowalczyk, and Adam Wysokiński, "Serum Levels of TNF-Alpha in Patients with Chronic Schizophrenia during Treatment Augmentation with Sarcosine (Results of the PULSAR Study)," *Psychiatry Research* 268 (October 2018): 447–53.

69. Soo Liang Ooi, Ruth Green, and Sok Cheon Pak, "N-Acetylcysteine for the Treatment of Psychiatric Disorders: A Review of Current Evidence," *BioMed Research International* 2018 (October 22, 2018): 2469486.

70. G. Paul Amminger et al., "Long-Chain ω-3 Fatty Acids for Indicated Prevention of Psychotic Disorders: A Randomized, Placebo-Controlled Trial," *Archives of General Psychiatry* 67, no. 2 (February 2010): 146–54.

    Nilufar Mossaheb et al., "Effect of Omega-3 Fatty Acids for Indicated Prevention of Young Patients at Risk for Psychosis: When Do They Begin to Be Effective?" *Schizophrenia Research* 148, nos. 1–3 (August 2013): 163–67.

    G. Paul Amminger et al., "Longer-Term Outcome in the Prevention of Psychotic Disorders by the Vienna Omega-3 Study," *Nature Communications* 6 (August 11, 2015): 7934.

71. Joshua L. Roffman et al., "Biochemical, Physiological and Clinical Effects of L-methylfolate in Schizophrenia: A Randomized Controlled Trial," *Molecular Psychiatry* 23, no. 2 (February 2018): 316–22.

    P. S. A. Godfrey et al., "Enhancement of Recovery from Psychiatric Illness by Methylfolate," *Lancet* 336, no. 8712 (August 18, 1990): 392–95.

72. Chun-Yuan Lin et al., "Adjunctive Sarcosine Plus Benzoate Improved Cognitive Function in Chronic Schizophrenia Patients with Constant Clinical Symptoms: A Randomised, Double-Blind, Placebo-Controlled Trial," *World Journal of Biological Psychiatry* 18, no. 5 (August 2017): 357–68.

73. Kamal Patel, "Melatonin," Examine.com, last updated September 30, 2018, https://examine.com/supplements/melatonin/.

    Patrick Lemoine et al., "Prolonged-Release Melatonin Improves Sleep Quality and Morning Alertness in Insomnia Patients Aged 55 Years and Older and Has No Withdrawal Effects," *Journal of Sleep Research* 16, no. 4 (December 2007): 372–80.

    Ingeborg M. van Geijlswijk et al., "Evaluation of Sleep, Puberty and Mental Health in Children with Long-Term Melatonin Treatment for Chronic Idiopathic Childhood Sleep Onset Insomnia," *Psychopharmacology (Berlin)* 216, no. 1 (July 2011): 111–20.

    Remy Luthringer et al., "The Effect of Prolonged-Release Melatonin on Sleep Measures and Psychomotor Performance in Elderly Patients with Insomnia," *International Clinical Psychopharmacology* 24, no. 5 (September 2009): 239–49.

74. Andrew Herxheimer and Keith J. Petrie, "Melatonin for the Prevention and Treatment of Jet Lag," *Cochrane Database of Systematic Reviews*, no. 2 (2002): CD001520.

75. Michael R. Lyon, Mahendra P. Kapoor, and Lekh R. Juneja, "The Effects of L-Theanine (Suntheanine) on Objective Sleep Quality in Boys with Attention Deficit Hyperactivity Disorder (ADHD): A Randomized, Double-Blind, Placebo-Controlled Clinical Trial," *Alternative Medicine Review* 16, no. 4 (December 2011): 348–54.

76. Behnood Abbasi et al., "The Effect of Magnesium Supplementation on Primary Insomnia in Elderly: A Double-Blind Placebo-Controlled Clinical Trial," *Journal of Research in Medical Sciences* 17, no. 12 (December 2012): 1161–69.

    Mariangela Rondanelli et al., "The Effect of Melatonin, Magnesium, and Zinc on Primary Insomnia in Long-Term Care Facility Residents in Italy: A Double-Blind, Placebo-Controlled Clinical Trial," *Journal of the American Geriatric Society* 59, no. 1 (January 2011): 82–90.

    Yingting Cao et al., "Magnesium Intake and Sleep Disorder Symptoms: Findings from the Jiangsu Nutrition Study of Chinese Adults at Five-Year Follow-Up," *Nutrients* 10, no. 10 (September 21, 2018): e1354.

77. Simin Taavoni et al., "Effect of Valerian on Sleep Quality in Postmenopausal Women:

A Randomized Placebo-Controlled Clinical Trial," *Menopause* (New York) 18, no. 9 (September 2011): 951–55.

M. Isabel Fernández-San-Martín et al., "Effectiveness of Valerian on Insomnia: A Meta-analysis of Randomized Placebo-Controlled Trials," *Sleep Medicine* 11, no. 6 (June 2010): 505–11.

78. M. Takada et al., "Beneficial Effects of *Lactobacillus casei* Strain Shirota on Academic Stress-Induced Sleep Disturbance in Healthy Adults: A Double-Blind, Randomised, Placebo-Controlled Trial," *Beneficial Microbes* 8, no. 2 (2017): 153–62.

79. Mariangela Rondanelli et al., "The Effect of Melatonin, Magnesium, and Zinc on Primary Insomnia in Long-Term Care Facility Residents in Italy: A Double-Blind, Placebo-Controlled Clinical Trial," *Journal of the American Geriatric Society* 59, no. 1 (January 2011): 82–90.

80. Amir Ghaderi et al., "Clinical Trial of the Effects of Vitamin D Supplementation on Psychological Symptoms and Metabolic Profiles in Maintenance Methadone Treatment Patients," *Progress in Neuro-Psychopharmacology and Biological Psychiatry* 79, part B (October 2017): 84–89.

81. Richard De la Garza et al., "Safety and Preliminary Efficacy of the Acetylcholinesterase Inhibitor Huperzine A as a Treatment for Cocaine Use Disorder," *International Journal of Neuropsychopharmacology* 19, no. 3 (March 2016): pyv098.

82. Michael Silvio Duailibi et al., "N-Acetylcysteine in the Treatment of Craving in Substance Use Disorders: Systematic Review and Meta-analysis," *American Journal on Addictions* 26, no. 7 (October 2017): 660–66.

Soo Liang Ooi, Ruth Green, and Sok Cheon Pak, "N-Acetylcysteine for the Treatment of Psychiatric Disorders: A Review of Current Evidence," *BioMed Research International* 2018 (October 22, 2018): 2469486.

83. Eduardo Prado et al., "*N*-Acetylcysteine for Therapy-Resistant Tobacco Use Disorder: A Pilot Study," *Redox Report* 20, no. 5 (September 2015): 215–22.

Gregory L. Powell et al., "Chronic Treatment with *N*-Acetylcysteine Decreases Extinction Responding and Reduces Cue-Induced Nicotine-Seeking," *Physiological Reports* 7, no. 1 (January 2019): e13958.

84. Lindsay M. Squeglia et al., "Alcohol Use during a Trial of *N*-Acetylcysteine for Adolescent Marijuana Cessation," *Addictive Behaviors* 63 (December 2016): 172–77.

85. Kevin M. Gray et al., "A Double-Blind Randomized Controlled Trial of *N*-Acetylcysteine in Cannabis-Dependent Adolescents," *American Journal of Psychiatry* 169, no. 8 (August 2012): 805–12.

86. Steven D. LaRowe et al., "Is Cocaine Desire Reduced by *N*-Acetylcysteine?" *American Journal of Psychiatry* 164, no. 7 (July 2007): 1115–17.

Steven D. LaRowe et al., "A Double-Blind Placebo-Controlled Trial of N-Acetylcysteine in the Treatment of Cocaine Dependence," *American Journal on Addictions* 22, no. 5 (September/October 2013): 443–52.

87. Seyed Ghafur Mousavi et al., "The Efficacy of N-Acetylcysteine in the Treatment of Methamphetamine Dependence: A Double-Blind Controlled, Crossover Study," *Archives of Iranian Medicine* 18, no. 1 (January 2015): 28–33.

88. Ritchy Hodebourg et al., "Heroin Seeking Becomes Dependent on Dorsal Striatal Dopaminergic Mechanisms and Can Be Decreased by N-Acetylcysteine," *European Journal of Neuroscience*, special issue, March 7, 2018, https://doi.org/10.1111/ejn.13894.

89. Jon E. Grant, Suck Won Kim, and Brian L. Odlaug, "N-Acetyl Cysteine, a Glutamate-Modulating Agent, in the Treatment of Pathological Gambling: A Pilot Study," *Biological Psychiatry* 62, no. 6 (September 15, 2007): 652–57.

Jon E. Grant et al., "A Randomized, Placebo-Controlled Trial of *N*-Acetylcysteine Plus Imaginal Desensitization for Nicotine-Dependent Pathological Gamblers," *Journal of Clinical Psychiatry* 75, no. 1 (January 2014): 39–45.

90. Stephen D. Anton et al., "Effects of Chromium Picolinate on Food Intake and Satiety," *Diabetes Technology and Therapeutics* 10, no. 5 (2008): 405–12.

Kimberly A. Brownley et al., "A Double-Blind, Randomized Pilot Trial of Chromium Picolinate for Binge Eating Disorder: Results of the Binge Eating and Chromium (BEACh) Study," *Journal of Psychosomatic Research* 75, no. 1 (July 2013): 36–42.

91. Dnyanraj Choudhary, Sauvik Bhattacharyya, and Kedar Joshi, "Body Weight Management in Adults under Chronic Stress through Treatment with Ashwagandha Root Extract: A Double-Blind, Randomized, Placebo-Controlled Trial," *Journal of Evidence-Based Complementary and Alternative Medicine* 22, no. 1 (2017): 96–106.

92. Rachel L. Tomko, et al., "*N*-Acetylcysteine: A Potential Treatment for Substance Use Disorders," *Current Psychiatry* 17, no. 6 (June 2018): 30–55.

93. John A. Chalmers et al., "Anxiety Disorders Are Associated with Reduced Heart Rate Variability: A Meta-Analysis," *Frontiers in Psychiatry* 5 (July 11, 2014): 80.

94. Massachusetts General Hospital, "Physical Activity as a Preventive Strategy against Depression: Genetic Data Suggests Physical Activity Can Protect against the Risk of Depression," ScienceDaily, January 23, 2019, https://www.sciencedaily.com/releases /2019/01/190123112333.htm.

95. Daniel G. Amen and Tana Amen, *The Brain Warrior's Way* (New York: New American Library, 2016), 179.

CHAPTER 17: YOU CANNOT CHANGE WHAT YOU DO NOT MEASURE

1. Daniel G. Amen, *Feel Better Fast and Make It Last* (Carol Stream, IL: Tyndale, 2018), 309–10.

2. Gina Kolata, "Under New Guidelines, Millions More Americans Will Need to Lower Blood Pressure," *New York Times*, November 13, 2017, https://www.nytimes.com/2017/11/13 /health/blood-pressure-treatment-guidelines.html?_r=0.

Susan Scutti, "Nearly Half of Americans Now Have High Blood Pressure, Based on New Guidelines," Health, CNN, November 14, 2017, https://www.cnn.com/2017/11/13/health /new-blood-pressure-guidelines/index.html.

3. Penelope Elias et al., "Serum Cholesterol and Cognitive Performance in the Framingham Heart Study," *Psychosomatic Medicine* 67, no. 1 (January/February 2005): 24–30.

4. M. M. Mielke et al., "High Total Cholesterol Levels in Late Life Associated with a Reduced Risk of Dementia," *Neurology* 64, no. 10 (May 24, 2005): 1689–95.

Annelies W. E. Weverling-Rijnsburger et al., "Total Cholesterol and Risk of Mortality in the Oldest Old," *Lancet* 350, no. 9085 (October 18, 1997): 1119–23.

5. Amen, *Feel Better Fast*, 313.

6. Daniel G. Amen, *Change Your Brain, Change Your Life*, rev. ed. (New York: Harmony Books, 2015), 83–84.

7. Daniel G. Amen, *Unleash the Power of the Female Brain* (New York: Harmony Books, 2013), 80–81.

8. Amen, *Feel Better Fast*, 309.

9. "Cancers Associated with Overweight and Obesity Make Up 40 Percent of Cancers Diagnosed in the United States," CDC Newsroom, Centers for Disease Control and Prevention, last updated October 3, 2017, https://www.cdc.gov/media/releases/2017 /p1003-vs-cancer-obesity.html.

10. Amen, *Change Your Brain*, 80.

CHAPTER 18: FOOD MADE INSANELY SIMPLE

1. T. S. Sathyanarayana Rao et al., "Understanding Nutrition, Depression and Mental Illnesses," *Indian Journal of Psychiatry* 50, no. 2 (April–June 2008): 77–82.

2. Jerome Sarris et al., "Nutritional Medicine as Mainstream in Psychiatry," *Lancet* 2, no. 3 (2015): 271–74.

3. Felice N. Jacka et al., "Western Diet Is Associated with a Smaller Hippocampus: A Longitudinal Investigation," *BMC Medicine* 13 (September 8, 2015): 215.

4. Felice N. Jacka et al., "Dietary Patterns and Depressive Symptoms over Time: Examining the Relationships with Socioeconomic Position, Health Behaviours and Cardiovascular Risk," *PLOS One* 9, no. 1 (January 29, 2014): e87657.

   Behnaz Shakersain et al., "Prudent Diet May Attenuate the Adverse Effects of Western Diet on Cognitive Decline," *Alzheimer's and Dementia* 12, no. 2 (February 2016): 100–109.

   Amber L. Howard et al., "ADHD Is Associated with a 'Western' Dietary Pattern in Adolescents," *Journal of Attention Disorders* 15, no. 5 (July 2011): 403–11.

   Giovanni Tarantino, Vincenzo Citro, and Carmine Finelli, "Hype or Reality: Should Patients with Metabolic Syndrome-Related NAFLD be on the Hunter-Gatherer (Paleo) Diet to Decrease Morbidity?" *Journal of Gastrointestinal and Liver Diseases* 24, no. 3 (September 2015): 359–68.

5. National Center for Chronic Disease Prevention and Health Promotion, *The Power of Prevention: Chronic Disease . . . the Public Health Challenge of the 21st Century*, US Department of Health and Human Services, Centers for Disease Control and Prevention, 2009, https://www.cdc.gov/chronicdisease/pdf/2009-Power-of-Prevention.pdf.

6. Maximus Berger et al., "Cross-Sectional Association of Seafood Consumption, Polyunsaturated Fatty Acids and Depressive Symptoms in Two Torres Strait Communities," *Nutritional Neuroscience*, August 3, 2018, https://doi.org/10.1080/10284 15X.2018.1504429.

7. Lawrence E. Armstrong et al., "Mild Dehydration Affects Mood in Healthy Young Women," *Journal of Nutrition* 142, no. 2 (February 2012): 382–88.

   Matthew S. Ganio et al., "Mild Dehydration Impairs Cognitive Performance and Mood of Men," *British Journal of Nutrition* 106, no. 10 (November 28, 2011): 1535–43.

8. Ana Adan, "Cognitive Performance and Dehydration," *Journal of the American College of Nutrition* 31, no. 2 (2012): 71–78.

9. Kunio Nakamura et al., "Correlation between Brain Volume Change and T2 Relaxation Time Induced by Dehydration and Rehydration: Implications for Monitoring Atrophy in Clinical Studies," *NeuroImage: Clinical* 6 (2014): 166–70.

10. Paul D. Lindseth et al., "Effects of Hydration on Cognitive Function of Pilots," *Military Medicine* 178, no. 7 (July 2013): 792–98.

11. Daniel G. Amen and Tana Amen, *The Brain Warrior's Way* (New York: New American Library, 2016), 113.

12. Rosebud O. Roberts et al., "Relative Intake of Macronutrients Impacts Risk of Mild Cognitive Impairment or Dementia," *Journal of Alzheimer's Disease* 32, no. 2 (2012): 329–39.

13. Lenore Arab, Rong Guo, and David Elashoff, "Lower Depression Scores among Walnut Consumers in NHANES," *Nutrients* 11, no. 2 (January 26, 2019): e275.

14. James E. Gangwisch et al., "High Glycemic Index Diet as a Risk Factor for Depression: Analyses from the Women's Health Initiative," *American Journal of Clinical Nutrition* 102, no. 2 (August 2015): 454–63.

15. Kara L. Breymeyer et al., "Subjective Mood and Energy Levels of Healthy Weight and Overweight/Obese Healthy Adults on High- and Low-Glycemic Load Experimental Diets," *Appetite* 107 (December 1, 2016): 253–59.

16. Daniel G. Amen, *Feel Better Fast and Make It Last* (Carol Stream, IL: Tyndale, 2018), 212–13.

17. Bayani Uttara et al., "Oxidative Stress and Neurodegenerative Diseases: A Review of Upstream and Downstream Antioxidant Therapeutic Options," *Current Neuropharmacology* 7, no. 1 (March 2009): 65–74.

18. Gora Dadheech et al., "Evaluation of Antioxidant Deficit in Schizophrenia," *Indian Journal of Psychiatry* 50, no. 1 (January–March 2008): 16–20.

19. Tao Liu et al., "A Meta-Analysis of Oxidative Stress Markers in Depression," *PLOS One* 10, no. 10 (October 7, 2015): e0138904.

20. Medhavi Gautam et al., "Role of Antioxidants in Generalised Anxiety Disorder and Depression," *Indian Journal of Psychiatry* 54, no. 3 (July–September 2012): 244–47.

21. See "List of Foods," ORAC Database, accessed August 25, 2019, https://oracdatabase.com/list-of-foods/list-of-foods/. Numbers have been rounded down.

22. University of Warwick, "Fruit and Veggies Give You the Feel-Good Factor," ScienceDaily, July 10, 2016, https://www.sciencedaily.com/releases/2016/07/160710094239.htm.

23. Daniel G. Amen, *Change Your Brain, Change Your Life*, rev. ed. (New York: Harmony Books, 2015), 137.

24. Amen and Amen, *Brain Warrior's Way*, 142.

25. Lidy M. Pelsser et al., "A Randomised Controlled Trial into the Effects of Food on ADHD," *European Child and Adolescent Psychiatry* 18, no. 1 (January 2009): 12–19.

26. Lidy M. Pelsser et al., "Effects of Food on Physical and Sleep Complaints in Children with ADHD: A Randomised Controlled Pilot Study," *European Journal of Pediatrics* 169, no. 9 (September 2010): 1129–38.

27. Donna McCann et al., "Food Additives and Hyperactive Behavior in 3-Year-Old and 8/9-Year-Old Children in the Community: A Randomised, Double-Blinded, Placebo-Controlled Trial," *Lancet* 370, no. 9598 (November 3, 2007): 1560–67.

28. Rachel B. Acton et al., "Added Sugar in the Packaged Foods and Beverages Available at a Major Canadian Retailer in 2015: A Descriptive Analysis," *CMAJ Open* 5, no. 1 (January 12, 2017): e1–6.

29. Michelle Pearlman, Jon Obert, and Lisa Casey, "The Association between Artificial Sweeteners and Obesity," *Current Gastroenterology Reports* 19, no. 12 (2017): 64.

30. Jessica R. Jackson et al., "Neurologic and Psychiatric Manifestations of Celiac Disease and Gluten Sensitivity," *Psychiatric Quarterly* 83, no. 1 (March 2012): 91–102.

31. Megan Anne Arroll, Lorraine Wilder, and James Neil, "Nutritional Interventions for the Adjunctive Treatment of Schizophrenia: A Brief Review," *Nutrition Journal* 13 (September 16, 2014): 91.

    Elena Lionetti et al., "Gluten Psychosis: Confirmation of a New Clinical Entity," *Nutrients* 7, no. 7 (July 8, 2015): 5532–39.

32. Helmut Niederhofer, "Association of Attention-Deficit/Hyperactivity Disorder and Celiac Disease: A Brief Report," *Primary Care Companion to CNS Disorders* 13, no. 3 (2011): e1–31.

    Paul Whiteley et al., "The ScanBrit Randomised, Controlled, Single-Blind Study of a Gluten- and Casein-Free Dietary Intervention for Children with Autism Spectrum Disorders," *Nutritional Neuroscience* 13, no. 2 (2010): 87–100.

    Antonio Di Sabatino et al., "Small Amounts of Gluten in Subjects with Suspected Nonceliac Gluten Sensitivity: A Randomized, Double-Blind, Placebo-Controlled, Cross-Over Trial," *Clinical Gastroenterology and Hepatology* 13, no. 9 (September 2015): 1604–12.e3.

    S. L. Peters et al., "Randomised Clinical Trial: Gluten May Cause Depression in Subjects with Non-coeliac Gluten Sensitivity—An Exploratory Clinical Study," *Alimentary Pharmacology and Therapeutics* 39, no. 10 (May 2014): 1104–12.

33. Eleanor Busby et al., "Mood Disorders and Gluten: It's Not All in Your Mind! A Systematic Review with Meta-Analysis," *Nutrients* 10, no. 11 (November 8, 2018): e1708.

34. Paola Bressan and Peter Kramer, "Bread and Other Edible Agents of Mental Disease," *Frontiers in Human Neuroscience* 10 (March 29, 2016): 130.

35. Leo Pruimboom and Karin de Punder, "The Opioid Effects of Gluten Exorphins: Asymptomatic Celiac Disease," *Journal of Health, Population and Nutrition* 33 (November 24, 2015): 24.

36. Bressan and Kramer, "Bread and Other Edible Agents," 130.

37. P. Usai et al., "Frontal Cortical Perfusion Abnormalities Related to Gluten Intake and Associated Autoimmune Disease in Adult Coeliac Disease: 99mTc-ECD Brain SPECT Study," *Digestive and Liver Disease* 36, no. 8 (August 2004): 513–18.

    A. De Santis et al., "Schizophrenic Symptoms and SPECT Abnormalities in a Coeliac Patient: Regression after a Gluten-Free Diet," *Journal of Internal Medicine* 242, no. 5 (November 1997): 421–23.

38. Giovanni Addolorato et al., "Regional Cerebral Hypoperfusion in Patients with Celiac Disease," *American Journal of Medicine* 116, no. 5 (March 1, 2004): 312–17.

    Maurizio Gabrielli et al., "Association between Migraine and Celiac Disease: Results from a Preliminary Case-Control and Therapeutic Study," *American Journal of Gastroenterology* 98, no. 3 (March 2003): 625–29.

39. M. Hadjivassiliou et al., "Dietary Treatment of Gluten Ataxia," *Journal of Neurology, Neurosurgery and Psychiatry* 74, no. 9 (September 2003): 1221–24.

40. F. C. Dohan et al., "Is Schizophrenia Rare if Grain Is Rare?" *Biological Psychiatry* 19, no. 3 (March 1984): 385–99.

41. F. C. Dohan and J. C. Grasberger, "Relapsed Schizophrenics: Earlier Discharge from the Hospital after Cereal-Free, Milk-Free Diet," *American Journal of Psychiatry* 130, no. 6 (1973): 685–88.

42. Robin Mesnage et al., "Potential Toxic Effects of Glyphosate and Its Commercial Formulations below Regulatory Limits," *Food and Chemical Toxicology* 84 (October 2015): 133–53.

43. K. R. Fluegge and K. R. Fluegge, "Glyphosate Use Predicts ADHD Hospital Discharges in the Healthcare Cost and Utilization Project Net (HCUPnet): A Two-Way Fixed-Effects Analysis," *PLOS One* 10, no. 8 (August 21, 2015): e0133525, retraction August 21, 2015, *PLOS One*, https://doi.org/10.1371/journal.pone.0137489.

44. "15 Health Problems Linked to Monsanto's Roundup," EcoWatch, January 23, 2015, https://www.ecowatch.com/15-health-problems-linked-to-monsantos-roundup -1882002128.html.

45. Abdulaziz Farooq et al., "A Prospective Study of the Physiological and Neurobehavioral Effects of Ramadan Fasting in Preteen and Teenage Boys," *Journal of the Academy of Nutrition and Dietetics* 115, no. 6 (June 2015): 889–97.

46. N. M. Hussin et al., "Efficacy of Fasting and Calorie Restriction (FCR) on Mood and Depression among Ageing Men," *Journal of Nutrition, Health and Aging* 17, no. 8 (2013): 674–80.

    Kathryn C. Fitzgerald et al., "Effect of Intermittent vs. Daily Calorie Restriction on Changes in Weight and Patient-Reported Outcomes in People with Multiple Sclerosis," *Multiple Sclerosis and Related Disorders* 23 (July 2018): 33–39.

47. Tatiana Moro et al., "Effects of Eight Weeks of Time-Restricted Feeding (16/8) on Basal Metabolism, Maximal Strength, Body Composition, Inflammation, and Cardiovascular Risk Factors in Resistance-Trained Males," *Journal of Translational Medicine* 14, no. 1 (October 13, 2016): 290.

48. M. E. Faris et al., "Intermittent Fasting during Ramadan Attenuates Proinflammatory Cytokines and Immune Cells in Healthy Subjects," *Nutrition Research* 32, no. 12 (December 2012): 947–55.

49. Andrea R. Vasconcelos et al., "Intermittent Fasting Attenuates Lipopolysaccharide-Induced Neuroinflammation and Memory Impairment," *Journal of Neuroinflammation* 11 (May 6, 2014): 85.

50. Ben Spencer, "Why You Should NEVER Eat after 7pm: Late Night Meals 'Increases the Risk of Heart Attack and Stroke,'" Daily Mail, August 31, 2016, https://www.dailymail .co.uk/health/article-3767231/Why-NEVER-eat-7pm-Late-night-meals-increases-risk -heart-attack-stroke.html.

51. Ameneh Madjd et al., "Beneficial Effect of High Energy Intake at Lunch Rather Than Dinner on Weight Loss in Healthy Obese Women in a Weight-Loss Program:

A Randomized Clinical Trial," *American Journal of Clinical Nutrition* 104, no. 4 (October 2016): 982–89.

52. I published a similar list in *Memory Rescue* (Tyndale, 2017), but this list is narrowed down to the foods that will help or hurt mental health issues.

53. Coreyann Poly et al., "The Relation of Dietary Choline to Cognitive Performance and White-Matter Hyperintensity in the Framingham Offspring Cohort," *American Journal of Clinical Nutrition* 94, no. 6 (December 2011): 1584–91.

54. Xiaoshuang Dai et al., "Consuming *Lentinula edodes* (Shiitake) Mushrooms Daily Improves Human Immunity: A Randomized Dietary Intervention in Healthy Young Adults," *Journal of the American College of Nutrition* 34, no. 6 (2015): 478–87.

J. M. Gaullier et al., "Supplementation with a Soluble β-glucan Exported from Shiitake Medicinal Mushroom, *Lentinus edodes* (Berk.) Singer Mycelium: A Crossover, Placebo-Controlled Study in Healthy Elderly," *International Journal of Medical Mushrooms* 13, no. 4 (2011): 319–26.

55. Lawrance C. Chandra et al., "White Button, Portabella, and Shiitake Mushroom Supplementation Up-Regulates Interleukin-23 Secretion in Acute Dextran Sodium Sulfate Colitis C57BL/6 Mice and Murine Macrophage J.744.1 Cell Line," *Nutrition Research* 33, no. 5 (May 2013): 388–96.

APPENDIX B: 10 COMMON GENES THAT MAY INFLUENCE BRAIN HEALTH/MENTAL HEALTH

1. Simon Gilbody, Tracy Lightfoot, and Trevor Sheldon, "Is Low Folate a Risk Factor for Depression? A Meta-analysis and Exploration of Heterogeneity," *Journal of Epidemiology and Community Health*, 61, no. 7 (2007): 631–37.

2. Odette L. J. Peerbooms et al., "Meta-Analysis of MTHFR Gene Variants in Schizophrenia, Bipolar Disorder and Unipolar Depressive Disorder: Evidence for a Common Genetic Vulnerability?" *Brain, Behavior, and Immunity* 25, no. 8 (November 2011): 1530–43.

3. Naushad Shaik Mohammad et al., "Aberrations in Folate Metabolic Pathway and Altered Susceptibility to Autism," *Psychiatric Genetics* 19, no. 4 (2009): 171–76.

Robin P. Goin-Kochel et al., "The *MTHFR* 677C→T Polymorphism and Behaviors in Children with Autism: Exploratory Genotype–Phenotype Correlations," *Autism Research* 2, no. 2 (April 2009): 98–108.

4. Priya Rajagopalan et al., "Common Folate Gene Variant, *MTHFR* C677T, Is Associated with Brain Structure in Two Independent Cohorts of People with Mild Cognitive Impairment," *NeuroImage: Clinical* 1, no. 1 (2012): 179–87.

5. Arnold W. Mech and Andrew Farah, "Correlation of Clinical Response with Homocysteine Reduction during Therapy with Reduced B Vitamins in Patients with MDD Who Are Positive for *MTHFR* C677T or A1298C Polymorphism: A Randomized, Double-Blind, Placebo-Controlled Study," *Journal of Clinical Psychiatry* 77, no. 5 (May 2016): 668–71.

6. Steven Taylor, "Association between *COMT Val158Met* and Psychiatric Disorders: A Comprehensive Meta-analysis," *American Journal of Medical Genetics Part B: Neuropsychiatric Genetics* 177, no. 2, special issue (March 2018): 199–210.

7. Avshalom Caspi et al., "Moderation of the Effect of Adolescent-Onset Cannabis Use on Adult Psychosis by a Functional Polymorphism in the Catechol-O-Methyltransferase Gene: Longitudinal Evidence of a Gene X Environment Interaction," *Biological Psychiatry* 57, no. 10 (May 15, 2005): 1117–27.

8. Taylor, "Association between *COMT Val158Met* and Psychiatric Disorders," 199–210.

9. Eva Asselmann et al., "Interplay between *COMT* Val158Met, Childhood Adversities and Sex in Predicting Panic Pathology: Findings from a General Population Sample," *Journal of Affective Disorders* 234 (July 2018): 290–96.

10. Kirk I. Erickson et al., "The Brain-Derived Neurotrophic Factor Val66Met Polymorphism Moderates an Effect of Physical Activity on Working Memory Performance," *Psychological Science* 24, no. 9 (September 2013): 1770–79.

11. Romain Colle et al., "Brain-Derived Neurotrophic Factor Val66Met Polymorphism and 6-Month Antidepressant Remission in Depressed Caucasian Patients," *Journal of Affective Disorders* 175 (April 1, 2015): 233–40.

12. M. Kato and A. Serretti, "Review and Meta-Analysis of Antidepressant Pharmacogenetic Findings in Major Depressive Disorder," *Molecular Psychiatry* 15, no. 5 (May 2010): 473–500.

    A. Serretti et al., "Meta-Analysis of Serotonin Transporter Gene Promoter Polymorphism (5-HTTLPR) Association with Selective Serotonin Reuptake Inhibitor Efficacy in Depressed Patients," *Molecular Psychiatry* 12, no. 3 (March 2007): 247–57.

    Stefano Porcelli, Chiara Fabbri, and Alessandro Serretti, "Meta-analysis of Serotonin Transporter Gene Promoter Polymorphism (5-HTTLPR) Association with Antidepressant Efficacy," *European Neuropsychopharmacology* 22, no. 4 (April 2012): 239–58.

13. Davide Seripa et al., "Role of the Serotonin Transporter Gene Locus in the Response to SSRI Treatment of Major Depressive Disorder in Late Life," *Journal of Psychopharmacology* 29, no. 5 (2015): 623–33.

14. Srijan Sen, Margit Burmeister, and Debashis Ghosh, "Meta-Analysis of the Association between a Serotonin Transporter Promoter Polymorphism (5-HTTLPR) and Anxiety-Related Personality Traits," *American Journal of Medical Genetics Part B: Neuropsychiatric Genetics* 127B, no. 1 (May 15, 2004): 85–89.

15. Ahmad R. Hariri et al., "A Susceptibility Gene for Affective Disorders and the Response of the Human Amygdala," *Archives of General Psychiatry* 62, no. 2 (February 2005): 146–52.

16. Manuel A. R. Ferreira et al., "Collaborative Genome-Wide Association Analysis Supports a Role for *ANK3* and *CACNA1C* in Bipolar Disorder," *Nature Genetics* 40, no. 9 (September 2008): 1056–58.

17. Ferreira et al., "*ANK3* and *CACNA1C* in Bipolar Disorder," 1056–58.

    Fei Wang et al., "The Association of Genetic Variation in *CACNA1C* with Structure and Function of a Frontotemporal System," *Bipolar Disorders* 13, nos. 7–8 (November/ December 2011): 696–700.

    Daixing Zhou et al., "AnkyrinG Is Required for Clustering of Voltage-Gated Na Channels at Axon Initial Segments and for Normal Action Potential Firing," *Journal of Cell Biology* 143, no. 5 (1998): 1295–304.

    T. G. Schulze et al., "Two Variants in *Ankyrin 3 (ANK3)* Are Independent Genetic Risk Factors for Bipolar Disorder," *Molecular Psychiatry* 14, no. 5 (May 2009): 487–91.

18. Sabrina Schilling et al., "*APOE* Genotype and MRI Markers of Cerebrovascular Disease: Systematic Review and Meta-analysis," *Neurology* 81, no. 3 (July 16, 2013): 292–300.

19. Madhav Thambisetty et al., "APOE ε4 Genotype and Longitudinal Changes in Cerebral Blood Flow in Normal Aging," *Archives of Neurology* 67, no. 1 (January 2010): 93–98.

Index

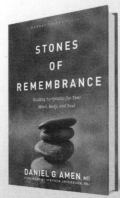